Nutrition and Well-Being A to Z

Nutrition and Well-Being A to Z

VOLUME 1 A–H

Delores C. S. James, Editor in Chief

MACMILLAN REFERENCE USA

An imprint of Thomson Gale, a part of The Thomson Corporation

THOMSON
★
™
GALE

Detroit • New York • San Francisco • San Diego • New Haven, Conn. • Waterville, Maine • London • Munich

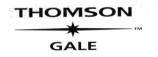

Nutrition and Well-Being A to Z

Delores C. S. James, Editor in Chief

LIBRARY OF CONGRESS CATALOGING-IN-PUBLICATION DATA

Nutrition and well being A to Z / Delores C.S. James, editor in chief.
    p. cm.
    Includes bibliographical references and index.
    ISBN 0-02-865707-1 (set hardcover)—ISBN 0-02-865708-X (volume 1)—
    ISBN 0-02-865709-8 (volume 2)
    1. Nutrition—Encyclopedias.   2. Health—Encyclopedias.
    I. James, Delores C.S., 1961–

RA784.N838 2004
613.2′03—dc22
                                  2004006088

This title is also available as an e-book
ISBN 0-02-865990-2 (set)
Contact your Gale sales representative for ordering information

Printed in the United States of America
10 9 8 7 6 5

Table of Contents

Volume 2

Preface

Nutrition is one of the most important factors that impact health in all areas of the lifecycle. Pregnant women need adequate food and health care to deliver a healthy baby who has a good birth weight and a fighting chance for survival. In many regions of the world, the infant mortality rate is very high, meaning that many infants will not live to see their first birthday. Breastfeeding is the ideal method of feeding and nurturing infants, because breast milk contains many immunologic agents that protect the infant against bacteria, viruses, and parasites. Yet, less than 40 percent of infants worldwide are exclusively breastfed (no other food or drink, not even water) for the first four months of life. Children need adequate nutrition to develop and grow to their full potential.

Malnutrition, both undernutrition and overnutrition, is at an all time high, with close to one-third of the world's children suffering from it. The number of undernourished people in the world continues to increase because of little or no progress to reduce poverty. Thousands of children die daily from hunger and its effects, even in technologically advanced countries. Without adequate nutrition, a person's cognitive ability is diminished, which adversely affects their ability to get a good paying job and contribute to their local economy. Paradoxically, childhood and adult obesity in many parts of the developed world are also near epidemic proportions. There are 300 million obese people in the world. In the United States, about 34 percent of Americans are overweight and 30.5 percent are obese.

Life expectancy has increased in many countries and the population of older adults is growing at an unprecedented rate in the United States and other technologically advanced countries. In the United States the average life expectancy is 70, while globally, the average rose to 67 years in 1998, up from 61 in 1980. These countries are unsure of how they will provide adequate health care for this growing segment of the population. Cardiovascular disease (coronary heart disease, hypertension, stroke) and cancer are top killers in many countries and HIV/AIDS continue to ravage our societies, taking individuals in the productive years of their lives.

Arrangement of the Material

Nutrition and Well-Being A to Z is a two-volume set that provides timely information on the personal, cultural, and global issues that affect (or have an impact on) health and nutritional status. Users will find detailed coverage of topics covered in general nutrition, food science, and personal and family courses. This encyclopedia explains fundamental concepts such as amino acids, cutting-edge ideas such as functional foods, social issues such as food insecurity, and political issues such as bioterrorism.

The set was also designed to meet consumer needs. Users will be able to spot a quack health-care provider, discriminate between reliable and unreliable health claims, as well as understand the role of government in keeping food safe. The set also profiles individuals who have made a social, historical, or scientific impact on health, nutrition, and food trends. Most entries are written from a global perspective, and dietary patterns from different regions of the world are discussed. Many professional health organizations are described.

The information in *Nutrition and Well-Being A to Z* is clearly presented and easy to find. Professionals in the field of nutrition, dietetics, food science, agriculture, medicine, health education, and public health wrote with the student in mind. Students and teachers can use the set to reinforce classroom topics on food, nutrition, and health, and to expand discussions on special or new topics. The extensive use of illustrations enhances the learning of the material. Entries are arranged alphabetically and an extensive cross-referencing system encourages the user to further explore other entries. All topics in a volume can be found in the index at the back of the book.

Acknowledgements and Thanks

A project of this magnitude would not be possible without the dedication and hard work of many people. I wish to thank the associate editors, Dr. Catherine Christie and Dr. Ranjita Misra, for the many hours they spent recruiting authors and editing entries. Thank you for your timely turnaround of the materials. The project would not have been possible without the many authors who wrote, and sometimes rewrote, the entries. Thank you for sharing your expertise and time. Amanda Foote, Senior Secretary in the Department of Health Science Education, was extremely valuable in copying and mailing the edited materials to the publishers. I wish to thank the many people at Macmillan Reference USA and the Gale Group for conceiving the project and providing direction throughout the entire project, especially the copyeditors and illustrators. I also send special thanks to Mr. Raymond Abruzzi.

Delores C. S. James

Topical Outline

American Dietary Habits

African Americans, Diet of
Asian Americans, Diets of
Dietary Trends, American
Hispanics and Latinos, Diet of
Native Americans, Diet of
Pacific Islander Americans, Diet of
Regional Diets, American

Biographies

Battle Creek Sanitarium
Brillat-Savarin, Jean Anthelme
Funk, Casimir
Glisson, Francis
Goldberger, Joseph
Graham, Sylvester
Johnson, Howard
Kellogg, John Harvey
Krock, Ray
Mellanby, Edward
Pasteur, Louis
Pauling, Linus
Pemberton, John S.
Rosenstein, Nils Rosén von
Stark, William
Tulp, Nicholaas
White, Ellen G.
Wilson, Owen

Body Function and Processes

Digestion and Absorption
Immune System
Insulin
Metabolism

Dieting, Weight Management, Exercise, Eating Disorders

Addiction, Food
Anorexia Nervosa
Appetite
Binge Eating
Body Image
Bulimia Nervosa
Cravings
Diet
Dieting
Eating Disorders
Eating Disturbances
Eating Habits
Ergogenic Aids
Exercise
Exercise Addiction
Fad Diets
Female Athlete Triad
Grazing
Mood-Food Relationships
Pica
Satiety
Sports Nutrition
Weight Loss Diets
Weight Management
Yo-Yo Dieting

Diseases and Disorders

Arteriosclerosis
Atherosclerosis
Bezoars
Cancer
Cardiovascular Disease
Diabetes Mellitus
Heart Disease
HIV/AIDS
Hyperglycemia
Hypertension
Hypoglycemia
Obesity

Food Habits, Trends, and Alternative Choices

Alternative Medicines and Therapies
Fat Substitutes
Legumes
Macrobiotic Diet
Plant-Based Diets
Popular Culture, Food and
Quackery
Soy
Vegan
Vegetarianism
Whole Foods Diet

Food Industry, Technology, and Food Safety

Additives and Preservatives
Artificial Sweeteners
Biotechnology
Commodity Foods
Convenience Foods
Fast Foods
Fat Substitutes
Food Safety
Fortification
Generally Recognized as Safe
Genetically Modified Foods
Green Revolution
Illnesses, Food-Borne
Irradiation
Marketing Strategies
Meat Analogs
Organic Foods
Organisms, Food-Borne
Pasteurization
Pesticides
Probiotics
Regulatory Agencies

For Your Reference

TABLE 1. SELECTED METRIC CONVERSIONS

WHEN YOU KNOW	MULTIPLY BY	TO FIND
Temperature		
Celsius (˚C)	1.8 (˚C) +32	Fahrenheit (˚F)
Celsius (˚C)	˚C +273.15	Kelvin (K)
degree change (Celsius)	1.8	degree change (Fahrenheit)
Fahrenheit (˚F)	[(˚F) −32] / 1.8	Celsius (˚C)
Fahrenheit (˚F)	[(˚F −32) / 1.8] +273.15	Kelvin (K)
Kelvin (K)	K −273.15	Celsius (˚C)
Kelvin (K)	1.8(K −273.15) +32	Fahrenheit (˚F)

WHEN YOU KNOW	MULTIPLY BY	TO FIND
Distance/Length		
centimeters	0.3937	inches
kilometers	0.6214	miles
meters	3.281	feet
meters	39.37	inches
meters	0.0006214	miles
microns	0.000001	meters
millimeters	0.03937	inches

WHEN YOU KNOW	MULTIPLY BY	TO FIND
Capacity/Volume		
cubic kilometers	0.2399	cubic miles
cubic meters	35.31	cubic feet
cubic meters	1.308	cubic yards
cubic meters	8.107×10^{-4}	acre-feet
liters	0.2642	gallons
liters	33.81	fluid ounces

WHEN YOU KNOW	MULTIPLY BY	TO FIND
Area		
hectares (10,000 square meters)	2.471	acres
hectares (10,000 square meters)	107,600	square feet
square meters	10.76	square feet
square kilometers	247.1	acres
square kilometers	0.3861	square miles

WHEN YOU KNOW	MULTIPLY BY	TO FIND
Weight/Mass		
kilograms	2.205	pounds
metric tons	2205	pounds
micrograms (μg)	10^{-6}	grams
milligrams (mg)	10^{-3}	grams
nanograms (ng)	10^{-9}	grams

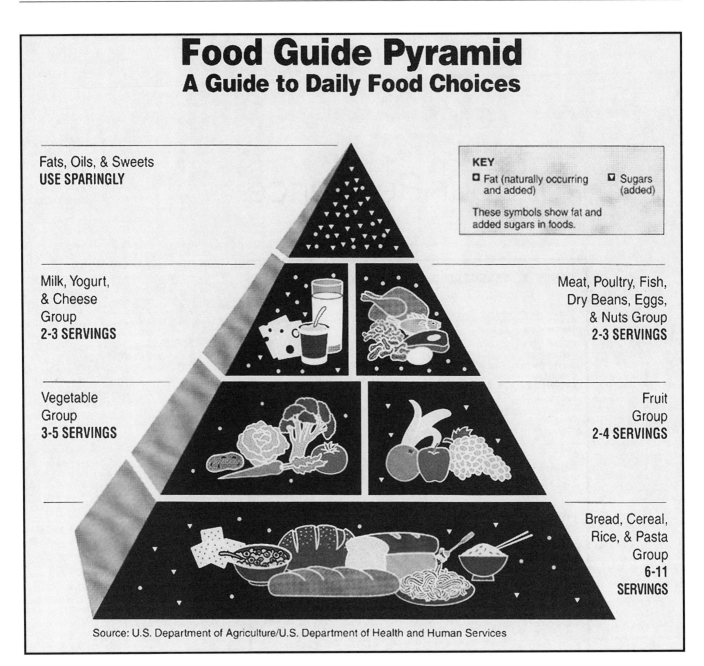

Food Guide Pyramid
A Guide to Daily Food Choices

Fats, Oils, & Sweets
USE SPARINGLY

KEY
▢ Fat (naturally occurring and added)   ▣ Sugars (added)

These symbols show fat and added sugars in foods.

Milk, Yogurt, & Cheese Group
2-3 SERVINGS

Meat, Poultry, Fish, Dry Beans, Eggs, & Nuts Group
2-3 SERVINGS

Vegetable Group
3-5 SERVINGS

Fruit Group
2-4 SERVINGS

Bread, Cereal, Rice, & Pasta Group
6-11 SERVINGS

Source: U.S. Department of Agriculture/U.S. Department of Health and Human Services

VITAMINS IN FOODS

Vitamin A	liver, carrots, kale, red peppers, milk, spinach, eggs, butter
Vitamin B_6	meat, whole grains, cabbage, peanuts, potatoes, soybeans, liver, fish, beans, milk
Vitamin B_{12}	liver, fish, eggs, milk
Vitamin B_9 (Folate)	tomatoes, spinach, beets, asparagus, potatoes, liver, wheat germ, soybeans, cabbage, whole grains, eggs, milk, meats
Vitamin C	tomatoes, potatoes, most fruits and vegetables
Vitamin D	milk, liver, fatty fish like herring, chicken skin, egg yolks
Vitamin E	most vegetable oils
Vitamin K	broccoli, turnip greens, lettuce, liver, cauliflower, spinach, cabbage, asparagus, Brussels sprouts
Thiamin	meats, whole grains, potatoes, fish, liver, legumes (like beans and peas)
Biotin	liver, soybeans, egg yolks, peanuts, cauliflower, carrots, oatmeal
Riboflavin	eggs, asparagus, liver, milk, fish, meat, whole grains
Pantothenic Acid	liver, fish, eggs, milk, whole grains, meats, legumes (like beans and peas)
Niacin	meats, whole grains, eggs, fish, milk, legumes (like beans and peas)

SOURCE: Adapted from "The Vitamins" by G. F. Coombs Jr.

RECOMMENDED PYRAMID SERVINGS FOR INDIVIDUALS

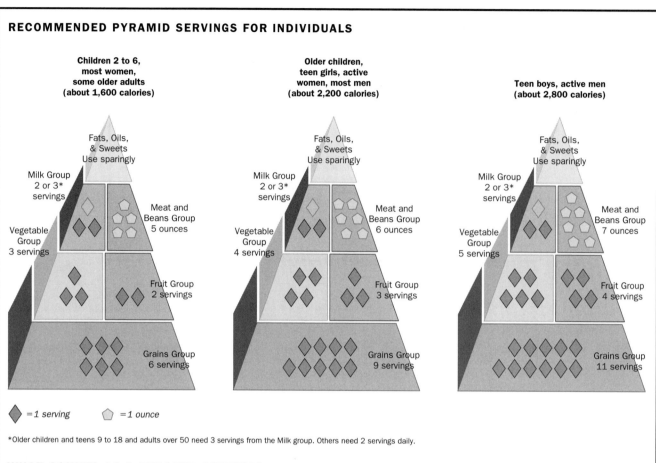

Children 2 to 6, most women, some older adults (about 1,600 calories)

Fats, Oils, & Sweets Use sparingly

Milk Group 2 or 3* servings

Meat and Beans Group 5 ounces

Vegetable Group 3 servings

Fruit Group 2 servings

Grains Group 6 servings

Older children, teen girls, active women, most men (about 2,200 calories)

Fats, Oils, & Sweets Use sparingly

Milk Group 2 or 3* servings

Meat and Beans Group 6 ounces

Vegetable Group 4 servings

Fruit Group 3 servings

Grains Group 9 servings

Teen boys, active men (about 2,800 calories)

Fats, Oils, & Sweets Use sparingly

Milk Group 2 or 3* servings

Meat and Beans Group 7 ounces

Vegetable Group 5 servings

Fruit Group 4 servings

Grains Group 11 servings

◆ = 1 serving   ⬠ = 1 ounce

*Older children and teens 9 to 18 and adults over 50 need 3 servings from the Milk group. Others need 2 servings daily.

WHAT COUNTS AS A PYRAMID SERVING?

Grains Group
• 1 slice of bread
• About 1 cup of ready to eat cereal flakes
• ½ cup of cooked cereal, rice, or pasta

Vegetable Group
• 1 cup of raw leafy vegetables
• ½ cup of other vegetables—cooked or raw*
• ¾ cup of vegetable juice

Fruit Group
• 1 medium apple, banana, orange, pear
• ½ cup of chopped, cooked or canned fruit
• ¾ cup of fruit juice

Milk Group
• 1 cup of milk of yogurt
• 1½ ounces of natural cheese (such as Cheddar)
• 2 ounces of processed cheese (such as American)

Meat and Beans Group
The Pyramid recommends 2 to 3 servings for a total of 5 to 7 ounces. The following all count as 1 ounce equivalent:

• 1 ounce of cooked lean meat, poultry, or fish
• ½ cup of cooked, dry beans*
• ½ cup of tofu or 2½-ounce soyburger
• 1 egg
• 2 tablespoons of peanut butter
• ⅓ cup of nuts

*Dry beans, peas, and lentils can be counted as servings in either the Meat and Beans group of the Vegetable group. As a vegetable, ½ cup of cooked, dry beans counts as 1 serving. As a meat substitute, ½ cup of cooked, dry beans counts as 1 ounce of meat.

SOURCE: Adapted from *Home and Garden Bulletin* 267–3. USDA.

BODY MASS INDEX TABLE

		Normal					Overweight					Obese										Extreme Obesity														
BMI	19	20	21	22	23	24	25	26	27	28	29	30	31	32	33	34	35	36	37	38	39	40	41	42	43	44	45	46	47	48	49	50	51	52	53	54
Height (inches)															Body Weight (pounds)																					
58	91	96	100	105	110	115	119	124	129	134	138	143	148	153	158	162	167	172	177	181	186	191	196	201	205	210	215	220	224	229	234	239	244	248	253	258
59	94	99	104	109	114	119	124	128	133	138	143	148	153	158	163	168	173	178	183	188	193	198	203	208	212	217	222	227	232	237	242	247	252	257	262	267
60	97	102	107	112	118	123	128	133	138	143	148	153	158	163	168	174	179	184	189	194	199	204	209	215	220	225	230	235	240	245	250	255	261	266	271	276
61	100	106	111	116	122	127	132	137	143	148	153	158	164	169	174	180	185	190	195	201	206	211	217	222	227	232	238	243	248	254	259	264	269	275	280	285
62	104	109	115	120	126	131	136	142	147	153	158	164	169	175	180	186	191	196	202	207	213	218	224	229	235	240	246	251	256	262	267	273	278	284	289	295
63	107	113	118	124	130	135	141	146	152	158	163	169	175	180	186	191	197	203	208	214	220	225	231	237	242	248	254	259	265	270	278	282	287	293	299	304
64	110	116	122	128	134	140	145	151	157	163	169	174	180	186	192	197	204	209	215	221	227	232	238	244	250	256	262	267	273	279	285	291	296	302	308	314
65	114	120	126	132	138	144	150	156	162	168	174	180	186	192	198	204	210	216	222	228	234	240	246	252	258	264	270	276	282	288	294	300	306	312	318	324
66	118	124	130	136	142	148	155	161	167	173	179	186	192	198	204	210	216	223	229	235	241	247	253	260	266	272	278	284	291	297	303	309	315	322	328	334
67	121	127	134	140	146	153	159	166	172	178	185	191	198	204	211	217	223	230	236	242	249	255	261	268	274	280	287	293	299	306	312	319	325	331	338	344
68	125	131	138	144	151	158	164	171	177	184	190	197	203	210	216	223	230	236	243	249	256	262	269	276	282	289	295	302	308	315	322	328	335	341	348	354
69	128	135	142	149	155	162	169	176	182	189	196	203	209	216	223	230	236	243	250	257	263	270	277	284	291	297	304	311	318	324	331	338	345	351	358	365
70	132	139	146	153	160	167	174	181	188	195	202	209	216	222	229	236	243	250	257	264	271	278	285	292	299	306	313	320	327	334	341	348	355	362	369	376
71	136	143	150	157	165	172	179	186	193	200	208	215	222	229	236	243	250	257	265	272	279	286	293	301	308	315	322	329	338	343	351	358	365	372	379	386
72	140	147	154	162	169	177	184	191	199	206	213	221	228	235	242	250	258	265	272	279	287	294	302	309	316	324	331	338	346	353	361	368	375	383	390	397
73	144	151	159	166	174	182	189	197	204	212	219	227	235	242	250	257	265	272	280	288	295	302	310	318	325	333	340	348	355	363	371	378	386	393	401	408
74	148	155	163	171	179	186	194	202	210	218	225	233	241	249	256	264	272	280	287	295	303	311	319	326	334	342	350	358	365	373	381	389	396	404	412	420
75	152	160	168	176	184	192	200	208	216	224	232	240	248	256	264	272	279	287	295	303	311	319	327	335	343	351	359	367	375	383	391	399	407	415	423	431
76	156	164	172	180	189	197	205	213	221	230	238	246	254	263	271	279	287	295	304	312	320	328	336	344	353	361	369	377	385	394	402	410	418	426	435	443

SOURCE: Adapted from Clinical Guidelines on the Identification, Evaluation, and Treatment of Overweight and Obesity in Adults: The Evidence Report.

Contributors

Karen Ansel
Walnut Creek, California

Katherine Beals
Ball State University
Muncie, Indiana

Mindy Benedict
Ponte Vedra Beach, Florida

Frances Berg
Healthy Weight Network and University of North Dakota School of Medicine
Hellinger, North Dakota

Linda B. Bobroff
University of Florida
Gainesville, Florida

Leslie Bonci
University of Pittsburgh Medical Center
Pittsburgh, Pennsylvania

Susan T. Borra
International Food Information Council Foundation
Washington, DC

Karen Bryla
University of Kentucky
Lexington, Kentucky

Lori Keeling Buhi
Bryan-College Station Community Health Center
Bryan, Texas

Slande Celeste
University of Florida
Gainesville, Florida

Nilesh Chatterjee
Texas A&M University
College Station, Texas

Sara Chelland
Department of Nutrition, Food and Exercise Science
Tallahassee, Florida

Catherine Christie
University of North Florida
Jacksonville, Florida

Sonja Connor
Portland, Oregon

William Connor
Oregon Health Sciences University
Portland, Oregon

Marilyn Dahl
Preferred Nutrition Services
Jacksonville Beach, Florida

Raju Das
University of Dundee
Dundee, UK

Ruth DeBusk
Private Practice
Tallahassee, Florida

Sharon Doughten
Cuyahoga Community College
Cleveland, Ohio

Karen Drummond
Yardley, Pennsylvania

M. Cristina Flaminiano Garces
University of North Carolina at Chapel Hill

Beth Fontenot
McNeese State University
Lake Charles, Louisiana

John P. Foreyt
Baylor College of Medicine
Houston, Texas

Mohammed Forouzesh
California State University at Long Beach
Long Beach, California

Marion J. Franz
Nutrition Concepts by Franz, Inc.
Minneapolis, Minnesota

Marjorie Freedman
San Jose, California

Keri M. Gans
New York, New York

Chandak Ghosh
Harvard Medical School
Boston, Massachusetts

Gita C. Gidwani
Johns Hopkins University
Baltimore, Maryland

Emil Ginter
Institute of Preventive and Clinical Medicine
Bratislava, Slovak Republic

Diane Golzynski
California State University
Fresno, California

Leslene E. Gordon
Pasco County Health Department Nutrition Division
New Port Ritchey, Florida

Marcus Harding
International Medical Volunteers Association
Woodville, Massachusetts

Karen Hare
Nutrition Services, Inc.
Fort Collins, Colorado

Beth Hensleigh
Texas A&M University
College Station, Texas

Kirsten Herbes
University of Florida
Gainesville, Florida

Susan Himburg
Florida International University
Miami, Florida

Lenore S. Hodges
Florida Hospital
Orlando, Florida

Steve Hohman
Ohio University
Athens, Ohio

Elissa M. Howard-Barr
Coastal Carolina University
Conway, South Carolina

Delores C. S. James
University of Florida
Gainesville, Florida

Sunitha Jasti
University of North Carolina,
Chapel Hill, North Carolina

Warren B. Karp
The Medical College of Georgia
Augusta, Georgia

Susan Kim
Williams College
Williamstown, Massachusetts

Seema Pania Kumar
Alexandria Primary Care Associates
Alexandria, Virginia

M. Elizabeth Kunkel
Clemson University
Clemson, South Carolina

Julie Lager
Texas A&M University
College Station, Texas

Jens Levy
University of North Carolina
Chapel Hill, North Carolina

Kheng Lim
*University of Medicine and
Dentistry of New Jersey*
Camden, New Jersey

Nadia Lugo
University of Florida
Gainesville, Florida

Teresa Lyles
University of Florida
Gainesville, Florida

Carole Mackey
*Agency for Health Care
Administration*
St. Petersburg, Florida

Amy N. Marlow
New York, New York

Cindy Martin
Texas A&M University
College Station, Texas

Toni Martin
Duval County Health Department
Jacksonville, Florida

Kiran Misra
Texas A&M University
College Station, Texas

Ranjita Misra
San Diego State University
San Diego, California

Braxton D. Mitchell
University of Maryland
Baltimore, Maryland

Susan Mitchell
Practicalories, Inc.
Winter Park, Florida

Robert J. Moffatt
Florida State University
Tallahassee, Florida

Melissa Morris
University of Florida
Gainesville, Florida

Kweethai C. Neill
University of North Texas
Denton, Texas

Laura Nelson
Texas A&M University
College Station, Texas

Virginia Noland
University of Florida
Gainesville, Florida

Neelima Pania
New York University Hospital
New York, New York

Mary Parke
*Duval County Health Department,
UIC and Nutrition Program*
Jacksonville, Florida

Isabel Parraga
Case Western Reserve University
Cleveland, Ohio

Gita Patel
Nutrition Consultant
Etna, New Hampshire

Nadine Pazder
Morton Plant Hospital
Clearwater, Florida

Judy E. Perkin
University of North Florida
Jacksonville, Florida

Jeffrey Radecki
*Robert Wood Johnson Medical
School*
Piscataway, New Jersey

Sheah Rarback
*University of Miami School
Medicine*
Miami, Florida

Catherine Rasberry
Texas A&M University
College Station, Texas

Barbara L. Rice
Enterprise Advisory Services, Inc.
Houston, Texas

Carlos Robles
University of the Virgin Islands

Judy Rodriguez
University of North Florida
Jacksonville, Florida

Kim Schenck
Colorado Springs, Colorado

Claire D. Schmelzer
*Virginia Polytechnic Institute and
State University*
Blacksburg, Virginia
University of Kentucky
Lexington, Kentucky

Louise Schneider
Lorna Linda University
Lorna Linda, California

Jessica Schulman
University of Florida
Gainesville, Florida

Kyle Shadix
Art Institute of New York City

Jackie Shank
Southeast Nutrition Consultants
St. Augustine, Florida

Heidi J. Silver
*National Policy and Resource Center
on Nutrition and Aging*
Miami, Florida

Donna Staton
*International Medical Volunteers
Association*

Tanya Sterling
Duval County Health Department
Jacksonville, Florida

Milton Stokes
New York, New York

Lisa A. Sutherland
University of North Carolina
Chapel Hill, North Carolina

Marie Boyle Struble
College of Saint Elizabeth
Morristown, New Jersey

D. Michelle Swords
Gainesville, Florida

Patricia Thomas
San Antonio, Texas

Delores Truesdell
Florida State University
Tallahassee, Florida

Katherine Tucker
*USDA/HNRCA at Tufts
University*
Boston, Massachusetts

Simin Vaghefi
University of North Florida
Jacksonville, Florida

Pauline Vickery
*Suwannee River Area Health
Education Center*

Ruth Waibel
Ohio University
Athens, Ohio

Daphne C. Watkins
Texas A&M University
College Station, Texas

Sally Weerts
University of North Florida
Jacksonville, Florida

Paulette Weir
Elmont, New York

Katherine Will
Ohio University
Athens, Ohio

Heidi Williams
Gainesville, Florida

Addiction, Food

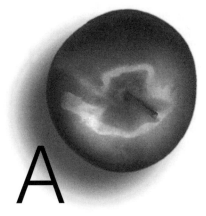

Food addiction is a nonmedical term that refers to a compulsion to eat specific foods, usually those that are high in sugar or starch. Although this term is used to describe intense cravings to seek out specific foods, these foods are not, in and of themselves, physically addictive in the way a drug might be. Instead, the need to pursue and consume these foods may be representative of a **psychological** disturbance, extreme **anxiety**, or emotional distress. SEE ALSO EATING DISORDERS; EATING DISTURBANCES.

Karen Ansel

psychological: related to thoughts, feelings, and personal experiences

anxiety: nervousness

Bibliography

Cassell, Dana, and Gleaves, David (2000). *The Encyclopedia of Eating Disorders*, 2nd edition. New York: Facts on File.

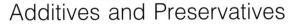

Additives and Preservatives

Additives are defined by the United States Food and Drug Administration (FDA) as "any substance, the intended use of which results or may reasonably be expected to result, directly or indirectly, in its becoming a component or otherwise affecting the characteristics of any food." In other words, an additive is any substance that is added to food. Direct additives are those that are intentionally added to foods for a specific purpose. Indirect additives are those to which the food is exposed during processing, packaging, or storing. Preservatives are additives that inhibit the growth of **bacteria**, yeasts, and molds in foods.

bacteria: single-celled organisms without nuclei, some of which are infectious

Additives and preservatives have been used in foods for centuries. When meats are smoked to preserve them, compounds such as butylated hydroxyanisole (BHA) and butyl gallate are formed and provide both **antioxidant** and **bacteriostatic** effects. Salt has also been used as a preservative for centuries. Salt lowers the water activity of meats and other foods and inhibits bacterial growth. Excess water in foods can enhance the growth of bacteria, yeast, and fungi. Pickling, which involves the addition of acids such as vinegar, lowers the **pH** of foods to levels that retard bacterial growth. Some herbs and spices, such as curry, cinnamon, and chili pepper, also contain antioxidants and may provide **bactericidal** effects.

antioxidant: substance that prevents oxidation, a damaging reaction with oxygen

bacteriostatic: a state that prevents growth of bacteria

pH: level of acidity, with low numbers indicating high acidity

bactericidal: a substance that kills bacteria

1

leavening: yeast or other agents used for rising bread

food additive: substance added to foods to improve nutrition, taste, appearance, or shelf-life

microorganisms: bacteria and protists; single-celled organisms

oxygen: O₂, atmospheric gas required by all animals

nutrient: dietary substance necessary for health

vitamin: necessary complex nutrient used to aid enzymes or other metabolic processes in the cell

mineral: an inorganic (non-carbon-containing) element, ion, or compound

enrichment: addition of vitamins and minerals to improve the nutritional content of a food

fortification: addition of vitamins and minerals to improve the nutritional content of a food

fortified: altered by addition of vitamins or minerals

vitamin D: nutrient needed for calcium uptake and therefore proper bone formation

niacin: one of the B vitamins, required for energy production in the cell

Uses of Additives and Preservatives in Foods

Additives and preservatives are used to maintain product consistency and quality, improve or maintain nutritional value, maintain palatability and wholesomeness, provide **leavening**, control pH, enhance flavor, or provide color. **Food additives** may be classified as:

1. *Antimicrobial agents,* which prevent spoilage of food by mold or **microorganisms.** These include not only vinegar and salt, but also compounds such as calcium propionate and sorbic acid, which are used in products such as baked goods, salad dressings, cheeses, margarines, and pickled foods.

2. *Antioxidants,* which prevent rancidity in foods containing fats and damage to foods caused by **oxygen.** Examples of antioxidants include vitamin C, vitamin E, BHA, BHT (butylated hydroxytolene), and propyl gallate.

3. *Artificial colors,* which are intended to make food more appealing and to provide certain foods with a color that humans associate with a particular flavor (e.g., red for cherry, green for lime).

4. *Artificial flavors and flavor enhancers,* the largest class of additives, function to make food taste better, or to give them a specific taste. Examples are salt, sugar, and vanilla, which are used to complement the flavor of certain foods. Synthetic flavoring agents, such as benzaldehyde for cherry or almond flavor, may be used to simulate natural flavors. Flavor enhancers, such as monosodium glutamate (MSG) intensify the flavor of other compounds in a food.

5. *Bleaching agents,* such as peroxides, are used to whiten foods such as wheat flour and cheese.

6. *Chelating agents,* which are used to prevent discoloration, flavor changes, and rancidity that might occur during the processing of foods. Examples are citric acid, malic acid, and tartaric acid.

7. ***Nutrient*** additives, including **vitamins** and **minerals,** are added to foods during **enrichment** or **fortification.** For example, milk is **fortified** with **vitamin D,** and rice is enriched with thiamin, riboflavin, and **niacin.**

8. *Thickening and stabilizing agents,* which function to alter the texture of a food. Examples include the emulsifier lecithin, which, keeps oil and vinegar blended in salad dressings, and carrageen, which is used as a thickener in ice creams and low-calorie jellies.

Regulating Safety of Food Additives and Preservatives

Based on the 1958 Food Additives Amendment to the Federal Food, Drug, and Cosmetic (FD&C) Act of 1938, the FDA must approve the use of all additives. The manufacturer bears the responsibility of proving that the additive is safe for its intended use. The Food Additives Amendment excluded additives and preservatives deemed safe for consumption prior to 1958, such as salt, sugar, spices, vitamins, vinegar, and monosodium glutamate. These substances are considered "generally recognized as safe" (GRAS) and may be used in any food, though the FDA may remove additives from the GRAS list if safety concerns arise. The 1960 Color Additives Amendment to the FD&C Act required the FDA to approve synthetic coloring agents used in

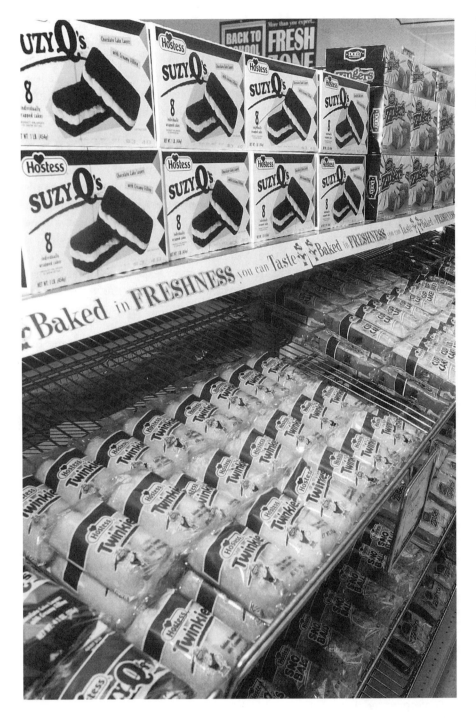

The legendary longevity of some packaged foods such as Twinkies, is attributable in part to food additives that stabilize ingredients and prevent spoilage. Additives also enhance the nutrition, flavor, and consistency of foods. [Photograph by Orlin Wagner. AP/Wide World Photos. Reproduced by permission.]

foods, **drugs**, cosmetics, and certain medical devices. The Delaney Clause, which was included in both the Food Additives Amendment and Color Additives Amendment, prohibited approval of any additive that had been found to cause **cancer** in humans or animals. However, in 1996 the Delaney Clause was modified, and the commissioner of the FDA was charged with assessing the risk from consumption of additives that may cause cancer and making a determination as to the use of that additive.

The FDA continually monitors the safety of all food additives as new scientific evidence becomes available. For example, use of erythrosine (FD&C Red No. 3) in cosmetics and externally applied drugs was banned

drugs: substances whose administration causes a significant change in the body's function

cancer: uncontrolled cell growth

3

nitrite: NO_2^-, used for preservatives

amine: compound containing nitrogen linked to hydrogen

carcinogen: cancer-causing substance

fermentation: reaction performed by yeast or bacteria to make alcohol

asthma: respiratory disorder marked by wheezing, shortness of breath, and mucus production

toxicant: harmful substance

The Discovery of Canning

During the late eighteenth century the French army was suffering from scurvy, malnourishment, and outright starvation, and the French government offered a prize of 12,000 francs to anyone who could discover a way to preserve food for the troops. Nicholas Appert, a candymaker, brewer, and baker, reasoned that he should be able to preserve food in bottles, like wine. After fourteen years of experimentation, he finally discovered that if he put food in glass jars reinforced with wire, sealed them with wax, and applied heat, the food didn't spoil. Appert was presented with the 12,000-franc prize by Napoleon himself. However, the secret of preserved food soon leaked to the English, who proceeded to invent the can, and the armies that faced off at Waterloo were both fortified by preserved rations.

—*Paula Kepos*

in 1990 after it was implicated in the development of thyroid tumors in male rats. However, the cancer risk associated with FD&C Red No. 3 is about 1 in 100,000 over a seventy-year lifetime, and its use in some foods, such as candies and maraschino cherries, is still allowed. Tartrazine (FD&C Yellow No. 5) has been found to cause dermatological reactions ranging from itching to hives in a small population subgroup. Given the mild nature of the reaction, however, it still may be used in foods.

Nitrites are also a controversial additive. When used in combination with salt, nitrites serve as antimicrobials and add flavor and color to meats. However, nitrite salts can react with certain **amines** in food to produce nitrosamines, many of which are known **carcinogens**. Food manufacturers must show that nitrosamines will not form in harmful amounts, or will be prevented from forming, in their products. The flavoring enhancer MSG is another controversial food additive. MSG is made commercially from a natural **fermentation** process using starch and sugar. Despite anecdotal reports of MSG triggering headaches or exacerbating **asthma**, the Joint Expert Committee on Food Additives of the United Nations Food and Agriculture Organization, the World Health Organization, the European Community's Scientific Committee for Food, the American Medical Association, and the National Academy of Sciences have all affirmed the safety of MSG at normal consumption levels.

In the United States, food additives and preservatives play an important role in ensuring that the food supply remains the safest and most abundant in the world. A major task of the FDA is to regulate the use and approval of thousands of approved food additives, and to evaluate their safety. Despite consumer concern about use of food additives and preservatives, there is very little scientific evidence that they are harmful at the levels at which they are used.

In Europe, food additives and preservatives are evaluated by the European Commission's Scientific Committee on Food. Regulations in European Union countries are similar to those in the United States. The Food and Agricultural Organization (FAO) of the United Nations and the World Health Organization (WHO) Expert Committee on Food Additives work together to evaluate the safety of food additives, as well as contaminants, naturally occurring **toxicants**, and residues of veterinary drugs in foods. Acceptable Daily Intakes (ADIs) are established on the basis of toxicology and other information. SEE ALSO ARTIFICIAL SWEETENERS; FAT SUBSTITUTES.

M. Elizabeth Kunkel
Barbara H. D. Luccia

Bibliography

Branen, A. Larry (2002). *Food Additives*, 2nd edition. New York: Marcel Dekker.

Clydesdale, Fergus M. (1997). *Food Additives: Toxicology, Regulation, and Properties.* Boca Raton, FL: CRC Press.

Potter, Norman N., and Hotchkiss, Joseph H. (1995) *Food Science*, 5th edition. New York: Chapman & Hall.

Adolescent Nutrition

Adolescence is the transition period between childhood and adulthood, a time of life that begins at **puberty**. For girls, puberty typically occurs be-

puberty: time of onset of sexual maturity

tween ages 12 and 13, while for boys it occurs between ages 14 and 15. It is one of the fastest growth periods of a person's life. During this time, physical changes affect the body's nutritional needs, while changes in one's lifestyle may affect eating habits and food choices. Nutritional health during adolescence is important for supporting the growing body and for preventing future health problems.

Increased Nutritional Needs

The physical changes of adolescence have a direct influence on a person's nutritional needs. Teenagers need additional **calories**, **protein**, **calcium**, and **iron**.

Calories. Adolescents need additional calories to provide **energy** for growth and activity. Boys ages 11 to 18 need between 2,500 and 2,800 calories each day. Adolescent girls need approximately 2,200 calories each day. This is a significant increase from childhood requirements. To meet these calorie needs, teens should choose a variety of healthful foods, such as lean protein sources, low-fat dairy products, whole grains, fruits, and vegetables.

Protein. Protein is important for growth and maintenance of muscle. Adolescents need between 45 and 60 grams of protein each day. Most teens easily meet this requirement with their intake of beef, pork, chicken, eggs, and dairy products. Protein is also available from certain vegetable sources, including **tofu** and other soy foods, beans, and nuts.

Calcium. Adequate calcium intake is essential for development of strong and dense bones during the adolescent growth spurt. Inadequate calcium intake during adolescence and young adulthood puts individuals at risk for developing **osteoporosis** later in life. In order to get the required 1,200 milligrams of calcium, teens are encouraged to consume three to four servings of calcium-rich foods each day. Good sources include milk, yogurt, cheese, calcium-fortified juices, and calcium-fortified cereals.

Iron. As adolescents gain muscle mass, more iron is needed to help their new muscle cells obtain **oxygen** for energy. A deficiency of iron causes **anemia**, which leads to **fatigue**, confusion, and weakness. Adolescent boys need 12 milligrams of iron each day, while girls need 15 milligrams. Good sources of iron include beef, chicken, pork, **legumes** (including beans and peanuts), enriched or whole grains, and leafy green vegetables such as spinach, collards, and kale.

Eating and Snacking Patterns

Adolescents tend to eat differently than they did as children. With afterschool activities and active social lives, teens are not always able to sit down for three meals a day. Busy schedules may lead to meal skipping, snacking throughout the day, and more eating away from home. Many teens skip breakfast, for example, but this meal is particularly important for getting enough energy to make it through the day, and it may even lead to better academic performance. When teens skip meals, they are more likely to grab fast food from a restaurant, vending machine, or convenience store. These foods are high in fat and sugar and tend to provide little nutritional value. In addition, eating too many fast foods can lead to weight gain and, in some cases, **diabetes** and **heart disease**.

calorie: unit of food energy

protein: complex molecule composed of amino acids that performs vital functions in the cell; necessary part of the diet

calcium: mineral essential for bones and teeth

iron: nutrient needed for red blood cell formation

energy: technically, the ability to perform work; the content of a substance that allows it to be useful as a fuel

tofu: soybean curd, similar in consistency to cottage cheese

osteoporosis: weakening of the bone structure

oxygen: O$_2$, atmospheric gas required by all animals

anemia: low level of red blood cells in the blood

fatigue: tiredness

legumes: beans, peas, and related plants

diabetes: inability to regulate level of sugar in the blood

heart disease: any disorder of the heart or its blood supply, including heart attack, atherosclerosis, and coronary artery disease

Dietary decisions made in adolescence may have lasting health effects. For example, in the United States, more than 85 percent of teen girls and about 65 percent of teen boys do not include enough calcium in their diets. Such deficiency increases their chances of developing osteoporosis as adults. *[AP/Wide World Photos. Reproduced by permission.]*

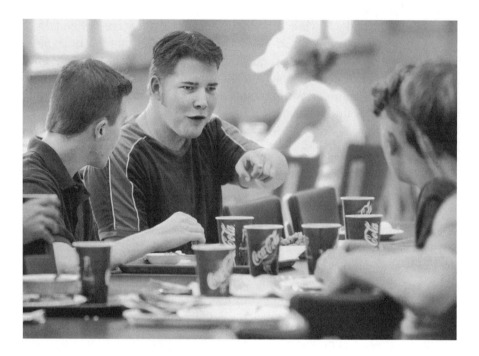

Eating meals and snacking away from home puts the responsibility for good food choices right in adolescents' hands. Snacks should be low in both fat and added sugar. Some healthful snack ideas include fresh fruit, sliced vegetables with low-fat dip, low-fat yogurt, low-fat string cheese, peanut butter and crackers, baked chips, granola bars, and graham crackers. Juices, fruit drinks, and sodas are usually very high in calories from natural or added sugar, so they should be consumed in moderation. The Food Guide Pyramid is an appropriate guide for adolescents' food choices, even when snacking.

Potential Nutrition-Related Problems

obesity: the condition of being overweight, according to established norms based on sex, age, and height

chronic: over a long period

Adolescents are at risk for **obesity**, obesity-related **chronic** diseases, and eating disorders.

Obesity, Diabetes, and Heart Disease. All over the world, adolescent obesity is on the rise. This has led to an increase in obesity-related diseases like diabetes and heart disease. Experts believe this rise in obesity is due to lack of physical activity and an increase in the amount of fast food and "junk food" available to adolescents. Staying active and eating foods that are low in fat and sugar promote a healthy weight for teens.

Eating Disorders. Adolescents tend to be very conscious of appearances and may feel pressure to be thin or to look a certain way. Fear of gaining weight may lead to overly restrictive eating habits. Some teens resort to self-induced vomiting or laxative use to control their weight. Both boys and girls are affected by eating disorders. Teens who suspect they have a problem with body image or eating habits should talk to a trusted adult.

High-Risk Groups

Certain groups of adolescents may be at risk for nutritional inadequacies.

Pregnant Teens. When a teenager becomes pregnant, she needs enough **nutrients** to support both her baby and her own continued growth and physical development. If her nutritional needs are not met, her baby may be born with low birth weight or other health problems. For the best outcome, pregnant teens need to seek prenatal care and nutrition advice early in their pregnancy.

nutrient: dietary substance necessary for health

Athletes. Adolescents involved in athletics may feel pressure to be at a particular weight or to perform at a certain level. Some young athletes may be tempted to adopt unhealthful behaviors such as crash dieting, taking supplements to improve performance, or eating unhealthful foods to fulfill their hearty appetites. A balanced nutritional outlook is important for good health and athletic performance.

Vegetarians. A vegetarian **diet** can be a very healthy option. However, adolescents who follow a vegetarian diet, whether for religious or personal reasons, need to carefully plan their intake to get the protein and **minerals** they need. Strict vegetarians (those who do not eat eggs or dairy products), also known as **vegans,** may need nutritional supplements to meet their needs for calcium, vitamin B$_{12}$, and iron.

diet: the total daily food intake, or the types of foods eaten

mineral: an inorganic (non-carbon-containing) element, ion, or compound

vegan: person who consumes no animal products, including milk and honey

Conclusion

Adolescence is a time of growing up both physically and socially. During these years, the nutrition choices people make will affect not only their current health, but their future health as well. SEE ALSO EATING DISORDERS; EATING DISTURBANCES; SCHOOL-AGED CHILDREN, DIET OF.

Amy N. Marlow

Bibliography

Bode, Janet (1999). *Food Fight: A Guide to Eating Disorders for Preteens and Their Parents.* New York: Aladdin Paperbacks.

Duyff, Roberta Larson (2002). *American Dietetic Association Complete Food and Nutrition Guide.* New York: Wiley.

Krizmanic, Judy (1999). *The Teen's Vegetarian Cookbook.* New York: Viking.

Adult Nutrition

The science of **nutrition** is dedicated to learning about foods that the human body requires at different stages of life in order to meet the nutritional needs for proper growth, as well as to maintain health and prevent disease. A baby is born with a very high requirement for **energy** and **nutrient** intake per unit of body weight to provide for rapid growth. The rate of growth is the highest during the first year and declines slowly after the age of two, with a corresponding decrease in nutrient and energy requirements. During **puberty,** however, **nutritional requirements** increase sharply until this period of fast growth is completed. Adulthood begins at about the age of fourteen or fifteen for girls, and eighteen or nineteen for boys.

nutrition: the maintenance of health through proper eating, or the study of same

energy: technically, the ability to perform work; the content of a substance that allows it to be useful as a fuel

nutrient: dietary substance necessary for health

puberty: time of onset of sexual maturity

nutritional requirements: the set of substances needed in the diet to maintain health

fat: type of food molecule rich in carbon and hydrogen, with high energy content

wellness: related to health promotion

An adult individual needs to balance energy intake with his or her level of physical activity to avoid storing excess body **fat.** Dietary practices and food choices are related to **wellness** and affect health, fitness, weight

chronic: over a long period

osteoporosis: weakening of the bone structure

cardiovascular: related to the heart and circulatory system

cancer: uncontrolled cell growth

diabetes: inability to regulate level of sugar in the blood

physiological: related to the biochemical processes of the body

basal metabolic rate: rate of energy consumption by the body during a period of no activity

vitamin: necessary complex nutrient used to aid enzymes or other metabolic processes in the cell

mineral: an inorganic (non-carbon-containing) element, ion, or compound

protein: complex molecule composed of amino acids that performs vital functions in the cell; necessary part of the diet

obesity: the condition of being over-weight, according to established norms based on sex, age, and height

carbohydrate: food molecule made of carbon, hydrogen, and oxygen, including sugars and starches

fiber: indigestible plant material that aids digestion by providing bulk

diet: the total daily food intake, or the types of foods eaten

constipation: difficulty passing feces

hemorrhoids: swollen blood vessels in the rectum

diverticulosis: presence of abnormal small sacs in the lining of the intestine

appendicitis: inflammation of the appendix

management, and the prevention of **chronic** diseases such as **osteoporosis**, **cardiovascular** diseases, **cancer**, and **diabetes**.

For adults (ages eighteen to forty-five or fifty), weight management is a key factor in achieving health and wellness. In order to remain healthy, adults must be aware of changes in their energy needs, based on their level of physical activity, and balance their energy intake accordingly.

As teenagers reach adulthood, the basal energy needs for maintaining the body's **physiological** functions (**basal metabolic rate**, or BMR) stabilize, and so energy requirements also stabilize. BMR is defined as the energy required by the body to keep functioning. These functions include the pumping of blood by the heart, respiration, kidney function, and maintaining muscle tone and a constant body temperature, among others. BMR is directly related to the amount of lean body muscle mass, size, and gender. Physical activity, especially weight-training exercises, help increase and maintain lean body mass.

It is very important to reduce one's energy intake at the onset of adulthood, and to make sure that all of one's nutritional needs are met. This can be accomplished by making sure that an adequate amount of energy is consumed (this will vary by body weight, degree of physical fitness, and muscle vs. body fat), and that this amount of energy is adjusted to one's level of physical activity. Foods that are chosen to provide the energy must be highly nutritious, containing high amounts of essential nutrients such as **vitamins**, **minerals**, and essential **proteins**.

It is usually at this age that young adults start gaining body fat and reducing their physical activity, resulting in an accumulation of fat in the abdominal areas. This is an ever-increasing risk factor in the population of the United States, where **obesity** is not only a problem in adults, but also in children. It is believed that the high level of obesity in the United States is mostly due to bad dietary practices such as eating a high-fat, low-complex **carbohydrate** (low **fiber**) **diet**, including excessive amounts of meat. The indulgence in fast foods and a lack of regular physical activity are major factors. Obesity is a risk factor for other degenerative diseases, such as type II (adult onset) diabetes, diseases of heart and circulation, and certain cancers. Another nutritional problem related to eating such a diet is **constipation**, due to low-fiber diets. This may result in **hemorrhoids**, **diverticulosis**, **appendicitis**, and other more serious diseases of the lower intestine. Increasing the number of servings of fruits, vegetables, and whole grains in the diet will prevent these diseases. In the United States, the Dietary Guidelines for Americans (as summarized in the Food Guide Pyramid) provide practical guidelines for healthful eating.

At the onset of adulthood, energy requirements usually reach a plateau that will last until one's mid-forties, after which they begin to decline, primarily because activity levels and lean muscle mass (amount of muscle vs. body fat), which represents the BMR, decrease. It is believed that the changes in body composition and reduced lean muscle mass occur at a rate of about 5 percent per decade, and energy requirements decrease accordingly. However, these changes in body composition and decreased energy requirements can be prevented by maintaining regular physical activity, including resistance training, which helps maintain lean muscle mass and prevent deposition of excess body fat.

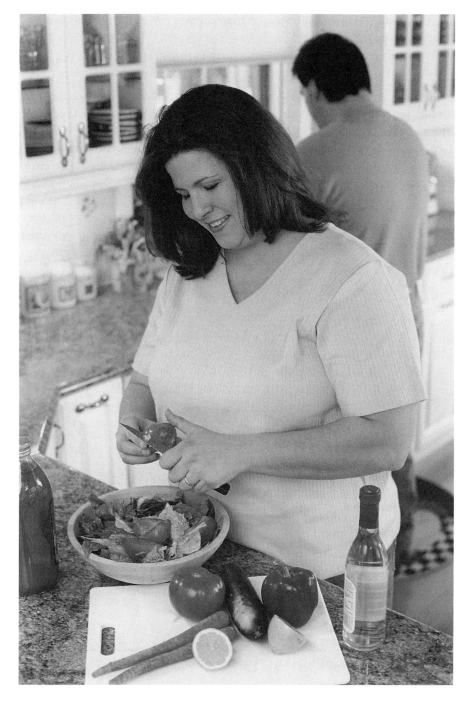

The basal metabolic rate—the number of calories a person's body uses while at rest—generally decreases with age. Good health requires adults to adapt their diets to the body's changing needs by eating low-fat and nutrient-rich foods. *[Photograph by Michael Keller. Corbis. Reproduced by permission.]*

By preventing normal age-related decline in lean muscle mass, one can prevent obesity and prolong one's physiological age. The result is that a person is less vulnerable to degenerative diseases, such as cardiovascular diseases, cancer, and diabetes, and can usually perform at a higher level than his or her chronological age would otherwise allow.

Older adults who are not physically active or who have poor nutritional practices will have a decline in BMR, a change in body composition, an increasing percentage of body fat, and a decrease in lean body muscle mass. In addition, they will show the signs of aging and will be more likely to develop degenerative diseases.

hypertension: high blood pressure

absorption: uptake by the digestive tract

calcium: mineral essential for bones and teeth

vitamin D: nutrient needed for calcium uptake and therefore proper bone formation

menopause: phase in a woman's life during which ovulation and menstruation ends

Many older adults need to take medications to control the advance of diabetes, **hypertension**, and cardiovascular disease. Medications can interfere with proper nutrition, however, as they affect appetite, the digestion and **absorption** of nutrients, and normal function of the digestive system.

As women age, they may develop osteoporosis if they have not built up strong bones by eating foods high in **calcium** and adequate **vitamin D**. Women start losing calcium from bones during and after the onset of **menopause** at the rate of 1 percent per year for about five years, after which the rate of calcium loss is reduced until about age seventy-five or eighty. Therefore, it is important for women to eat foods high in calcium up to the age of thirty-five. The recommended daily intake of calcium is 1,200 milligrams. This requirement can be met by consuming four servings of dairy products and two servings of green vegetables each day. It is well established that calcium from foods is much better absorbed than calcium from supplements. It is beneficial, therefore, to choose foods with a high calcium content, such as low-fat or skim dairy products. This regimen builds a bone density high enough so that, at menopause, losing approximately 5 percent of bone density in five years does not place a woman in the "fracture zone," where bones can break as a result of osteoporosis. SEE ALSO AGING AND NUTRITION; NUTRIENT-DRUG INTERACTIONS; OSTEOPOROSIS.

Simin B. Vaghefi

Bibliography

Poehlman, E. T., and Horton, E. S. (1999). "Energy Needs: Assessment and Requirements in Humans." In *Modern Nutrition in Health and Disease*, 9th edition, edited by M. E. Shils, J. A. Olson, M. Shike, and A. C. Ross. Baltimore, MD: Williams & Wilkins.

Pi-Suunyer, F. X. (1999). "Obesity." In *Modern Nutrition in Health and Disease*, 9th edition, edited by M. E. Shils, J. A. Olson, M. Shike, and A. C. Ross. Baltimore, MD: Williams & Wilkins.

Internet Resources

National Institutes of Health (2000). "Osteoporosis Prevention, Diagnosis, and Therapy." NIH Consensus Statement. Available from <http://odp.od.nih.gov>

U.S. Department of Agriculture. "The Food Guide Pyramid." Available from <http://www.nal.usda.gov>

African Americans, Diet of

The 2000 U.S. Census revealed that there were almost 35 million African Americans, or about 13 percent of the total U.S. population. This small percentage of the populace has had a significant influence on American cuisine, not only because African-American food is diverse and flavorful, but also because of its historical beginnings. Despite their cultural, political, economic, and racial struggles, African Americans have retained a strong sense of their culture, which is, in part, reflected in their food.

Origins of the African-American Diet: The Aftereffects of Slavery

diversity: the variety of cultural traditions within a larger culture

The roots of the **diversity** of African-American cuisine may be traced back to 1619, when the first African slaves were sold in the New World. In a quest to build new cities in America, Europeans actively transported Africans and West Indians (people from the West Indies) to the new land. The West Indies (in the Caribbean Sea) was part of the slave route to America. Because the West Indians' skin color was similar to that of Africans, they were not treated any differently. As a result, some West Indian food traditions are similar to those of African Americans.

It is not surprising that African-American food has a distinctive culinary heritage with diverse flavors, as it includes traditions drawn from the African continent, the West Indies, and from North America. While the European nations were busy establishing new societies, they did not realize that the African and West Indian slaves who worked for them brought their own vibrant and and rich culture—a culture that would withstand and adapt to the harsh centuries of slavery.

Food historian Karen Hess writes about the struggle of African Americans to maintain some of their original culture through food. "The only thing that Africans brought with them [from Africa] was their memories." Slave traders attempted to craft culturally sensitive rations for the Africans by including yams, rice, corn, plantains, coconuts, and scraps of meat in the slaves' provisions.

Southern slaves established their own cooking culture using foods that were similar to foods that were part of their African and West Indian heritages, and many popular foods in the African-American diet are directly associated with foods in Africa. For instance, the African yam is similar to the American sweet potato. White rice is also popular because it was a major part of the diet in West Africa. African Americans infuse plain rice dishes with their own savory ingredients (popular rice dishes include gumbo and "hoppin' John," a dish made with rice, black-eyed peas, and salt pork or bacon).

The Legacy of African-American Cuisine

Popular southern foods, such as the vegetable okra (brought to New Orleans by African slaves), are often attributed to the importation of goods from Africa, or by way of Africa, the West Indies, and the slave trade. Okra, which is the principal ingredient in the popular Creole stew referred to as gumbo, is believed to have spiritual and healthful properties. Rice and seafood (along with sausage or chicken), and filé (a sassafras powder inspired by the Choctaw Indians) are also key ingredients in gumbo. Other common foods that are rooted in African-American culture include black-eyed peas, benne seeds (sesame), eggplant, sorghum (a grain that produces sweet syrup and different types of flour), watermelon, and peanuts.

Though southern food is typically known as "soul food," many African Americans contend that soul food consists of African-American recipes that have been passed down from generation to generation, just like other African-American **rituals**. The legacy of African and West Indian culture is imbued in many of the recipes and food traditions that remain popular today. The staple foods of African Americans, such as rice, have remained largely unchanged since the first Africans and West Indians set foot in the New World, and the southern United States, where the slave population was most dense, has developed a cooking culture that remains true to the African-American tradition. This cooking is aptly named *southern cooking*,

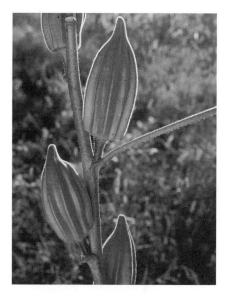

A major ingredient in cuisine of African origin, okra traveled to the eastern Mediterranean, Arabia, and India long before it came to the New World with African slaves. The thickening characteristic of its sticky substance is put to good use in the preparation of gumbos and stews. *[Photograph by Robert J. Huffman/Field Mark Publications. Reproduced by permission.]*

ritual: ceremony or frequently repeated behavior

the food, or *soul food*. Over the years, many have interpreted the term *soul food* based on current social issues facing the African-American population, such as the civil rights movement. Many civil rights advocates believe that using this word perpetuates a negative connection between African Americans and slavery. However, as Doris Witt notes in her book *Black Hunger* (1999), the "soul" of the food refers loosely to the food's origins in Africa.

In his 1962 essay "Soul Food," Amiri Baraka makes a clear distinction between southern cooking and soul food. To Baraka, soul food includes chitterlings (pronounced chitlins), pork chops, fried porgies, potlikker, turnips, watermelon, black-eyed peas, grits, hoppin' John, hushpuppies, okra, and pancakes. Today, many of these foods are limited among African Americans to holidays and special occasions. Southern food, on the other hand, includes only fried chicken, sweet potato pie, collard greens, and barbecue, according to Baraka. The idea of what soul food is seems to differ greatly among African Americans.

General Dietary Influences

In 1992 it was reported that there is little difference between the type of foods eaten by whites and African Americans. There have, however, been large changes in the overall quality of the diet of African Americans since the 1960s. In 1965, African Americans were more than twice as likely as whites to eat a diet that met the recommended guidelines for **fat**, **fiber**, and fruit and vegetable intakes. By 1996, however, 28 percent of African Americans were reported to have a poor-quality diet, compared to 16 percent of whites, and 14 percent of other racial groups. The diet of African Americans is particularly poor for children two to ten years old, for older adults, and for those from a low socioeconomic background. Of all racial groups, African Americans have the most difficulty in eating diets that are low in fat and high in fruits, vegetables, and whole grains. This represents an immense change in diet quality. Some explanations for this include: (1) the greater market availability of packaged and **processed foods**; (2) the high cost of fresh fruit, vegetables, and lean cuts of meat; (3) the common practice of frying food; and (4) using fats in cooking.

Regional differences. Although there is little overall variability in diets between whites and African Americans, there are many notable regional influences. Many regionally influenced **cuisines** emerged from the interactions of Native American, European, Caribbean, and African cultures. After emancipation, many slaves left the south and spread the influence of soul food to other parts of the United States. Barbecue is one example of African-influenced cuisine that is still widely popular throughout the United States. The Africans who came to colonial South Carolina from the West Indies brought with them what is today considered signature southern cookery, known as *barbacoa*, or barbecue. The original barbecue recipe's main ingredient was roasted pig, which was heavily seasoned in red pepper and vinegar. But because of regional differences in livestock availability, pork barbecue became popular in the eastern United States, while beef barbecue became popular in the west of the country.

Other Ethnic Influences. Cajun and Creole cooking originated from the French and Spanish but were transformed by the influence of African

fat: type of food molecule rich in carbon and hydrogen, with high energy content

fiber: indigestible plant material that aids digestion by providing bulk

processed food: food that has been cooked, milled, or otherwise manipulated to change its quality

cuisine: types of food and traditions of preparation

cooks. African chefs brought with them specific skills in using various spices, and introduced okra and native American foodstuffs, such as crawfish, shrimp, oysters, crabs, and pecans, into both Cajun and Creole cuisine. Originally, Cajun meals were bland, and nearly all foods were boiled. Rice was used in Cajun dishes to stretch out meals to feed large families. Today, Cajun cooking tends to be spicier and more robust than Creole. Some popular Cajun dishes include pork-based sausages, jambalayas, gumbos, and coush-coush (a creamed corn dish). The symbol of Cajun cooking is, perhaps, the crawfish, but until the 1960s crawfish were used mainly as bait.

More recently, the immigration of people from the Caribbean and South America has influenced African-American cuisine in the south. New spices, ingredients, combinations, and cooking methods have produced popular dishes such as Jamaican jerk chicken, fried plantains, and bean dishes such as Puerto Rican *habichuelas* and Brazilian *feijoada*.

Holidays and Traditions. African-American meals are deeply rooted in traditions, holidays, and celebrations. For American slaves, after long hours working in the fields the evening meal was a time for families to gather, reflect, tell stories, and visit with loved ones and friends. Today, the Sunday meal after church continues to serve as a prime gathering time for friends and family.

Kwanzaa, which means "first fruits of the harvest," is a holiday observed by more than 18 million people worldwide. Kwanzaa is an African-American celebration that focuses on the traditional African values of family, community responsibility, commerce, and self-improvement. The Kwanzaa Feast, or Karamu, is traditionally held on December 31. This symbolizes the celebration that brings the community together to exchange and to give thanks for their accomplishments during the year. A typical menu includes a black-eyed pea dish, greens, sweet potato pudding, cornbread, fruit cobbler or compote dessert, and many other special family dishes.

Folk beliefs and remedies. Folk beliefs and remedies have also been passed down through generations, and they can still be observed today. The majority of African-American beliefs surrounding food concern the medicinal uses of various foods. For example, yellow root tea is believed to cure illness and lower blood sugar. The bitter yellow root contains the antihistamine berberine and may cause mild low **blood pressure**. One of the most popular folk beliefs is that excess blood will travel to the head when one eats large amounts of pork, thereby causing **hypertension**. However, it is not the fresh pork that should be blamed for this rise in blood pressure, but the salt-cured pork products that are commonly eaten. Today, folk beliefs and remedies are most often held in high regard and practiced by the elder and more traditional members of the population.

Effects of Socioeconomic Status: Poverty and Health

Many of the foods commonly eaten by African Americans, such as greens, yellow vegetables, **legumes**, beans, and rice, are rich in **nutrients**. Because of cooking methods and the consumption of meats and baked goods, however, the diet is also typically high in fat and low in fiber, **calcium**, and

blood pressure: measure of the pressure exerted by the blood against the walls of the blood vessels

hypertension: high blood pressure

legumes: beans, peas, and related plants

nutrient: dietary substance necessary for health

calcium: mineral essential for bones and teeth

Diet-Related Disease by Race	Obesity (%)	Diabetes (%)	Hypertension (%)
African Americans			
Male	21.1	7.6	36.7
Female	37.4	11.2	36.6
Total	**33.4**	**10.8**	**36.6**
Whites			
Male	20.0	4.7	24.6
Female	22.4	5.4	20.5
Total	**21.3**	**7.8**	**22.1**
Hispanics			
Male	23.1	8.1	NA
Female	33.0	11.4	NA
Total	**26.2**	**9.0**	**NA**

SOURCE: Centers for Disease Control and Prevention, National Center for Health Statistics (2002).

obesity: the condition of being overweight, according to established norms based on sex, age, and height

type II diabetes: Inability to regulate the level of sugar in the blood due to a reduction in the number of insulin receptors on the body's cells

heart disease: any disorder of the heart or its blood supply, including heart attack, atherosclerosis, and coronary artery disease

diabetes: inability to regulate level of sugar in the blood

high blood pressure: elevation of the pressure in the bloodstream maintained by the heart

prevalence: describing the number of cases in a population at any one time

potassium. In 1989, 9.3 million of the black population (30.1%) had incomes below the poverty level. Individuals who are economically disadvantaged may have no choice but to eat what is available at the lowest cost. In comparison to other races, African Americans experience high rates of **obesity**, hypertension, **type II diabetes**, and **heart disease**, which are all associated with an unhealthful diet.

Obesity and hypertension are major causes of heart disease, **diabetes**, kidney disease, and certain cancers. African Americans experience disproportionately high rates of obesity and hypertension, compared to whites.

High blood pressure and obesity have known links to poor diet and a lack of physical activity. In the United States, the **prevalence** of high blood pressure in African Americans is among the highest in the world. The alarming rates of increase of obesity and high blood pressure, along with the deaths from diabetes-related complications, heart disease, and kidney failure, have spurred government agencies to take a harder look at these problems. As a result, many U.S. agencies have created national initiatives to improve the diet quality and the overall health of African Americans.

Looking Forward to a Healthier Tomorrow

African-American food and its dietary evolvement since the beginning of American slavery provide a complicated, yet extremely descriptive, picture of the effects of politics, society, and the economy on culture. The deep-rooted dietary habits and economic issues that continue to affect African Americans present great challenges regarding changing behaviors and lowering disease risk. In January 2000, the U.S. Department of Health and Human Services launched Healthy People 2010, a comprehensive, nationwide health promotion and disease prevention agenda. The overarching goal of this program is to increase quality and years of healthy life and eliminate health disparities between whites and minority populations, specifically African Americans. As national health initiatives and programs continue to improve and target African Americans and other populations in need, preventable diseases will be lowered, creating a healthier U.S. society. SEE ALSO AFRICANS, DIETS OF; CARIBBEAN ISLANDERS, DIET OF; DIETARY TRENDS, AMERICAN.

M. Cristina F. Garces
Lisa A. Sutherland

Bibliography

Basiotis, P. P.; Lino, M; and Anand, R. S. (1999). "Report Card on the Diet Quality of African Americans." *Family Economics and Nutrition Review* 11:61–63.

de Wet, J. M. J. (2000). "Sorghum." In *The Cambridge World History of Food*, Vol. 1, ed. Kenneth F. Fiple and Kriemhil Conee Ornelas. Cambridge, UK: Cambridge University Press.

Dirks, R. T., and Duran, N. (2000). "African American Dietary Patterns at the Beginning of the 20th Century." *Journal of Nutrition* 131(7):1881–1889.

Foner, Eric, and Garraty, John A., eds. (1991). *The Reader's Companion to American History*. Boston: Houghton Mifflin.

Genovese, Eugene D. (1974). *Roll, Jordan, Roll: The World the Slaves Made*. New York: Vintage.

Harris, Jessica (1995). *A Kwanzaa Keepsake: Celebrating the Holiday with New Traditions and Feasts*. New York: Simon & Schuster.

Harris, Jessica (1999). *Iron Pots and Wooden Spoons: Africa's Gift to the New World Cooking*. New York: Simon & Schuster.

Kittler, Pamela Goyan, and Sucher, Kathryn, eds. (1989). "Black Americans." In *Food and Culture in America*. New York: Van Nostrand and Reinhold.

Popkin, B. M.; Siega-Riz, A. M.; and Haines, P. S. (1996). "A Comparison of Dietary Trends among Racial and Socioeconomic Groups in the United States." *New England Journal of Medicine* 335:716–720.

Thompson, Becky W. (1994). *A Hunger So Wide and So Deep: American Women Speak Out on Eating Problems*. Minneapolis: University of Minnesota Press.

Wilson, C. R., and Ferris, W. (1989). *The Encyclopedia of Southern Culture*. Chapel Hill: University of North Carolina Press.

Witt, Doris (1999). *Black Hunger*. New York: Oxford University Press.

Zinn, Howard (1980). "Drawing the Color Line." In *A People's History of the United States*. New York: HarperCollins.

Internet Resources

Centers for Disease Control and Prevention, National Center for Health Statistics (2002). "Monitoring the Nation's Health." Available from <http://www.cdc.gov/nchs/>

U.S. Census Bureau (2001). "General Demographic Characteristics for the Black or African American Population." Available from <http://www.census.gov>

U.S. Census Bureau (2001). "Profile of General Demographic Characteristics." Available from <http://factfinder.census.gov>

U.S. Department of Health and Human Services. *Healthy People 2010*. Available from <http://health.gov/healthypeople>

Africans, Diets of

Africa, the second largest continent in the world, is rich in geographic and cultural **diversity**. It is a land populated by peoples with histories dating to ancient times and cultures shaped by innumerable tribes, languages, and traditions. Because it is the birthplace of *Homo sapiens* and the land of origin for much of the world's population, the culture of food and eating in the different regions of Africa is important to people throughout the world.

Early History of Africa

The early history of man is the story of food in Africa. *Homo sapiens* evolved apart from other apes in Africa, and the adaptation of humans has been shaped by adaptations to **diet**. For example, some anthropologists believe

diversity: the variety of cultural traditions within a larger culture

diet: the total daily food intake, or the types of foods eaten

15

that the selection pressure that led to bipedalism (walking on two legs) was an adaptation to changing environments that involved travel in search of tubers (rounded underground plant stems, such as potatoes). Africa's history includes some of humankind's earliest food production, with one of the most fertile centers located in Northern Africa, the Nile Valley. The Nile Valley historically was and continues to be a rich source of fish, animal, and plant food. In the drier African savannas, especially after the Sahara region became arid after 6000 B.C.E., nomad tribes raised cattle, goats, or sheep, which served as part of the tribes' food source. Crops that were less affected by extreme weather like cereals (such as wheat, barley, millet, and sorghum) and tubers (such as yams) slowly became popular throughout the continent and have remained important **staples** in the African diet today.

staples: essential foods in the diet

The African Climate and Terrain. The historic influences on the African diet began in ancient times and continue to the present day. Great geographic differences across the African continent caused much of the variety in the African diet. In addition, many tribes and peoples migrated or traded, bringing spices and foods from each other's culture into their own. However, though each region of Africa has its distinct **cuisines**, African food has its basic staples.

cuisine: types of food and traditions of preparation

The African Diet

Throughout Africa, the main meal of the day is lunch, which usually consists of a mixture of vegetables, **legumes**, and sometimes meat. However, though different meats are considered staples in many areas, many Africans are not able to eat meat often, due to economic constraints. Beef, goat, and sheep (mutton) are quite expensive in Africa, so these foods are reserved for special days. However, fish is abundant in coastal regions and in many lakes.

legumes: beans, peas, and related plants

The combination of various foods is called stew, soup, or sauce, depending on the region. This mixture is then served over a porridge or mash made from a root vegetable such as cassava or a grain such as rice, corn, millet, or teff. Regional differences are reflected in variations on this basic meal, primarily in the contents of the stew. The greatest variety of ingredients occurs in coastal areas and in the fertile highlands. Flavorings and spiciness have varied principally due to local histories of trade. In the traditional African diet, meat and fish are not the focus of a meal, but are instead used to enhance the stew that accompanies the mash or porridge. Meat is rarely eaten, though it is well-liked among carnivorous (meat-eating) Africans.

Traditional Cooking Methods. Traditional ways of cooking involve steaming food in leaf wrappers (banana or corn husks), boiling, frying in oil, grilling beside a fire, roasting in a fire, or baking in ashes. Africans normally cook outdoors or in a building separate from the living quarters. African kitchens commonly have a stew pot sitting on three stones arranged around a fire. In Africa, meals are normally eaten with the hands.

North Africa

The countries of North Africa that border the Mediterranean Sea are largely Muslim countries. As a result, their diet reflects Islamic traditions. The religion of Islam does not permit eating pork or any animal product that has

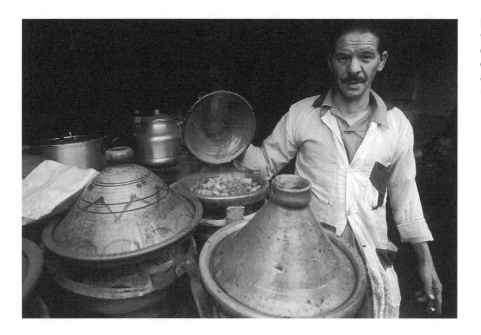

North African cuisine reflects the Islamic traditions of the region. Here, a man cooks with traditional Moroccan *tajines,* conical clay pots used for lamb stews and curries. *[Photograph by Owen Franken. Corbis. Reproduced by permission.]*

not been butchered in accordance with the traditions of the faith. Like other regions of Africa, much of the diet is based on grains. However, cooking with olive oil, onions, and garlic is more common in the countries of North Africa. Notable spices include cumin, caraway, clove, and cinnamon. Flat breads are a common staple and can accompany any meal, including breakfast, which is usually porridge prepared from millet or chickpea flour. *Couscous* (made from hard wheat and millet) is often the main dish at lunch, which is the primary meal. This may be accompanied by vegetable salads. Other main dishes include *tajine,* named for the conical clay pot in which a whole meal is prepared. Lamb is cooked in tajines as well as on kabobs (roasted on a skewer). Vegetables include okra, meloukhia (spinach-like greens), and radishes. Common fruits are oranges, lemons, pears, and mandrakes. Legumes such as broad beans (fava beans), lentils, yellow peas, and black-eyed peas are also important staples. Alcoholic drinks are forbidden by Islamic tradition. Mint tea and coffee are very popular beverages in this region.

West Africa

Within West Africa, there is considerable variation in the staple food. Rice is predominant from Mauritania to Liberia and across to the Sahel, a region that stretches across the continent between the Sahara and the southern savannas. Couscous is the prevalent dish in the Sahara. Along the coast from Côte d'Ivoire (Ivory Coast) to Nigeria and Cameroon, root crops, primarily varieties of yam and cassava, are common. Cassava, imported from Brazil by the Portuguese, is boiled and then pounded into a nearly pure starch. Yam is the chief crop in West Africa and is served in a variety of dishes, including *amala* (pounded yam) and *egwansi* (melon) sauce. Millet is also used for making porridge or beer.

Palm oil is the base of stew in the Gambia, southern, and eastern regions. In the Sahalian area, groundnut paste (peanut butter) is the main ingredient for stew. Other stews are based on okra (a vegetable native to the

Biotechnology and Africa

Many scientists believe that biotechnology is the most promising route to fighting and possibly eradicating chronic malnutrition among the 800 million people in the developing world who live in poverty. Researchers are working to develop improved versions of African staples, including a strain of sweet potato that is resistant to a virus that regularly devastates the crop, cassava that is resistant to the cassava mosaic virus, and corn that is resistant to the maize streak virus. Also under development is cotton that is less susceptible to insect infestation. However, genetically modified crops are controversial in some African countries. Zambia has banned donations of genetically modified food, and Zimbabwe has raised concerns about donations of corn from the United States that is not certified to be free of genetic modifications.

—*Paula Kepos*

rainforests of Africa), beans, sweet potato leaves, or cassava. Other vegetables are eggplant, cabbage, carrots, chilies, french beans, lettuce, okra, onions, and cherry tomatoes. All the stews in this territory tend to be heavily spiced, often with chilies.

West African Fruit. Plantain, a variety of banana, is abundant in the more tropical West Africa. Sweet plantains are normally fried, while hard plantains are boiled or pounded into *fufu*. Dates, bananas, guava, melons, passionfruit, figs, jackfruit, mangos, pineapples, cashews, and wild lemons and oranges are also found here.

Protein Sources. Meat sources of protein include cattle, sheep, chicken, and goat, though beef is normally reserved for holidays and special occasions. Fish is eaten in the coastal areas. Because of the Islamic influence, pork is localized to non-Muslim areas. In these regions, "bush meat" is widely eaten, including bush rat, a large herbivorous rodent, antelope, and monkey. Giant snails are also eaten in various parts of West Africa.

East Africa

Extensive trade and migrations with Arabic countries and South Asia has made East African culture unique, particularly on the coast. The main staples include potatoes, rice, *matake* (mashed plantains), and a maize meal that is cooked up into a thick porridge. Beans or a stew with meat, potatoes, or vegetables often accompany the porridge. Beef, goat, chicken, or sheep are the most common meats. Outside of Kenya and the horn of Africa, the stew is not as spicy, but the coastal area has spicy, coconut-based stews. This is quite unique in comparison to the central and southern parts of Africa.

Two herding tribes, the Maasai and Fulbe, have a notably different eating pattern. They do not eat very much meat, except for special occasions. Instead, they subsist on fresh and soured milk and butter as their staples. This is unusual because very few Africans consume milk or dairy products, primarily due to **lactose intolerance**.

The horn of Africa, which includes modern-day Somalia and Ethiopia, is characterized by its remarkably spicy food prepared with chilies and garlic. The staple grain, teff, has a considerably higher **iron** and **nutrient** content than other grain staples found in Africa. A common traditional food here is *injera*, a spongy flat bread that is eaten by tearing it, then using it to scoop up the meat or stew.

Southern Africa

Outside of the **temperate zones**, in the southern part of the continent, a greater variety of fruits and vegetables are available. Fruits and vegetables in southern Africa include bananas, pineapples, pau-pau (papaya), mangoes, avocadoes, tomatoes, carrots, onions, potatoes, and cabbage. Nonetheless, the traditional meal in southern Africa is centered on a staple crop, usually rice or maize, served with a stew. The most common dish made from cornmeal is called *mealie meal*, or *pap* in South Africa. Also known as *nshima* or *nsima* further north, it is usually eaten with stew poured over it. The stew may include a few boiled vegetables, such as cabbage, spinach, or turnips, or on more special occasions, fish, beans, or chicken.

lactose intolerance: inability to digest lactose, or milk sugar

iron: nutrient needed for red blood cell formation

nutrient: dietary substance necessary for health

temperate zone: region of the world between the tropics and the arctic or Antarctic

18

Nutrition and Disease

White South Africans (Dutch descendants called Afrikaaners), Europeans, and Asian Indians in Africa have diets similar to their countries of origin. In urban areas, however, the diet of (black) Africans is increasingly dependent on meat, much like the diet of some West African pastoral tribes, as well as on empty **calories** from prepackaged foods similar to those found in the West. The result is an unbalanced diet. In many parts of Africa, the traditional diets of indigenous peoples are often inadequate in essential **vitamins**, **minerals**, and protein, which can lead to a variety of diseases. **Micronutrient** deficiencies, particularly vitamin A, iodine, and iron deficiencies, which can result in vision impairment, goiter, and **anemia**, respectively, are prevalent throughout much of Africa, particularly in the arid areas where the soil is deficient either naturally or due to overuse.

Food Security

A far greater threat comes from increasingly insecure food sources (a lack of consistent and affordable food staples) arising from adverse weather (drought and floods) and war. During the late 1900s, **famine** became increasingly frequent in Africa. In addition, a new threat to the food supply emerged due to the worsening HIV/AIDS epidemic. As adults fall ill and die, agricultural production declines. Rural communities are the hardest hit, and women are particularly at risk given their unique physiologic needs tied to their roles as mothers, as well as their vulnerability due to lower economic and social status.

With its immense population, resources, and growing population, Africa is a continent that struggles to keep its people and cultures healthy. African history, the proliferation of foods and spices across the land, and the preservation of land that can still be farmed, will continue to be important. Weather, geography, politics, culture, and religion are forces that have caused strife within Africa for centuries, and will continue to do so. A land that was once pure and fertile can only be restored through land preservation and food availability. SEE ALSO AFRICAN AMERICANS, DIET OF; CARIBBEAN ISLANDERS, DIET OF.

Jens Levy
M. Cristina F. Garces

calorie: unit of food energy

vitamin: necessary complex nutrient used to aid enzymes or other metabolic processes in the cell

mineral: an inorganic (non-carbon-containing) element, ion, or compound

micronutrient: nutrient needed in very small quantities

anemia: low level of red blood cells in the blood

famine: extended period of food shortage

Bibliography

Carr, Marilyn, ed. (1991). *Women and Food Security: The Experience of the SADCC Countries.* London: IT Publications.

Eles, Dale, and Fitzpatrick, Mary. (2000). *Lonely Planet West Africa.* Singapore: Lonely Planet.

Finlay, Hugh (2000). *Lonely Planet East Africa.* Singapore: Lonely Planet.

Fiple, Kenneth F., and Ornelas, Kriemhil Coneè, eds. (2000). *The Cambridge World History of Food,* Volumes 1 and 2. Cambridge, UK: Cambridge University Press.

Harris, Jessica B. (1998). *The Africa Cookbook: Tastes of a Continent.* New York: Simon & Schuster.

Lentz, Carola, ed. (1999). *Changing Food Habits: Case Studies from Africa, South America, and Europe.* Sydney, Australia: Harwood Academic Publishers.

Von Braun, Joachim; Teklue, Tesfaye; and Webb, Patrick (1999). *Famine in Africa: Causes, Responses, and Prevention.* Baltimore: Johns Hopkins University Press.

Internet Resource

Haslwimmer, Martina (1996). "AIDS and Agriculture in Sub-Saharan Africa." Available from <http://www.fao.org>

Aging and Nutrition

Aging Americans will make up an unprecedented proportion of the population as the 78 million baby boomers reach age 50. The baby boomers, those born between 1946 and 1964, will first reach age 65 in 2011, transforming the 35 million people over age 65 in 2000 to an estimated 69 million by 2030. With improved health care, **socioeconomic status**, and health behaviors, people 85 and over are expected to be the fastest-growing group of elderly persons, tripling from 4 million in 2000 to about 14 million by 2040. Growth in the elderly population has led to two subgroups: the young-old (55 to 74 years) and the old-old (75 and older). Still, elderly people remain the most diverse segment of American society.

A nutritious daily **diet** is one factor that can assist people who are 55 and older in maintaining optimal levels of health and preventing or delaying the onset of disease. The **Dietary Reference Intakes** (DRI) are the quantities of **nutrients** that form the basis for planning and assessing diets. The DRIs include the **Recommended Dietary Allowances** (RDA), the nutrient levels that meet the requirement for nearly all (97–98%) healthy people. Two sets of RDAs exist for elderly individuals, one for those 51 to 70 years of age, and one for those over 70 years of age.

According to the RDAs, elderly people have the same nutrient requirements as their younger counterparts, yet most need fewer **calories**. **Vitamins** D and B$_6$, and **calcium**, are exceptions and are needed in greater amounts for those 51 years old and older. Therefore, a nutrient-dense diet, with fewer calorie-laden foods, becomes more crucial at older ages of the life cycle. In general, women have nutrient requirements similar to men, though they require fewer calories. Therefore, elderly women must be especially careful to select nutrient-dense foods.

The best way to establish a nutrient-dense diet is to balance a variety of food choices (in moderation) that are adequate to meet nutritional and caloric needs. The Food Guide Pyramid (FGP) is helpful to guide food selection and daily serving totals. An FGP specifically for those over 70 years of age recommends 1,200–1,600 calories from whole-grain foods, a variety of colored fruits and vegetables, low-fat dairy products, lean meats, fish and poultry, and eight glasses of fluid daily. Food labels help put single servings of food into the FGP. Results of national dietary surveys have led some experts to recommend calcium supplements and a one-a-day type of multiple vitamin. Other health food supplements are not generally needed and can be very expensive for those on fixed incomes.

Nutrition Screening Initiative

Elderly individuals are at increased risk for problems that affect their nutritional status. The nationwide Nutrition Screening Initiative (NSI) categorizes these problems as those affecting functional, social, or financial status and access to food and drink. These problems can affect quality of life and the

socioeconomic status: level of income and social class

diet: the total daily food intake, or the types of foods eaten

Dietary Reference Intakes: set of guidelines for nutrient intake

nutrient: dietary substance necessary for health

Recommended Dietary Allowances: nutrient intake recommended to promote health

calorie: unit of food energy

vitamin: necessary complex nutrient used to aid enzymes or other metabolic processes in the cell

calcium: mineral essential for bones and teeth

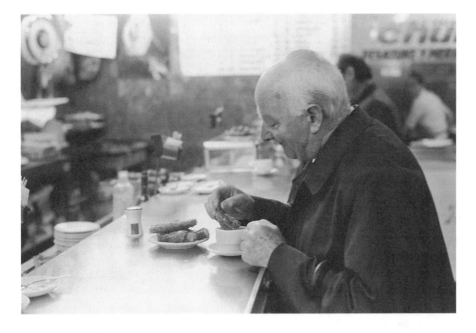

Elderly people face unique nutritional challenges. Although age can diminish appetite and physical mobility, the body still requires as many nutrients as a younger adult's. *[Photograph by Owen Franken. Corbis. Reproduced by permission.]*

ability to perform activities of daily living, including eating. The **DETER-MINE** checklist is the NSI tool used by physicians, registered dietitians, other health care providers and social service agencies to assess the impact of various dietary, medical, or physical and social problems:

Disease

Eating poorly

Tooth loss/mouth pain

Economic hardship

Reduced social contact

Multiple medications

Involuntary weight loss/gain

Needs assistance in self care

Elder years above age 80

Recognizing the risk posed by these factors can result in interventions to improve the quality of life and the ability to perform activities of daily living.

Dietary Problems

Some elderly individuals encounter dietary problems, making them less able to select, purchase, prepare, eat, digest, absorb, and use food. An inability to consume an adequate daily diet places the elderly person at increased risk for medical, physical, and functional problems. Therefore, it is important to intervene to correct any dietary problems that may exist. Examples of dietary problems, and interventions to improve the problems, are described below.

Difficulty Chewing or Swallowing. Choose more fruit and vegetable juices, soft canned fruits, and creamed or mashed cooked vegetables; eggs, milk dishes (like creamed soups), cheese, and yogurt; and cooked cereals when chewing meat or fresh fruits and vegetables are difficult. Chop, stew, steam, or grate hard foods.

DETERMINE: checklist used to identify nutritionally at-risk individuals

Difficulty Digesting. Choose more fruit and vegetable juices, soft canned fruits, and non-gas-forming vegetables rather than gas-producing vegetables like cabbage or broccoli. If digesting milk is a problem, use cultured dairy products like yogurt or add lactaid to milk. If milk continues to be problematic, consider a daily calcium supplement.

Difficulty Shopping. Shop by phone to find grocery stores that deliver in your area. Find volunteer or paid help in your area. Ask family or neighbors to help. See yellow pages under "Home Health Services" for assistance.

Difficulty Cooking. Use a microwave. Cook and freeze in batches. Relocate to a facility where other's cook, such as a family member's home or an **assisted-living** home **environment**.

Appetite Difficulties. Increase the flavor of food by adding spices and herbs, lemon juice, or meat sauces. Discuss medications with your physician, particularly if they are causing appetite or taste changes.

Financial Difficulty. Use coupons, unit pricing, and shopping lists. Plan and prepare ahead, freezing several meals at once. Buy more generic or store-brand foods and foods on sale. Find food assistance programs or sources for free and reduced-price meals, such as churches, Meals On Wheels, **Congregate Dining**, and Food Stamps. Buy more low-cost foods, such as dried beans and peas, rice, pasta, canned tuna, and peanut butter.

Social Problems

Loneliness. Invite a friend or neighbor over or have a standing date to eat out with friends or family. Buy smaller sizes to avoid the repetition of leftovers. Set the table attractively and play music softly. Participate in Congregate Dining in your area.

Living Alone. Research has shown a correlation between living alone and having lower quality diets. Men may be at greater risk because they are less experienced with planning, shopping, and preparing meals. Women may feel less motivated to prepare meals when there is no one to share them with. Ways to improve social interaction during meals and improve the experience of dining alone include: participating with others, such as at churches or Congregate Dining sites, eating by a window, using good china, eating in a park or on one's porch, garnishing meals, and trying various frozen or prepared dinners.

When living alone challenges an elderly person's health, he or she can investigate the continuum of care, including adult day care, in-home care, retirement communities, residential care or assisted living, intermediate care, and nursing homes or convalescent hospitals.

Medical, Physical, and Functional Problems

Many **chronic** medical conditions, such as **osteoporosis, arthritis, depression,** and **diabetes** have nutritional consequences. Loss of body water, lean body mass, and bone mass; decline of the immune response; over- and underweight; **malnutrition**; and declining taste, smell, and thirst are among the problems that affect physical strength, functional ability, and vitality. At times, specialized diets or medical nutrition therapy are needed; these are

assisted-living: facility that provides aid in meal preparation, cleaning, and other activities to help maintain independent living

environment: surroundings

Congregate Dining: a support service that provides a meal at a central location on a specified day

chronic: over a long period

osteoporosis: weakening of the bone structure

arthritis: inflammation of the joints

depression: mood disorder characterized by apathy, restlessness, and negative thoughts

diabetes: inability to regulate level of sugar in the blood

malnutrition: chronic lack of sufficient nutrients to maintain health

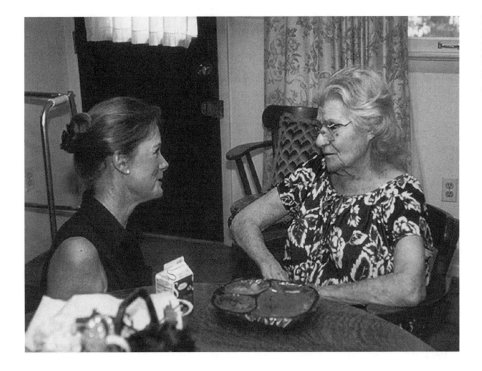

best planned with a registered dietitian. In addition, medications can affect the **absorption** and use of nutrients. Lists of food and drug interactions are available from a pharmacist or from a registered dietitian who can coordinate advice about medications with specialized dietary information. SEE ALSO DIETARY REFERENCE INTAKES; MEALS ON WHEELS; MENOPAUSE; NUTRIENT-DRUG INTERACTIONS; OSTEOPOROSIS; RECOMMENDED DIETARY ALLOWANCES.

Sally Weerts

absorption: uptake by the digestive tract

Bibliography

Davis, M. (2000). "Living Arrangements Affect Dietary Quality for U.S. Adults Aged 50 Years and Older: NHANES III 1988–1994." *The Journal of Nutrition* 130(9): 2256–2264.

Fletcher, R. H. (2002). "Vitamins for Chronic Disease Prevention in Adults: Clinical Applications." *Journal of the American Medical Association* 287(23): 3127–3129.

Alcohol and Health

Alcohol is a central-nervous-system depressant that affects judgment, coordination, and inhibition. Mild alcohol intoxication causes a relaxed and carefree feeling, as well as the loss of inhibitions. After several drinks a person will exhibit impaired judgment, poor coordination, and slurred speech, while consumption of alcohol in large amounts can lead to coma and even death. Blood alcohol concentration (BAC) is a measurement of the amount of alcohol in a person's blood. Most states consider a person to be legally drunk at a BAC between .08 and .10. At a BAC level of .40 to .50, a person may go into a coma, while a BAC level of .60 to .70 will cause death.

Alcoholic beverages can be divided into three categories: beer, wine, and distilled spirits. Beer includes beer, ale, and malt liquor; wine includes wine,

CALORIES IN ALCOHOLIC BEVERAGES AND MIXERS

Beverage	Number of Calories
Beer, 12 oz.	150
Martini, 3 oz.	145
Rum, 1 oz.	73
Sherry, 3 oz.	150
Wine, 5 oz.	100
Scotch, 1 oz.	73

vitamin: necessary complex nutrient used to aid enzymes or other metabolic processes in the cell

mineral: an inorganic (non-carbon-containing) element, ion, or compound

calorie: unit of food energy

dependence: a condition in which attempts to stop use leads to withdrawal symptoms, including irritability and insomnia

tolerance: development of a need for increased amount of drug to obtain a given level of intoxication

gene: DNA sequence that codes for proteins, and thus controls inheritance

lifestyle: set of choices about diet, exercise, job type, leisure activities, and other aspects of life

chronic: over a long period

high blood pressure: elevation of the pressure in the bloodstream maintained by the heart

heart disease: any disorder of the heart or its blood supply, including heart attack, atherosclerosis, and coronary artery disease

stroke: loss of blood supply to part of the brain, due to a blocked or burst artery in the brain

cancer: uncontrolled cell growth

hepatitis: liver inflammation

metabolize: processing of a nutrient

hypoglycemia: low blood sugar level

diet: the total daily food intake, or the types of foods eaten

energy: technically, the ability to perform work; the content of a substance that allows it to be useful as a fuel

enzyme: protein responsible for carrying out reactions in a cell

champagne, wine coolers, and vermouth; and examples of distilled spirits are gin, rum, vodka, and whiskey. Alcohol provides no **vitamins** or **minerals**, only **calories**. Small amounts of alcohol are absorbed from the mouth, approximately 20 percent is absorbed in the stomach, and the remaining 80 percent is absorbed in the small intestine.

About 7 percent of Americans abuse alcohol or suffer from alcoholism. Alcoholism can be identified through four symptoms: (1) a craving or strong urge to drink alcohol, (2) not being able to stop drinking, (3) physical **dependence**, and (4) **tolerance**. Physical dependence occurs when an individual depends on the presence of alcohol to function normally. Tolerance occurs when the same amount of alcohol results in a lesser effect; therefore, more alcohol must be consumed in order to feel the same effect. Alcohol abuse differs from alcoholism in that it does not include a strong craving for alcohol, the loss of control over one's drinking, or physical dependence. Individuals may have a problem with alcohol abuse if they exhibit one or more of the following symptoms: work and money problems, drinking while driving, being arrested due to drinking, exhibiting violent or aggressive behaviors, or continuing to drink despite the problems that result from drinking.

Alcoholism

Although there is a debate among experts over whether alcoholism should be considered a disease, the National Institute on Alcohol Abuse and Alcoholism recognizes alcoholism as a disease. The risk for developing alcoholism is influenced by a person's **genes** and **lifestyle** behaviors. Alcoholism is a **chronic** disease that lasts for a lifetime. If diagnosed and treated early, however, alcoholism may be completely cured and severe complications prevented. Chronic alcohol abuse increases a person's risk for developing serious health problems, such as liver disease, **high blood pressure**, **heart disease**, **stroke**, **cancer** (especially cancer of the esophagus, mouth, and throat), and pancreatitis.

Approximately two million Americans suffer from liver damage caused by alcohol abuse. About 10 to 20 percent of heavy drinkers will develop cirrhosis of the liver, which is characterized by scarring of the liver and causes irreversible damage. If heavy drinkers do not stop drinking, cirrhosis can cause poor health and, ultimately, death. In addition to cirrhosis, heavy drinkers may suffer from chronic liver disease or alcoholic **hepatitis**.

Damage to the liver can lead to problems with blood sugar levels. When alcohol is present in the body, the liver works to **metabolize** it. Because the liver is busy metabolizing alcohol, it is often not able to adequately maintain blood sugar levels, which may result in **hypoglycemia** (low levels of blood sugar). Hypoglycemia is most likely to occur in individuals who have not maintained an adequate **diet**. When it occurs, the brain is not able to receive the **energy** it needs to function, and symptoms such as hunger, weakness, headache, tremor, and even coma (in severe cases) may occur.

Chronic alcohol abuse can lead to poor nutritional status. Chronic heavy drinkers do not eat adequate amounts of food because of the high caloric content of alcohol. This prevents them from getting the required vitamins and minerals to maintain health and well-being. Furthermore, when a person consumes large amounts of alcohol, it impedes or halts the digestion of food, as alcohol decreases the secretion of digestive **enzymes** from the pan-

College Binge Drinking

Alcohol abuse is considered the most significant public health problem facing college students in the United States. It is estimated that more than 500,000 injuries and 70,000 cases of sexual assault a year result from alcohol abuse among students, and more than 1,400 students die each year as a result of their injuries. Two out of every five students report an episode of binge drinking—which is usually defined as five or more drinks in a row—in any given two-week period. During the 1990s, as government and health organizations began to recognize the magnitude of the problem, the U.S. Surgeon General set a goal of reducing binge drinking by 50 percent by the year 2010, and colleges sharply increased alcohol education programs and penalties for excessive or underage drinking. Nevertheless, the rate of binge drinking on college campuses remained virtually unchanged between 1993 and 2001, the year of the last comprehensive study.

—Paula Kepos

creas. Alcohol also inhibits the **absorption** of **nutrients** into the blood. This decrease in digestion and absorption over a long period of time can lead to **malnutrition**.

absorption: uptake by the digestive tract

nutrient: dietary substance necessary for health

malnutrition: chronic lack of sufficient nutrients to maintain health

High-Risk Groups

While alcohol abuse and alcoholism affect virtually every segment of the population, certain groups are at greater risk. Young adults between the ages of eighteen and twenty-nine have the highest **prevalence** of alcohol abuse, and persons who begin to drink at an early age, especially before the age of fourteen, have a greater risk for developing problems with alcohol. Persons with a family history of alcohol abuse or alcoholism are also more likely to experience alcohol-related problems. In the United States, American Indians and Alaska Natives (AI/ANs) have the highest rates of current and heavy drinking of all racial or ethnic groups. Deaths from chronic liver disease and cirrhosis are nearly four times greater among AI/ANs compared to the general U.S. population. They also have a higher prevalence of drunk driving compared to the general U.S. population.

prevalence: describing the number of cases in a population at any one time

The U.S. Department of Health and Human Services and the U.S. Department of Agriculture recommend that alcohol be consumed in moderation only. Moderation is considered two drinks per day for men and one drink per day for women (one drink is defined as twelve ounces of beer, five ounces of wine, or 1.5 ounces of a distilled spirit). Drinking alcohol is inappropriate for recovering alcoholics, persons under the age of twenty-one, persons taking medication, those who plan to drive, and women who are pregnant or plan to become pregnant.

There is no known safe level of alcohol consumption during pregnancy, as it could injure the fetus. Alcohol consumption during pregnancy may result in fetal alcohol syndrome (FAS) or fetal alcohol effects (FAE). FAS is characterized by growth retardation, facial abnormalities, and central-nervous-system dysfunction. FAS is irreversible and will affect children their entire life. If a fetus's exposure to alcohol during pregnancy is not severe enough to cause FAS, it may result in fetal alcohol effects (FAE), alcohol-related developmental disabilities (ARDD), or alcohol-related neurodevelopmental disabilities (ARND).

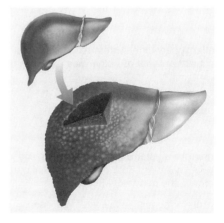

This illustration shows a healthy liver above, and a diseased liver below. Liver disease in alcoholics progresses from an enlargement of the liver to cirrhosis, which is characterized by liver scarring and is usually fatal unless alcohol consumption ceases. *[Custom Medical Stock Photo, Inc. Reproduced by permission.]*

In conclusion, knowing the effects of alcohol on the body and the consequences of alcohol abuse and misuse is very important. When consumed in large amounts or irresponsibly, alcohol can cause extensive damage to health and well-being, including liver damage, poor nutritional status, birth defects, and death. Therefore, if alcohol is consumed, it should be done so responsibly and in moderation only. SEE ALSO FETAL ALCOHOL SYNDROME; FRENCH PARADOX; MALNUTRITION; PREGNANCY.

Laura Nelson

Bibliography

Kinney, Jean (2000). *Loosening the Grip: A Handbook of Alcohol Information*, 6th edition. Boston: McGraw-Hill Higher Education.

Leone, Bruno, ed. (1998). *Alcohol: Opposing Viewpoints.* San Diego, CA: Greenhaven Press.

Marshall, Ronald (2001). *Alcoholism: Genetic Culpability or Social Irresponsibility?* New York: University Press of America.

Internet Resources

Centers for Disease Control and Prevention. "Fetal Alcohol Syndrome." Available from <http://www.cdc.gov/ncbddd>

National Institute on Alcohol Abuse and Alcoholism. "Alcohol and Minorities: An Update." Available from <http://www.niaaa.nih.gov/publications>

National Institute on Alcohol Abuse and Alcoholism. "Alcohol and Nutrition." Available from <http://www.niaaa.nih.gov/publications>

National Institute on Alcohol Abuse and Alcoholism. "Frequently Asked Questions on Alcohol Abuse and Alcoholism." Available from <http://www.niaaa.nih.gov/>

Robert Wood Johnson Foundation. "Substance Abuse: The Nation's Number One Health Problem." Available from <http://www.rwjf.org/resourcecenter>

U.S. Department of Health and Human Services, and U.S. Department of Agriculture. "Dietary Guidelines for Americans, 2000." Available from <http://www.health.gov/dietaryguidelines>

Allergies and Intolerances

Food **allergies** affect approximately 3 percent of children and 1 percent of adults in the United States. It is estimated that an even larger percentage of the population experiences problems with food intolerance. Worldwide, adverse reactions to food constitute a significant public health issue.

Definitions

The term *adverse reaction* is used to describe health problems linked to food. Food allergy and food intolerance are two types of adverse food reactions (food-borne illnesses caused by bacterial, viral, or other forms of contamination are also adverse reactions). A food allergy is said to exist when the health problem is linked to a malfunction of the **immune system**. It is believed that this malfunctioning occurs when the body identifies a food **protein** (**allergen**) as a harmful substance. *Food intolerance* occurs when the underlying problem causing the adverse reaction is not related to a malfunction of the immune system. One example of a food intolerance is **lactose intolerance**, a condition affecting people who cannot digest milk due to a deficiency of the **enzyme** lactase, which breaks down milk sugar (lactose).

allergy: immune system reaction against substances that are otherwise harmless

immune system: the set of organs and cells, including white blood cells, that protect the body from infection

protein: complex molecule composed of amino acids that performs vital functions in the cell; necessary part of the diet

allergen: a substance that provokes an allergic reaction

lactose intolerance: inability to digest lactose, or milk sugar

enzyme: protein responsible for carrying out reactions in a cell

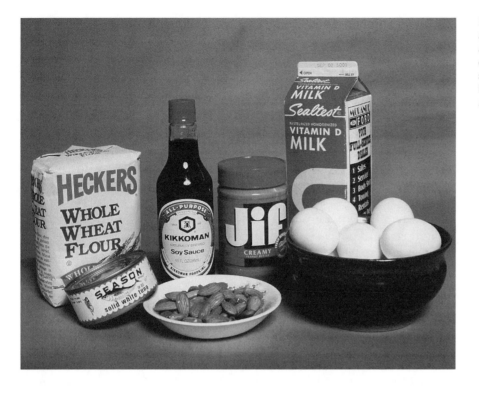

Food allergies can be triggered by almost any food. The most common food allergies are caused by wheat, nuts, fish, eggs, milk, and soy. Wheat, milk, and soy are also common causes of food intolerance. *[Erik Freeland/Corbis. Reproduced by permission.]*

Common Foods Associated with Food Allergy

Almost any food can cause an allergy, though the foods most commonly associated with an **allergic reaction** are those frequently consumed by a population. For example, an allergy to rice is common in Southeast Asia, while fish allergy is a problem in the Scandinavian countries, where fish is frequently consumed (even at breakfast). Age is also a factor influencing the types of foods to which a person might be allergic. In the United States, common foods to which adults are allergic include eggs, shrimp, lobster, peanuts, other nuts, and fish. U.S. children who have food allergies find their problems are most frequently linked to milk, soy, eggs, and peanuts. Infants may be allergic to cow's milk or soy formulas. Some food allergies may be outgrown, but allergies to peanuts, shrimp, and fish tend to last throughout life. In addition, some individuals are only allergic to one food, whereas some are allergic to several foods.

An allergic reaction can be triggered by a very small amount of a food. Persons with food allergies need to read food labels carefully and ask restaurant workers about food ingredients, and the food industry needs to ensure that **processed foods** are appropriately prepared so that people are not exposed to food allergens unknowingly. This may happen when improperly cleaned food equipment is used to prepare multiple types of food.

Food Allergy: Clinical Presentation and Diagnosis

Health problems associated with food allergies can involve the **gastrointestinal** system, the **respiratory system**, the skin, and the eyes. Persons with a food allergy may have difficulty breathing, or they may have problems with itching, rashes, swelling, **nausea**, or vomiting. A food allergy may also be a cause of **asthma**.

allergic reaction: immune system reaction against a substance that is otherwise harmless

processed food: food that has been cooked, milled, or otherwise manipulated to change its quality

gastrointestinal: related to the stomach and intestines

respiratory system: the lungs, throat, and muscles of respiration, or breathing

nausea: unpleasant sensation in the gut that precedes vomiting

asthma: respiratory disorder marked by wheezing, shortness of breath, and mucus production

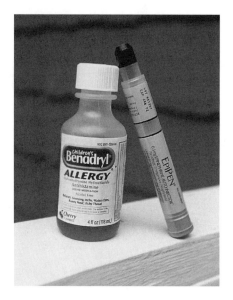

Antihistamines can give some relief of minor allergic reactions, such as skin irritation. For more severe reactions, administering a dose of epinephrine may halt life-threatening anaphylactic shock.
[Erik Freeland/Corbis. Reproduced by permission.]

anaphylaxis: life-threatening allergic reaction, involving drop in blood pressure and swelling of soft tissues especially surrounding the airways

diet: the total daily food intake, or the types of foods eaten

prevalence: describing the number of cases in a population at any one time

anxiety: nervousness

elimination diet: diet in which particular foods are eliminated to observe the effect

glucose: a simple sugar; the most commonly used fuel in cells

The symptoms of food allergy vary widely from person to person. Food allergies can also cause a severe clinical reaction known as **anaphylaxis**, which can result in death. Anaphylaxis may be characterized by throat and lip swelling, shortness of breath, sweating, itching, and feeling very faint.

Diagnosis of a food allergy usually involves a careful examination of the patient's symptom history. Other causes of symptoms must be ruled out, and in some instances the suspected food or foods will be eliminated from the **diet** to see if symptoms stop. Blood tests or skin tests may also be performed. One test sometimes used to diagnose food allergy is the double-blind, placebo-controlled food challenge. This test involves giving a patient a capsule containing a suspected food allergen and a capsule without the allergen (the placebo) and seeing if either causes symptoms in a controlled clinical setting. The test is called *double-blind* because neither the patient nor the physician evaluating the symptoms is aware of which capsule contains the allergen at the time the testing occurs.

Common Foods Associated with Intolerance

Foods associated with intolerance include: preserved foods, foods containing monosodium glutamate (MSG, a flavor enhancer), and specific foods such as milk, pickled herring, soy sauce, chili peppers, and nutmeg. Intolerance to lactose is a major problem for many populations. In the United States, lactose intolerance is common among those of African and Asian descent. The Native American population also has a high **prevalence** of lactose intolerance.

For many food intolerances, including those listed above, specific chemicals or enzyme abnormalities have been identified as being associated with the intolerance. Lactose intolerance is associated with problems with the enzyme lactase. Chemicals associated with food intolerance include sulfite (in preserved foods), tyramine (in pickled herring and soy sauce), capsaicin (in chili peppers), and myristicin (in nutmeg).

Food Intolerance: Clinical Presentation and Diagnosis

Health problems caused by food intolerance vary depending upon the food and chemical involved. The amount of a food eaten may also play a role. Lactose intolerance is usually characterized by gastrointestinal problems such as bloating and diarrhea. Sulfite intolerance is typically characterized by difficulty in breathing. Those sensitive to MSG may experience a variety of symptoms, such as headache, numbness, and rapid heartbeat. Tyramine, found in pickled herring, soy sauce, red wine, and other foods, has been linked to migraine headache. Capsaicin can cause a "burning" pain in the mouth and other problems, such as nausea and vomiting. Myristicin has been associated with **anxiety**, chest pressure, hallucinations, fever, and skin redness.

Diagnostic techniques for food intolerances vary depending upon the specific intolerance suspected. Symptom history and **elimination diets** are tools that are used, and the double-blind, placebo-controlled food challenge may also be helpful. Diagnosis of lactose intolerance in adults may involve measuring the blood to see if lactose is being broken down and showing up as blood sugar (**glucose**), or by measuring the level of hydrogen in the breath, which is increased in persons who are lactose intolerant (lactose produces hydrogen gas in the colon).

Peanut Allergies

Peanut allergies, which are among the most widespread food allergies, affect more than 1.5 million people in the United States. Symptoms of an allergic reaction may include a flushed face, hives, difficulty breathing or swallowing, vomiting, dizziness, chills, and loss of consciousness. The reaction of an allergic person to peanuts can be rapid and dramatic, sometimes causing death within minutes. The incidence of peanut allergies among children doubled in the United States between 1997 and 2002, prompting some schools to consider banning peanuts and peanut products from their premises. Proponents of a ban note that as little as half a peanut can be fatal in an allergic child, and that the risk of shared lunches or other accidental exposure is too great. Others argue that a peanut ban provides a false sense of security for children who inhabit a peanut-ridden world, and that educating students and school personnel about the problem, and preparing for the occasional incident, are more appropriate responses.

—*Paula Kepos*

Controversies Related to Food Allergies and Intolerances

Controversial issues in this area include the diagnosis of **brain allergy**, the diagnosis of **environmental illness** related to food allergy, and the diagnosis of **yeast allergy**. The connection of these problems to food allergies is not universally recognized. Some have also linked hyperactivity to food allergy or intolerance. Hyperactivity in children, in some instances, may be related to eating large amounts of **food additives**, but it is not accepted to be an allergic condition by the majority of the scientific community.

Other controversies relate to testing for food allergies. One controversial test is *cytotoxic* testing, which involves testing blood in the presence of the suspected food allergen to see if the blood cells are killed.

brain allergy: allergy whose symptoms affect brain function

environmental illness: illness due to substances in the environment

yeast allergy: allergy to yeasts used in baking or brewing

food additive: substance added to foods to improve nutrition, taste, appearance, or shelf-life

Treatment of Food Allergies and Intolerances

The major mode of treatment for food allergies and intolerances is for the person to avoid consuming the food or foods that seem to cause health problems. This involves a high degree of dietary awareness and careful food selection. When foods are eliminated from the diet, it is important to ensure the nutritional adequacy of the diet, and some individuals may need to take dietary supplements. There are some food intolerances, such as lactose intolerance, where individuals may be able to reduce the amount of the food consumed and not totally eliminate it from the diet. People with lactose intolerance do not have to completely eliminate milk products, though they must reduce their intake of lactose (milk sugar) to a manageable level. SEE ALSO ADDITIVES AND PRESERVATIVES.

Judy E. Perkin

Bibliography

Koerner, Celide B., and Munoz-Furlong, Anne (1998). *Food Allergies.* Minneapolis, MN: Chronimed.

Metcalfe, Dean D.; Sampson, Hugh A.; and Simon, Richard A. (1997). *Food Allergy: Adverse Reactions to Foods and Food Additives.* Cambridge, MA: Blackwell Science.

Trevino, Richard J., and Dixon, Hamilton S., eds. (1997). *Food Allergy.* New York, NY: Thieme Medical.

Internet Resources

American Academy of Allergy, Asthma, and Immunology. "Media Resources: Position Statement 14." Available from <http://www.aaaai.org/media>

National Digestive Diseases Information Clearinghouse. "Lactose Intolerance." Available from <http://www.niddk.nih.gov>

National Institute of Allergy and Infectious Diseases, and the National Institutes of Health. "Food Allergy and Intolerances Fact Sheet." Available from <http://www.niaid.nih.gov>

Alternative Medicines and Therapies

Alternatives to conventional medical care are increasingly popular in the United States, and their growing use by consumers represents a major trend in Western medicine. Alternative therapies appear to be used most frequently for medical conditions that are **chronic**, such as back pain, **arthritis**, sleep disorders, headache, and digestive problems. Surveys of U.S. consumers have shown that more people visit alternative practitioners each year than visit conventional primary-care physicians. Consumers do not necessarily reject conventional medicine, however. Many simply feel that alternative modalities offer complementary approaches that are more in line with their personal health philosophies.

Alternative Medicine, Complementary Medicine, and Integrative Medicine

The terms *alternative medicine* and *alternative therapies* refer to those medical practices that are not considered to be conventional medicine, as practiced in the United States. Other cultures, however, may use one or more of these approaches regularly, and, in fact, many have done so for thousands of years. Most people in the United States who use alternative medicine do so to complement conventional approaches. For example, in addition to using anti-inflammatory **drugs** to ease muscle pain, they may also use massage, **chiropractic**, and/or **osteopathic** manipulation. This practice of complementing conventional medicine with alternative approaches has given rise to the term *complementary medicine*. Presently, alternative medicine is most commonly referred to as *complementary and alternative medicine* (CAM). As conventional medical practitioners become familiar with alternative approaches, these approaches are being integrated into conventional medicine, which is giving rise to *integrative medicine*, in which a combination of therapies representing the best of conventional and alternative medicine is used.

Types of CAM Modalities

The National Center for Complementary and Alternative Medicine divides the various CAM *modalities* into five categories: (1) alternative medical systems, (2) mind-body interventions, (3) biologically-based treatments, (4) manipulative and body-based methods, and (5) **energy** therapies. These modalities include a wide variety of approaches, from **acupuncture** to **nutrition** to **meditation** to chiropractic.

Alternative medical systems include medical practices that are traditional in other cultures, such as the **ayurvedic** medical system of India, Chinese traditional medicine, and traditional Native American and Hawaiian medicine.

chronic: over a long period

arthritis: inflammation of the joints

drugs: substances whose administration causes a significant change in the body's function

chiropractic: manipulation of the spine and other bones for healing

osteopathic: related to the practice of osteopathy, which combines standard medical therapy with manipulation of the skeleton to correct problems

energy: technically, the ability to perform work; the content of a substance that allows it to be useful as a fuel

acupuncture: insertion of needles into the skin at special points to treat disease

nutrition: the maintenance of health through proper eating, or the study of same

meditation: stillness of thought, practiced to reduce tension and increase inner peace

ayurvedic: an Indian healing system

COMPLEMENTARY AND ALTERNATIVE THERAPIES POPULAR IN THE UNITED STATES

CAM Category	Examples
Alternative medical systems	Acupuncture, Ayurveda, homeopathy, naturopathy, traditional medical systems, such as aboriginal, African, Middle Eastern, Native American, Chinese, Tibetan, Central and South American
Mind-body interventions	Art therapy, dance therapy, hypnosis, meditation, mental healing, music therapy, prayer
Biologically-based treatments	Special diets and nutrition therapy, such as macrobiotic diet; herbal (botanical) therapy, vitamin/mineral therapy, orthomolecular therapy
Manipulative and body-based methods	Chiropractic, massage therapy, osteopathic manipulation
Energy therapies	Biofield therapies, such as Qi gong, Reiki, and Therapeutic Touch; bioelectromagnetic therapies, which involve the unconventional use of electromagnetic fields, such as pulsed fields, magnetic fields, or alternating current or direct current fields

SOURCE: National Center for Complementary and Alternative Medicine

Mind-body interventions recognize the connection between the physical body and the spiritual self, and include practices such as meditation, prayer, and music therapy. Biologically-based modalities are primarily nutrition-related and vary from special diets such as the **macrobiotic diet** to the inclusion of dietary supplements in the diet. Body-based methods involve hands-on manipulation of the body, and include such modalities as massage and chiropractic. The energy therapies are based on the concept that the body has an energy field that can be manipulated to promote healing.

Included among the nutrition approaches that make up the biologically-based modalities is the use of dietary supplements. Dietary supplements may be **botanical** (**herbal**) supplements or nutritional supplements, which include **vitamins, minerals, antioxidants, enzymes, metabolites,** nonprescription **hormones,** glandular extracts, and various **amino acids, fatty acids,** and other **nutrients**.

The Dietary Supplement Health and Education Act of 1994

Dietary supplement usage in the United States has increased significantly since the passage in 1994 of the Dietary Supplement Health and Education Act (DSHEA, pronounced Dee-shay). This legislation defined *dietary supplements* as distinct from food and drugs, and it allowed them to be sold without a prescription. The passage of DSHEA provided consumers with the right to purchase dietary supplements that they felt would help them attain their personal health goals. At the same time, DSHEA transferred to consumers the responsibility for making informed choices about the supplements that they used. In contrast to prescription and **over-the-counter** drugs, where effectiveness and safety must be demonstrated prior to marketing of the drugs, premarket approval is not required of manufacturers of dietary supplements. As a result, there is a greater potential risk that dietary supplements may be ineffective, or even harmful, as compared with drugs.

The dietary supplements industry is not unregulated, it is just not regulated to the extent that U.S. consumers have come to expect for prescrip-

macrobiotic: related to a specific dietary regimen based on balancing of vital principles

diet: the total daily food intake, or the types of foods eaten

botanical: related to plants

herbal: related to plants

vitamin: necessary complex nutrient used to aid enzymes or other metabolic processes in the cell

mineral: an inorganic (non-carbon-containing) element, ion, or compound

antioxidant: substance that prevents oxidation, a damaging reaction with oxygen

enzyme: protein responsible for carrying out reactions in a cell

metabolite: the product of metabolism, or nutrient processing within the cell

hormone: molecules produced by one set of cells that influence the function of another set of cells

amino acid: building block of proteins, necessary dietary nutrient

fatty acids: molecules rich in carbon and hydrogen; a component of fats

nutrient: dietary substance necessary for health

over-the-counter: available without a prescription

The rising popularity of alternative medicine has revived ancient techniques such as acupuncture. In the United States, the requirements for acupuncture licensure may vary from state to state. *[Photograph by Yoav Levy. Phototake NYC. Reproduced by permission.]*

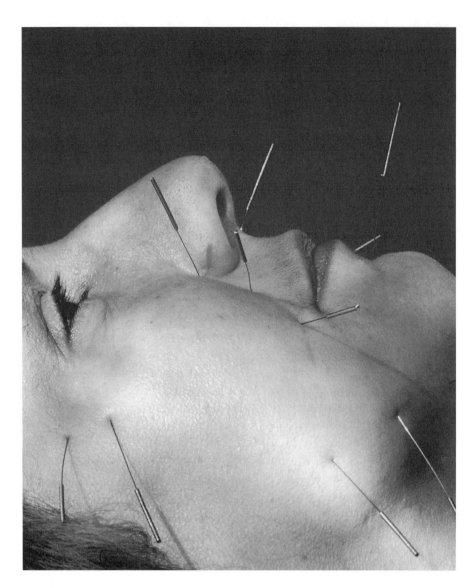

tion drugs. Instead of the drug manufacturer and the physician working to insure that a drug meets the needs of the patient and that it is both safe and effective, consumers must provide these services for themselves with dietary supplements. It is, therefore, important to know the appropriate use of a dietary supplement, the dose at which it is effective, and whether it is likely to interfere with other medications or dietary supplements being taken. It is also important to know that the manufacturer adheres to high quality standards in the preparation of its products.

Supplement Facts Label

To help consumers make informed choices, dietary supplements now contain a supplement facts panel that clearly labels the product as a dietary supplement and gives information such as the amount of a standard dose, the number of recommended doses per day, the list of components (and how much of each is present in a standard dose), and, if the product is a botanical, the Latin name of the plant and the part of the plant used to prepare the product. This latter information is important because the components responsible for a certain health effect may be in one part of the plant but not in other parts. For example, a consumer purchasing ginger to protect against seasickness would want a product prepared from the roots of the plant, where the active components are, and not the leaves.

In addition, DSHEA established standards for terms, such as **high potency** and antioxidant, and for the types of claims that could be made for a product. Claims that a dietary supplement may help to prevent or cure a disease cannot be made. Such claims are considered health claims and must be reviewed by the Food and Drug Administration for scientific accuracy prior to approval for use on a product label. Manufacturers may, however, use structure/function claims that state that a product can, for example, "help to promote healthy blood levels of **cholesterol**," but they may not state that a product "helps to prevent **heart disease**." All structure/function claims must be accompanied by the following disclaimer: "This statement has not been evaluated by the Food and Drug Administration. This product is not intended to diagnose, treat, cure, or prevent any disease."

Selecting a CAM Modality

When selecting a CAM modality, it is important to have clearly defined health goals. In other words, what are you trying to accomplish, and is this modality an appropriate fit for you? If selecting a therapy, determine if the practitioner of the therapy being considered is a licensed health care practitioner. Licensure does not guarantee the modality will successfully meet one's needs, but it does provide some assurance of training and competency on the part of the practitioner. This information can usually be obtained from the various state boards of medicine, which are responsible for licensing health care professionals.

Selecting quality dietary supplements can be a bit more challenging. Both the natural products industry and the Food and Drug Administration are working to develop uniform standards of quality for dietary supplements. Until these standards are in place, however, consumers must be proactive in determining for themselves what supplements are consistent with their health goals and what manufacturers offer quality products. It is important not to be fooled by **hype**. Be wary of supplements that sound too good to be true or that promise to cure a medical condition.

Quality natural ingredients and responsible product testing can add significantly to the cost of a dietary supplement. The cheapest supplement is not always the best buy, though a high price does not necessarily guarantee high quality. It is important to investigate the supplement manufacturer whose products are being considered. Manufacturer contact information appears on the supplement facts label. One should inquire whether the manufacturer uses Good Manufacturing Practices, how they ensure the purity of their ingredients, and whether they have their products tested by independent laboratories to verify that the label accurately reflects the product in the supplement container.

Alternative therapies are increasingly being used to complement conventional medicine. The consumer should be knowledgeable of the modality chosen, its intended purpose, and whether it is appropriate for that purpose. In the case of dietary supplements, consumers should educate themselves about the appropriate application for the supplement and the

high potency: a claim about vitamin or mineral content, defined as 100% or more of the Recommended Daily Intake

cholesterol: multi-ringed molecule found in animal cell membranes; a type of lipid

heart disease: any disorder of the heart or its blood supply, including heart attack, atherosclerosis, and coronary artery disease

hype: advertising and brash claims

33

dose that is known to be safe and effective. Although many reputable CAM practitioners and dietary supplement manufacturers exist, consumers should educate themselves about the hallmarks of a quality practitioner or dietary supplement. With CAM modalities in general, and dietary supplements in particular, it is helpful to identify health care professionals who are knowledgeable about CAM and who can provide help in using CAM effectively. SEE ALSO DIETARY SUPPLEMENTS; MACROBIOTIC DIET.

Ruth M. DeBusk

Bibliography

Astin, John A. (1998). "Why Patients Use Alternative Medicine: Results of a National Study." *Journal of the American Medical Association* 279:1548–1553.

Eisenberg, David M.; Davis, Roger B.; Ettner, Susan L.; Appel, Scott; Wilkey, Sonja; Van Rompay, Maria; Kessler, Ronald C. (1998). "Trends in Alternative Medicine Use in the United States, 1990–1997: Results of a Follow-Up National Survey." *Journal of the American Medical Association* 280:1569–1575.

Eisenberg, David M.; Kessler, Ronald C.; Foster, Cindy; Norlock, Frances E.; Calkins, David R.; and Delbanco, Thomas L. (1993). "Unconventional Medicine in the United States: Prevalence, Costs, and Patterns of Use." *New England Journal of Medicine* 328:246–252.

Internet Resources

Center for Food Safety and Applied Nutrition. "Dietary Supplements." Available from <http://www.cfsan.fda.gov>

Federation of State Medical Boards. "Member Medical Boards." Available from <http://www.fsmb.org/members.htm>

National Center for Complementary and Alternative Medicine. <http://www.nccam.nih.gov>

Office of Disease Prevention and Health Promotion (1997). "Report of the Commission on Dietary Supplement Labels." Available from <http://web.health.gov/dietsupp>

U.S. Food and Drug Administration (1995). "Dietary Supplement Health and Education Act." Available from <http://www.fda.gov>

American Dietetic Association

The American Dietetic Association (ADA) was founded in 1917, and its stated mission is to "promote optimal **nutrition** and well-being for all people by advocating for its members" (ADA).

The majority of ADA members are registered dietitians (RDs) or dietetic technicians, registered (DTRs). Membership includes membership in a state dietetic association and an option to join an ADA dietetic practice group representing employment or dietetic interests. Through its annual Food and Nutrition Conference and Exhibition (FNCE), members, students, and interested professionals can network and receive continuing education credits. In addition to the FNCE, ADA provides various member services including promoting dietetic professionals to the public, advocating for the profession, and providing resources for career development.

The Association publishes and has available online the *Journal of the American Dietetic Association*, as well as an online newsletter, the *Courier*. SEE ALSO CAREERS IN DIETETICS; DIETITIAN; DIETETIC TECHNICIAN, REGISTERED.

Susan P. Himburg

nutrition: the maintenance of health through proper eating, or the study of same

American Public Health Association

The American Public Health Association (APHA) is an association of individuals and organizations working to improve the public's health and to achieve equity in health status for all. Founded in 1872, APHA is the oldest and largest organization of public health professionals in the world. APHA members represent over fifty occupations of public health, including physicians, nurses, health educators, community dietitians, social workers, environmentalists, epidemiologists, and others. Members advocate for policies and practices that assure a healthy global society, emphasize health promotion and disease prevention, and seek to protect environmental and community health by addressing issues such as pollution control, **chronic** and **infectious diseases**, and the availability of professional education in public health.

Marie Boyle Struble

chronic: over a long period

infectious diseases: diseases caused by viruses, bacteria, fungi, or protozoa, which replicate inside the body

Internet Resource

American Public Health Association. <http://www.apha.org>

American School Food Service Association

The American School Food Service Association (ASFSA), founded in 1946, is dedicated to ensuring that "healthful meals and nutrition education are available to all children." Its stated mission is "to advance good nutrition for all children" (ASFSA).

The majority of ASFSA members are school food-service administrators, managers, educators, or personnel who advance the availability, quality, and acceptance of school nutrition programs as an integral part of education. Members can also join their state or local association, or pursue an option for professional certification. Through its annual national conference and state meetings, members, students, and interested professionals can network and receive continuing education credits. The association publishes *School Foodservice & Nutrition*. SEE ALSO SCHOOL FOOD SERVICE; SCHOOL-AGED CHILDREN, DIET OF.

Susan P. Himburg

Bibliography

Payne-Palacio, June, and Canter, Deborah D. (2000). *The Profession of Dietetics: A Team Approach*, 2nd edition. New York: Prentice Hall.

Internet Resource

American School Food Service Association. "About ASFSA." Available from <http://www.asfsa.org/>

American School Health Association

The American School Health Association (ASHA) was founded in 1927 by physicians who were members of the American Public Health Association. The main focus of the ASHA is to safeguard the health of school-age children. Over the years it has evolved into a multidisciplinary organization of administrators, counselors, dentists, health educators, physical educators, school nurses, and school physicians that advocates high-quality school health instruction, health services, and a healthful school **environment**.

The association's stated mission "is to protect and promote the health of children and youth by supporting coordinated school health programs as a foundation for school success." As part of its mission, the ASHA publishes the *Journal of School Health*. SEE ALSO SCHOOL FOOD SERVICE; SCHOOL-AGED CHILDREN, DIET OF.

Susan P. Himburg

Internet Resource

American School Health Association. <http://www.ashaweb.org/>

environment: surroundings

Amino Acids

Amino acids are the building blocks of **protein**. The body has twenty different amino acids that act as these building blocks. Nonessential amino acids are those that the body can synthesize for itself, provided there is enough nitrogen, carbon, hydrogen, and **oxygen** available. Essential amino acids are those supplied by the **diet**, since the human body either cannot make them at all or cannot make them in sufficient quantity to meet its needs. Under normal conditions, eleven of the amino acids are nonessential and nine are essential.

amino acid: building block of proteins, necessary dietary nutrient

protein: complex molecule composed of amino acids that performs vital functions in the cell; necessary part of the diet

oxygen: O_2, atmospheric gas required by all animals

diet: the total daily food intake, or the types of foods eaten

Structure

All amino acids have a similar chemical structure—each contains an amino group (NH_2), an acid group (COOH), a hydrogen atom (H), and a distinctive side group that makes proteins more complex than either **carbohydrates** or **lipids**. All amino acids are attached to a central carbon atom (C).

The distinctive side group identifies each amino acid and gives it characteristics that attract it to, or repel it from, the surrounding fluids and other amino acids. Some amino acid side groups carry electrical charges that are attracted to water **molecules** (hydrophilic), while others are neutral and are repelled by water (hydrophobic). Side-group characteristics (shape, size, composition, electrical charge, and **pH**) work together to determine each protein's specific function.

carbohydrate: food molecule made of carbon, hydrogen, and oxygen, including sugars and starches

lipid: fats, waxes, and steroids; important components of cell membranes

molecule: combination of atoms that form stable particles

pH: level of acidity, with low numbers indicating high acidity

---

TABLE OF ESSENTIAL AND NONESSENTIAL AMINO ACIDS

Essential amino acids	Nonessential amino acids
Histidine	Alanine
Isoleucine	Arginine
Leucine	Asparagine
Lysine	Aspartic acid
Methionine	Cysteine
Phenylalanine	Glutamic acid
Threonine	Glutamine
Tryptophan	Glycine
Valine	Proline
	Serine
	Tyrosine

The three-dimensional shape of proteins is derived from the sequence and properties of its amino acids and determines its function and interaction with other molecules. Each amino acid is linked to the next by a peptide bond, the name given to the link or attraction between the acid (COOH) end of one amino acid and the amino end (NH_2) of another. Proteins of various lengths are made when amino acids are linked together in this manner. A dipeptide is two amino acids joined by a peptide bond, while a tripeptide is three amino acids joined by peptide bonds.

The unique shapes of proteins enable them to perform their various tasks in the body. Heat, acid, or other conditions can disturb proteins, causing them to uncoil or lose their shape and impairing their ability to function. This is referred to as *denaturation*.

Functions of Proteins

Proteins act as **enzymes**, **hormones**, and **antibodies**. They maintain fluid balance and acid and base balance. They also transport substances such as oxygen, **vitamins**, and **minerals** to target cells throughout the body. Structural proteins, such as collagen and keratin, are responsible for the formation of bones, teeth, hair, and the outer layer of skin, and they help maintain the structure of blood vessels and other tissues. In contrast, motor proteins use **energy** and convert it into some form of mechanical work (e.g., dividing cells, contracting muscle).

Enzymes are proteins that facilitate chemical reactions without being changed in the process. The inactive form of an enzyme is called a proenzyme. Hormones (chemical messengers) are proteins that travel to one or more specific target tissues or organs, and many have important regulatory functions. **Insulin**, for example, plays a key role in regulating the amount of **glucose** in the blood. The body manufactures antibodies (giant protein molecules), which combat invading antigens. Antigens are usually foreign substances such as **bacteria** and **viruses** that have entered the body and could potentially be harmful. Immunoproteins, also called immunoglobulins or antibodies, defend the body from possible attack by these invaders by binding to the antigens and inactivating them.

Proteins help to maintain the body's fluid and **electrolyte** balance. This means that proteins ensure that the proper types and amounts of fluid and minerals are present in each of the body's three fluid compartments. These fluid compartments are *intracellular* (contained within cells), *extracellular* (existing outside the cell), and *intravascular* (in the blood). Without this balance, the body cannot function properly.

Proteins also help to maintain balance between acids and bases within body fluids. The lower a fluid's pH, the more acidic it is. Conversely, the higher the pH, the less acidic the fluid is. The body works hard to keep the pH of the blood near 7.4 (neutral). Proteins also act as carriers, transporting many important substances in the bloodstream for delivery throughout the body. For example, a *lipoprotein* transports **fat** and **cholesterol** in the blood.

Food Sources

Humans consume many foods that contain proteins or amino acids. One normally need not worry about getting enough protein or amino acids in

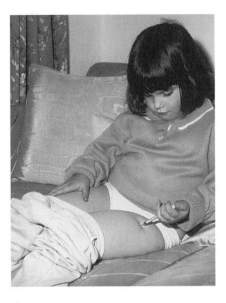

A diabetic child injects herself with insulin. Composed of 51 amino acids, insulin is a small protein used by the body to regulate glucose levels in the blood. *[Custom Medical Stock Photo. Reproduced by Permission.]*

enzyme: protein responsible for carrying out reactions in a cell

hormone: molecules produced by one set of cells that influence the function of another set of cells

antibody: immune system protein that protects against infection

vitamin: necessary complex nutrient used to aid enzymes or other metabolic processes in the cell

mineral: an inorganic (non-carbon-containing) element, ion, or compound

energy: technically, the ability to perform work; the content of a substance that allows it to be useful as a fuel

insulin: hormone released by the pancreas to regulate level of sugar in the blood

glucose: a simple sugar; the most commonly used fuel in cells

bacteria: single-celled organisms without nuclei, some of which are infectious

virus: noncellular infectious agent that requires a host cell to reproduce

electrolyte: salt dissolved in fluid

fat: type of food molecule rich in carbon and hydrogen, with high energy content

cholesterol: multi-ringed molecule found in animal cell membranes; a type of lipid

the typical American diet. Foods from animal sources are typically rich in essential amino acids. These include chicken, fish, eggs, dairy products, beef, and pork. With the increasing emphasis on vegetarian diets, plant sources of protein are gaining in popularity. Such sources include dried beans (black, kidney, northern, red, and white beans), peas, soy, nuts, and seeds. Although plant sources generally lack one or more of the essential amino acids, when combined with whole grains such as rice, or by eating nuts or seeds with **legumes**, all the amino acids can be obtained. SEE ALSO DIET; FATS; MAL-NUTRITION; NUTRIENTS; PLANT-BASED DIETS; PROTEIN.

Susan P. Himburg

Bibliography

Insel, Paul; Turner, R.; and Ross, Don (2001). *Nutrition*. Sudbury, MA: Jones and Bartlett.

Whitney, Eleanor N., and Rolfes, Sharon R. (2002). *Understanding Nutrition*, 9th edition. Belmont, CA: Wadsworth Group.

legumes: beans, peas, and related plants

Anemia

Anemia affects more than 30 percent of the world's population, and it is one of the most important worldwide health problems. It has a significant **prevalence** in both developing and industrialized nations. Causes of anemia include **nutritional deficiencies**, particularly of **iron**, vitamin B_{12}, and **folate** (folic acid); excess blood loss from menstruation or **chronic** illness and infection; ingestion of toxic substances, such as lead, ethanol, and other compounds; and **genetic** abnormalities such as **thalassemia** and **sideroblastosis**.

Anemia is caused by a deficiency in the intake and **absorption** elements required to make red blood cells. The condition is defined as one in which the blood is deficient in red blood cells, in **hemoglobin**, or in total volume. This results in blood that is incapable of meeting the **oxygen** needs of the body's tissues. Anemia is characterized by changes in the size and color of red blood cells. Red blood cells, or erythrocytes, are primarily responsible for oxygen transport from the lungs to the body's many cells. Hemoglobin is an oxygen-carrying **protein** in the red blood cell that incorporates iron into its structure. Therefore, iron is an essential building block of blood erythrocytes. When red blood cells are larger than normal, the anemia is termed *macrocytic*, and when they are smaller than normal, it is called *microcytic*. Normal red cell color is termed *normochromic*, and if the red cells appear pale, the anemia is called *hypochromic*. When extensive lab testing is not available for diagnosis, the use of a portable colorimeter can be used to detect anemia.

Iron-Deficiency Anemia

Anemia in the developing world is most commonly caused by an iron deficiency, which affects up to 50 percent of the population in some countries. Iron deficiency not only impairs the production of red cells in the blood, but also affects general cell growth and proliferation in tissues like the **nervous system** and the **gastrointestinal** tract. Red cells in a patient with iron-deficiency anemia are both microcytic and hypochromic.

anemia: low level of red blood cells in the blood

prevalence: describing the number of cases in a population at any one time

nutritional deficiency: lack of adequate nutrients in the diet

iron: nutrient needed for red blood cell formation

folate: one of the B vitamins, also called folic acid

chronic: over a long period

genetic: inherited or related to the genes

thalassemia: inherited blood disease due to defect in the hemoglobin protein

sideroblastosis: condition in which the blood contains an abnormally high number of sideroblasts, or red blood cells containing iron granules

absorption: uptake by the digestive tract

hemoglobin: the iron-containing molecule in red blood cells that carries oxygen

oxygen: O_2, atmospheric gas required by all animals

protein: complex molecule composed of amino acids that performs vital functions in the cell; necessary part of the diet

nervous system: the brain, spinal cord, and nerves that extend throughout the body

gastrointestinal: related to the stomach and intestines

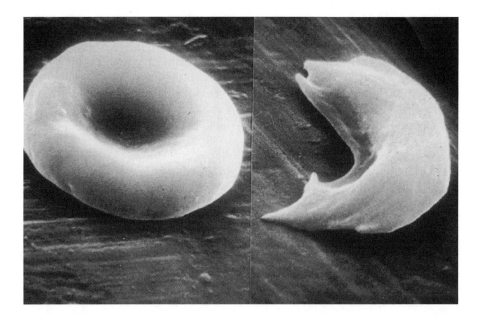

Sickle-cell anemia is a genetic disease that causes normal red blood cells (left) to become rigid and sickle-shaped (right). The misshapen cells can impede blood circulation, causing pain and possibly tissue damage. *[Photograph by Stanley Flegler. Visuals Unlimited. Reproduced by permission.]*

Iron deficiency affects young children, adolescents, and women of reproductive age—three periods of rapid growth during which the body's iron needs are higher than normal. In children, iron requirements are highest between the ages of six and eighteen months, and can be ten times the requirement of a normal adult. Iron is commonly absorbed from both human milk and cow's milk, and, if consumed in good quantities, these sources can meet the body's iron needs. A deficiency can result from inadequate intake, or it can occur if milk remains the sole source of a child's **nutrition** after the age of four months, when iron needs exceed that provided by milk alone. Research in Chile has shown that 40 percent of children whose main source of nutrition was breast milk developed iron-deficiency anemia. Such children can appear tired and inattentive, and they can suffer from delayed motor development. Some children can even develop mild to moderate mental retardation as a result of iron-deficiency anemia. Recent research has shown that iron-deficiency anemia can also contribute to emotional development problems, with **malnourished** children acting more irritable and fussy.

nutrition: the maintenance of health through proper eating, or the study of same

malnourished: lack of adequate nutrients in the diet

TYPES AND CAUSES OF ANEMIA

Type	Lab values	Causes
Macrocytic, normochromic	MCV: > 100fl MCHC: 34	Vitamin B$_{12}$ deficiency, folate deficiency, vitamin C deficiency, chemotherapy (megaloblastic marrow); aplastic anemia, hypothyroidism (normoblastic marrow)
Microcytic, hypochromic	MCV: < 80 MCHC: < 30	Iron deficiency, thalassemia, sideroblastic anemia, chronic lead poisoning, anemia of chronic illness
Normocytic, normochromic	MCV: 80–99fl MCHC: 34 +/−2	Iron deficiency (early), chronic disease

MCV: mean corpuscular volume
MCHS: mean corpuscular hemoglobin concentration
fl: femtoliter (one quadrillionth of a liter)

parasitic: feeding off another organism

hookworm: parasitic nematode that attaches to the intestinal wall

malaria: disease caused by infection with Plasmodium, a single-celled protozoon, transmitted by mosquitoes

DNA: deoxyribonucleic acid; the molecule that makes up genes, and is therefore responsible for heredity

RNA: ribonucleic acid, used in cells to create proteins from genetic information

bone marrow: dividing cells within the long bones that make the blood

congenital: present from birth

kwashiorkor: severe malnutrition characterized by swollen belly, hair loss, and loss of skin pigment

marasmus: extreme malnutrition, characterized by loss of muscle and other tissue

neural: related to the nervous system

cardiovascular: related to the heart and circulatory system

cancer: uncontrolled cell growth

Pregnant women can have up to double the requirement of iron for a normal adult, with the majority of the mother's iron being transferred to her growing fetus. Adult diets in most of the developing world tend to be iron-poor, and a low dietary intake can result in iron deficiency. Deficiency can also occur as a result of poor iron absorption due to gastrointestinal pathology, blood loss due to normal menstruation, blood loss from **parasitic** infections such as **hookworm** and **malaria**, and blood loss from chronic diarrhea—all of which are common in developing countries.

Other Causes

The two other primary causes of nutritional anemia are deficiencies in vitamin B_{12} and folic acid, both of which are necessary for the production of **DNA, RNA,** and protein. Without these necessary factors, red blood cells can develop abnormally, or even die prematurely in the **bone marrow** where they are made. This leads to what is known as *megaloblastic anemia.*

Folate deficiency is most often caused by poor intestinal absorption or low intake of folate-rich foods, such as human milk, cow's milk, fruits, green vegetables, and certain meats. It is also caused by **congenital** defects in intestinal absorption. Just as with iron, folic acid requirements are highest during periods of rapid growth, particularly infancy and pregnancy. Folate-deficient children present with common symptoms of anemia, as well as chronic diarrhea. Folate deficiency can also occur with **kwashiorkor** or **marasmus.** If it occurs during pregnancy, folate deficiency can lead to **neural** tube defects, spontaneous abortions, and prematurity.

Vitamin B_{12}, derived from a substance called *cobalamin*, is mainly found in meats and other animal products—humans cannot synthesize this vitamin on their own. A good amount of its absorption depends on the presence of a substance called *intrinsic factor* (see sidebar). It does not normally occur with kwashiorkor or marasmus. Both folate and vitamin B_{12} deficiencies have also been linked to **cardiovascular** disease, mood disorders, and increased frequency of chromosomal breaks (which may contribute to the development of **cancer**).

Treatment

Each of the important causes of nutritional anemia can be eradicated through prevention and treatment. Many countries have begun this process by instituting food supplementation programs in which grains and cereals are

Pernicious Anemia

Pernicious anemia is a common cause of cobalamin/vitamin B_{12} deficiency. It is primarily a disease of the elderly and caused by an abnormality in the immune system where the body creates antibodies to intrinsic factor (a substance that facilitates absorption of vitamin B_{12}) or to the cells in the stomach that secrete it. The lack of intrinsic factor B_{12} leads to vitamin B_{12} deficiency. It can also be caused by physiologic or anatomic disturbances of the stomach that might prevent intrinsic factor secretion. In children, an atypical and rare form of pernicious anemia can be inherited. It is an autosomal recessive disorder that results in an inability to secrete intrinsic factor, and it presents with anorexia, weakness, a painful red tongue, and neurologic abnormalities.

fortified with iron, folate, or vitamin B_{12}. Given adequate resources, these deficiencies can also be ameliorated with direct oral supplements of absorbable iron, vitamin B_{12}, and folic acid. Injectable forms of iron are also available. It has been found that the supplementation of vitamin A to at-risk populations improves anemia more efficiently than iron supplementation alone.

fortified: altered by addition of vitamins or minerals

Treatment plans must also focus on the causes of anemia and therefore must include sanitation, treatment of infections such as malaria and HIV, and, most important, treatment of intestinal **parasites**. Much work is needed to address general **malnutrition**—not only concerning these deficiencies, but also other commonly occurring ones (e.g., vitamin A, **zinc**, copper, **calcium**). Programs dedicated to decreasing the rates of infection and illness in developing countries—through health education, immunization, sanitation, and appropriate treatment—will also contribute to a lower **incidence** and prevalence of worldwide anemia. SEE ALSO KWASHIORKOR; MALNUTRITION; MARASMUS; NUTRITIONAL DEFICIENCY; VITAMINS, WATER SOLUBLE.

parasite: organism that feeds off of other organisms

malnutrition: chronic lack of sufficient nutrients to maintain health

zinc: mineral necessary for many enzyme processes

calcium: mineral essential for bones and teeth

incidence: number of new cases reported each year

Seema P. Kumar

Bibliography

Behrman, Robert E.; Kliegman, Robert M.; and Jenson, Hal B., eds. (2000). *Nelson Textbook of Pediatrics*, 16th edition. Philadelphia, PA: W. B. Saunders.

Hoffbrand, A. V., and Herbert, V. (1999). "Nutritional Anemias." *Seminars in Hematology* 36(4).

Isselbacher, Kurt J. (1994). *Harrison's Textbook of Internal Medicine*, 13th edition. New York: McGraw-Hill.

Pollitt, E. (2000). "Developmental Sequela from Early Nutritional Deficiencies: Conclusive and Probability Judgments." *Journal of Nutrition* 130.

Ramakrishnan, U., ed. (2001). *Nutritional Anemias*. Boca Raton, FL: CRC Press.

Rhoades, R. A., and Tanner, G. A. (1995). *Medical Physiology*. Boston: Little Brown.

Yip, R., and Ramakrishnan, U. (2002). "Experiences and Challenges in Developing Countries." *Journal of Nutrition* 132.

Anorexia Nervosa

Anorexia nervosa is an **eating disorder** characterized by an extreme reduction in food intake leading to potentially life-threatening weight loss. This syndrome is marked by an intense, irrational fear of weight gain or excess body fat, accompanied by a distorted perception of body weight and shape. The onset is usually in the middle to late teens and is rarely seen in females over age forty. Among women of menstruating age with this disorder, **amenorrhea** is common.

anorexia nervosa: refusal to maintain body weight at or above what is considered normal for height and age

eating disorder: behavioral disorder involving excess consumption, avoidance of consumption, self-induced vomiting, or other food-related aberrant behavior

amenorrhea: lack of menstruation

A clinical diagnosis of anorexia nervosa necessitates body weight less than 85 percent of average for weight and height. Subtypes of this disorder include the **binge** eating/purging type (bingeing and purging are present) or the restricting type (bingeing and purging are absent). SEE ALSO ADDICTION, FOOD; BODY IMAGE; BULIMIA NERVOSA; EATING DISORDERS; EATING DISTURBANCES.

binge: uncontrolled indulgence

Karen Ansel

Bibliography

American Dietetic Association (1998). *Nutrition Intervention in the Treatment of Anorexia Nervosa, Bulimia Nervosa, and Eating Disorder Not Otherwise Specified (EDNOS)*. Chicago: Author.

American Psychiatric Association (2000). *Diagnostic and Statistical Manual of Mental Disorders*, 4th edition. Washington, DC: Author.

Escott-Stump, Sylvia, and Mahan, L. Kathleen (1996). *Krause's Food, Nutrition, and Diet Therapy*, 9th edition. Philadelphia: W. B. Saunders.

Olson, James A.; Shike, Moshe; Shils, Maurice E. (1994). *Modern Nutrition in Health and Disease*. Media, PA: Williams & Wilkins.

Anthropometric Measurements

anthropometric: related to measurement of characteristics of the human body

The term **anthropometric** refers to comparative measurements of the body. Anthropometric measurements are used in nutritional assessments. Those that are used to assess growth and development in infants, children, and adolescents include length, height, weight, weight-for-length, and head circumference (length is used in infants and toddlers, rather than height, because they are unable to stand). Individual measurements are usually compared to reference standards on a growth chart.

body mass index: weight in kilograms divided by square of the height in meters; a measure of body fat

Anthropometric measurements used for adults usually include height, weight, **body mass index** (BMI), waist-to-hip ratio, and percentage of body fat. These measures are then compared to reference standards to assess weight status and the risk for various diseases. Anthropometric measurements require precise measuring techniques to be valid. SEE ALSO BODY MASS INDEX; NUTRITIONAL ASSESSMENT; WAIST-TO-HIP RATIO.

Delores C. S. James

Antioxidants

antioxidant: substance that prevents oxidation, a damaging reaction with oxygen

cancer: uncontrolled cell growth

heart disease: any disorder of the heart or its blood supply, including heart attack, atherosclerosis, and coronary artery disease

immune system: the set of organs and cells, including white blood cells, that protect the body from infection

free radical: highly reactive molecular fragment, which can damage cells

oxygen: O_2, atmospheric gas required by all animals

metabolism: the sum total of reactions in a cell or an organism

vitamin: necessary complex nutrient used to aid enzymes or other metabolic processes in the cell

carotenoid: plant-derived molecules used as pigments

water-soluble: able to be dissolved in water

diet: the total daily food intake, or the types of foods eaten

Americans spend several billion dollars a year on **antioxidants** in an effort to improve their health. Science has been looking at antioxidants and their role in everything from preventing **cancer** and **heart disease** to boosting the **immune system** and slowing the aging process. Antioxidants provide a layer of protection for the cells and tissues of the body, just as a thick coat of wax helps protect a car's finish. Specifically, antioxidants protect against free radical damage. What are **free radicals**?

People must breathe in **oxygen** to live. Continuously on the move in the blood stream and transported to every cell, oxygen is necessary for all essential bodily functions. However, a small amount of this oxygen gets loose and produces unstable by-products called free radicals. Body processes, such as **metabolism**, as well as environmental factors, including pollution and cigarette smoke, can produce free radicals. An overload of free radicals in the body causes damage to the cells, ultimately resulting in disease and accelerated aging.

Antioxidant-rich food may help prevent various cancers, heart disease, and diseases of aging. **Vitamins** C and E, **carotenoids** (including beta-carotene), and the mineral selenium are all powerful antioxidants found in food. Vitamin C, a **water-soluble** vitamin, is also known as ascorbic acid. Most of the vitamin C in the **diet** (90%) comes from fruits and vegetables. However, since vitamin C is water soluble, cooking can destroy the vitamin C in a food.

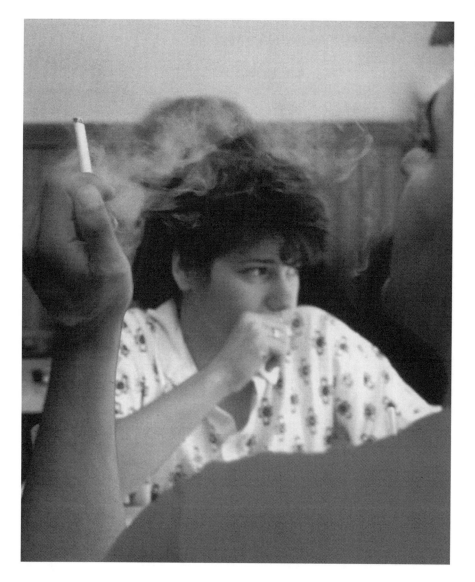

Cigarette smoke, including second-hand smoke, is a major source of free radicals. These volatile molecules can damage tissues and cause disease. [© 1993 Custom Medical Stock Photo, Inc. Reproduced by permission.]

Vitamin E, also known as alpha tocopherol, is a **fat**. Because vitamin E is found in oils, people who follow a low-fat diet may not get enough. Beta-carotene is a member of the carotenoid family. Found mainly in plants, carotenoids provide the vibrant red, yellow, green, and orange colors of fruits and vegetables, with carrots being a major contributor of beta-carotene. Typically, beta-carotene is a conditionally essential **nutrient**, but when one's intake of vitamin A is low, beta-carotene becomes an essential nutrient, meaning that it must be obtained from food and cannot be manufactured by the body.

Selenium is an essential **trace** mineral (*trace* **minerals** are needed only in small amounts). The amount of selenium found in food is directly related to the amount of selenium in the soil in which the food was grown. It is necessary for healthy immune function and is tied to **killer-cell** activity and **antibody** production. The many health benefits of the various antioxidants can be provided by a variety of food sources.

More and more **functional foods** contain combinations of various supplements. As popular as antioxidants are, an excess amount of them can be toxic. One reason to obtain antioxidants from food is that high doses may

fat: type of food molecule rich in carbon and hydrogen, with high energy content-soluble vitamin that is essential for human health

nutrient: dietary substance necessary for health

trace: very small amount

mineral: an inorganic (non-carbon-containing) element, ion, or compound

killer-cell: type of white blood cell that helps protect the body from infection

antibody: immune system protein that protects against infection

functional food: food whose health benefits are claimed to be higher than those traditionally assumed for similar types of foods

43

HEALTH BENEFITS OF ANTIOXIDANTS AND THEIR FOOD SOURCES

Antioxidant	Health benefits	Food sources
Selenium	Helps maintain healthy hair and nails, enhances immunity, works with vitamin E to protect cells from damage. Reduces the risk of cancer, particularly lung, prostate, and colorectal.	Garlic, seeds, Brazil nuts, meat, eggs, poultry, seafood, whole grains. The amount in plant sources varies according to the content of the soil.
Beta-carotene	Keeps skin healthy, helps prevent night blindness and infections, promotes growth and bone development.	Red, yellow-orange, and leafy green vegetables and fruits, including carrots, apricots, cantaloupe, peppers, tomatoes, spinach, broccoli, sweet potatoes, and pumpkin.
Vitamin E	Acts as the protector of essential fats in cell membranes and red blood cells. Reduces risk of cancer, heart disease, and other age-associated diseases.	Peanut butter, nuts, seeds, vegetable oils and margarine, wheat germ, avocado, whole grains, salad dressings.
Vitamin C	Destroys free radicals inside and outside cells. Helps in the formation of connective tissue, the healing of wounds, and iron absorption, and also helps to prevent bruising and keep gums healthy. May reduce risk of cataracts, heart disease, and cancer.	Peppers, tomatoes, citrus fruits and juices, berries, broccoli, spinach, cabbage, potatoes, mango, papaya.

SOURCE: The American Dietetic Association And WebMD.

stress: heightened state of nervousness or unease

calorie: unit of food energy

actually promote free radical production, also known as pro-oxidation, increasing the chance for health problems. Those who may benefit most from antioxidants include people dealing with a lot of **stress**, dieters limiting their **calories** to 1,200 per day or less, people on a low-fat diet, smokers, older adults, and people with a family history of heart disease or cancer. SEE ALSO FUNCTIONAL FOODS.

Susan Mitchell

Bibliography

Medical Economics Company (2001). *PDR for Nutritional Supplements*. Montvale, NJ: Author.

Internet Resources

American Dietetic Association. "Vitamin E: Disease Prevention for Your Good Health." Available from <http://www.eatright.org>

Doheny, Kathleen. "The Supplement Frenzy." Available from <http://www.webmd.com>

Appetite

Why do many people desire ice cream and pie or some other rich dessert after eating a huge Thanksgiving dinner? This desire is referred to as *appetite*, which is not the same as *hunger*. Appetite is a complicated phenomenon, linking biology with **environment**. It is a biopsychological system, meaning it is the result of both our biology (hunger) and psychology (desires and feelings).

environment: surroundings

Hunger, on the other hand, is purely **biological**. It is that nagging, irritating feeling that makes one think about food and the need to eat. It gets stronger the longer one goes without food, and it weakens after eating. Although the **physiological** reasons people feel hunger have not been clearly identified, the feeling of hunger rises and falls based on the activation of **neural** circuitry related to eating. There are many chemical agents in the human body that affect the sensation of hunger. Unfortunately for some people, eating behavior is not governed by hunger and satiety (feeling of fullness), but by a variety of other factors. For example, some people eat in response to their feelings of **anxiety**, **depression**, or **stress**. Eating temporarily helps lessen these feelings, and thus tends to become a coping response whenever they have these bad feelings.

biological: related to living organisms

physiological: related to the biochemical processes of the body

neural: related to the nervous system

anxiety: nervousness

depression: mood disorder characterized by apathy, restlessness, and negative thoughts

stress: heightened state of nervousness or unease

Weight gain may occur if people eat for reasons other than hunger. One strategy to help people manage their weight is for them to learn to differentiate between appetite and hunger, to learn to "listen to their bodies," and to eat only when they are hungry—and to stop when they are full. Hunger-control medications can help reduce the biological need to eat, but people still need to manage their psychological feelings about eating. SEE ALSO HUNGER; SATIETY; WEIGHT MANAGEMENT.

John P. Foreyt

Bibliography

Bray, George A. (1998). *Contemporary Diagnosis and Management of Obesity*. Newtown, PA: Handbooks in Health Care.

Fairburn, Christopher G., and Brownell, Kelly D. eds. (2002). *Eating Disorders and Obesity: A Comprehensive Handbook*, 2nd edition. New York: Guilford Press.

Arteriosclerosis

The term *arteriosclerosis* is used to describe several **cardiovascular** diseases, including those involving the blood vessels. In this instance, the **arteries** become hardened and blood vessels lose their "elastic" effect. Arteriosclerosis can begin in early childhood.

cardiovascular: related to the heart and circulatory system

artery: blood vessel that carries blood away from the heart toward the body tissues

The primary risk factors for arteriosclerosis include hypertension (**high blood pressure**), **diabetes** mellitus, smoking, and **obesity**. All of these risk factors are preventable by exercising regularly, smoking cessation, eating at least five servings of fruits and vegetables daily, and through proper **stress** management.

high blood pressure: elevation of the pressure in the bloodstream maintained by the heart

diabetes: inability to regulate level of sugar in the blood

obesity: the condition of being overweight, according to established norms based on sex, age, and height

stress: heightened state of nervousness or unease

Two types of arteriosclerosis include Monckeberg's arteriosclerosis, which usually involves restricted movement of the lower extremities, and arteriolar sclerosis, which can lead to decreased vision and peripheral vascular disease. Signs and symptoms of arteriosclerosis include high blood pressure, multiple kidney infections, and poor circulation in the toes and fingers. SEE ALSO ATHEROSCLEROSIS; CARDIOVASCULAR DISEASES; HEART DISEASE.

Teresa A. Lyles

Bibliography

Insel, P. M., and Roth, W. T. (2003). "Cardiovascular Disease and Cancer." In *Core Concepts in Health*, brief 9th edition. New York: McGraw-Hill

Internet Resources

Well-Net/Health Education Associates. "Arteriosclerosis." Available from <http://www.well-net.com/cardiov>

Health with Nutrition. "Arteriosclerosis/Atherosclerosis." Available from <http://www.healingwithnutrition.com>

Artificial Sweeteners

caries: cavities in the teeth

glucose: a simple sugar; the most commonly used fuel in cells

carbohydrate: food molecule made of carbon, hydrogen, and oxygen, including sugars and starches

metabolism: the sum total of reactions in a cell or an organism

insulin: hormone released by the pancreas to regulate level of sugar in the blood

Artificial sweeteners may assist in weight management, prevention of dental **caries**, and control of blood **glucose** for diabetics. It has also been suggested that low-calorie sweeteners may stimulate the appetite, but the bulk of evidence does not support this hypothesis. Conclusive research demonstrates that artificial sweeteners have no effect on **carbohydrate metabolism**, short- or long-term blood glucose control, or **insulin** secretion, and they are thus an excellent sugar alternative for diabetics. There have been a number of health concerns related with these products, though the Food and Drug Administration (FDA) approval process for artificial sweeteners involves a comprehensive analysis of scientific data to satisfy safety requirements. All "generally recognized as safe" (GRAS) sweeteners have undergone extensive safety testing and have been carefully reviewed by the FDA.

Five FDA-Approved (GRAS) Artificial Sweeteners

sucrose: table sugar

Acesulfame potassium (Acesulfame-K) was discovered in 1967 and approved for use in the United States in 1988. Its trade name is Sunette. Two hundred times sweeter than **sucrose**, this sweetener is stable when heated, making it suitable for cooking. However, when used in large amounts it has a bitter aftertaste. It is not broken down by the body, and it does not provide any calories. Over ninety scientific studies have been conducted by the FDA, and the World Health Organization's Joint Expert Committee on **Food Additives** (JECFA) has also endorsed Acesulfame K's safety.

food additive: substance added to foods to improve nutrition, taste, appearance, or shelf-life

Aspartame was discovered in 1969 and approved for use in the United States in 1981. Its trade name is NutraSweet. Also two hundred times sweeter than sugar, aspartame is not suitable in applications that require high temperatures, as it loses its sweetness when heated. It contains four calories per gram, but, because of its intense sweetness, the amount of **energy** derived from it is negligible. It is synthesized from aspartic acid and phenylalanine, two essential **amino acids**. Persons with the rare hereditary **metabolic** disorder **phenylketonuria** (PKU), an inborn error of metabolism, must control their intake of phenylalanine from all sources, including aspartame, and therefore all U.S. products containing aspartame are labeled "This product contains phenylalanine." Because it is impossible to know if an unborn child has PKU, it is recommended that pregnant women not use aspartame. The FDA states that aspartame is the most thoroughly tested food additive ever submitted to the agency.

energy: technically, the ability to perform work; the content of a substance that allows it to be useful as a fuel

amino acid: building block of proteins, necessary dietary nutrient

metabolic: related to processing of nutrients and building of necessary molecules within the cell

phenylketonuria: inherited disease marked by the inability to process the amino acid phenylalanine, causing mental retardation

Neotame was discovered in 1990 and was approved for use in the United States in 2002. Eight thousand times sweeter than sugar, this analog of aspartame can be used in both cooking and baking applications. Although neotame is a derivative of aspartame, it is not metabolized to phenylalanine, and

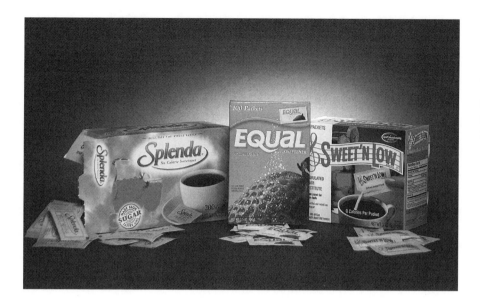

A few popular alternatives to table sugar include sucralose, aspartame, and saccharin. Despite controversy over potential health risks related to their consumption, each of these products has undergone a decade or more of scientific testing and is generally recognized as safe. *[Octane Photographic. Reproduced by permission.]*

no special PKU labeling is required. The FDA reviewed more than 113 human and animal studies before ruling on neotame.

Saccharin was discovered in 1879 and approved for use in the United States in 1879. Its trade name is Sweet'n Low. Three hundred to five hundred times sweeter than table sugar, saccharin provides no energy, as it is not metabolized by human beings. It has a bitter and somewhat metallic aftertaste. The largest population study to date, involving nine thousand individuals, showed that saccharin does not increase the risk of **cancer**, and on December 15, 2000, the U.S. Congress passed legislation to remove the warning label that had been required on foods and beverages containing saccharin since 1977 (warning labels were required because of findings that saccharin caused bladder tumors in mice when they were given high doses of the sweetener). Saccharin is approved in more than one hundred countries around the world and has been reviewed and determined safe by the Joint Expert Committee on Food Additives of the World Health Organization and the Scientific Committee for Food of the European Union.

cancer: uncontrolled cell growth

Sucralose was discovered in 1976 and approved for use in the United States in 1988. Its trade name is Splenda. Six hundred times sweeter than sugar, sucralose is not absorbed from the digestive tract, so it adds no calories to consumed food. It is made from rearranged sugar **molecules** that substitute three **atoms** of chlorine for three hydroxyl groups on the sugar molecule. Sucralose has been tested in more than one hundred studies.

molecule: combination of atoms that form stable particles

atoms: fundamental particles of matter

Sugar Alcohols (GRAS)

Sugar alcohols are not technically artificial sweeteners. Examples include sorbitol, xylitol, lactitol, mannitol, isomalt, and maltitol, which are used to sweeten "sugar-free" foods such as candy, cookies, and chewing gum. The alcohols have fewer calories than sugar, do not promote tooth decay, and do not cause a sudden increase in blood glucose because the bloodstream does not easily absorb them. They may cause, however, effects similar to a laxative if consumed in excess. Products containing large amounts of sugar alcohols must be labeled with the warning: "Excess consumption may have a laxative effect."

Artificial Sweeteners Pending FDA Approval

Alitame is two thousand times sweeter than sugar. An FDA petition was filed in 1986. Like neotame, alitame is a derivative of aspartame. It is approved for use in a variety of food and beverage products in Australia, New Zealand, Mexico, Colombia, Indonesia, and the People's Republic of China.

Cyclamate was discovered in 1937, banned in 1969, and a petition for approval was refiled in 1982. After being banned by the FDA in 1969, due to findings that high doses cause bladder tumors in mice, cyclamate has been approved for use in more than fifty countries. The sweetener is a derivative of cyclohexylsulfamic acid and is thirty times sweeter than sucrose. In May 2003, the European Union reduced the recommended average daily intake of this sweetener in soft drinks, juice, and milk-based drinks, based on evidence that the conversion rate of cyclamate in the body is higher than previously thought.

Stevioside (stevia) is obtained from the leaves of a South American shrub. Though it can impart a sweet taste to foods, it cannot be sold as a sweetener because the FDA considers it an unapproved food additive. Stevioside is a high-intensity low-calorie sweetener three hundred times sweeter than sucrose. It is approved in Japan, South Korea, Brazil, Paraguay, and Argentina. However, the World Health Organization (WHO) has determined that the data is insufficient to label it as a sweetener.

Artificial sweeteners taste sweet like sugar without the added calories. They do not promote tooth decay, and they are an acceptable alternative for people with **diabetes** or those wishing to decrease their use of sucrose. Artificial sweeteners, and their metabolic by-products and components, are not considered harmful to human beings at the levels normally used. When used in the context of a healthful **diet**, artificial sweeteners are generally safe for consumption. SEE ALSO GENERALLY RECOGNIZED AS SAFE; INBORN ERRORS OF METABOLISM; PHENYLKETONURIA.

Kyle Shadix

diabetes: inability to regulate level of sugar in the blood

diet: the total daily food intake, or the types of foods eaten

Bibliography

American Dietetic Association (1998). "Position of the American Dietetic Association: Use of Nutritive and Nonnutritive Sweeteners." *Journal of the American Dietetic Association* 98:580–587.

Drewnoski, A. (1995). "Intense Sweeteners and Control of Appetite." *Nutrition Review* 53:1–7.

Joint FAO/WHO Expert Committee on Food Additives (1993–2003). "Evaluation of Certain Food Additives and Contaminants." Geneva, Switzerland: World Health Organization.

Nabors, Lyn (2001). *Alternative Sweeteners*, 3rd edition. New York: Marcel Dekker.

Stegink, Lewis, and Filer, L. (1984). *Aspartame: Physiology and Biochemistry*. New York: Marcel Dekker.

Asian Americans, Diets of

Asian Americans represent a large and rapidly growing segment of the U.S. population. According to the U.S. Census Bureau, there were 11.9 million Asian Americans residing in the United States (4.2 percent of the total population) in the year 2000. Chinese Americans were the leading Asian group

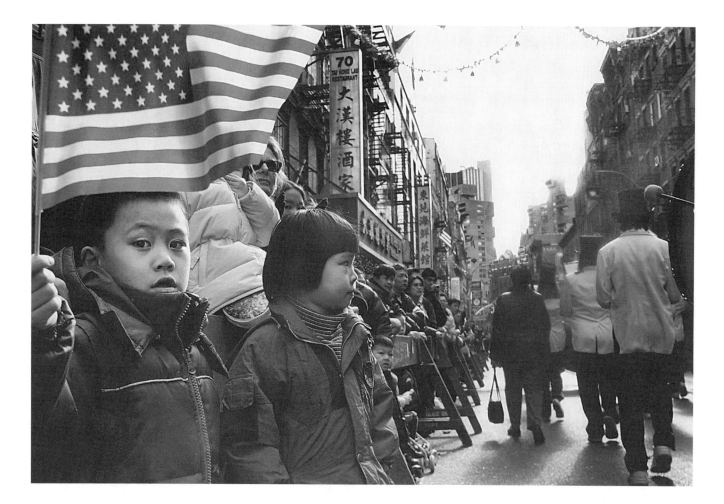

(not including Taiwanese Americans), followed by Filipinos (2.4 million) and Asian Indians (1.9 million). A U.S. Census estimate predicts a tripling of this population by 2050.

Asian Americans are exceedingly diverse, coming from nearly fifty countries and ethnic groups, each with distinct cultures, traditions, and histories, and they speak over 100 languages and dialects. Asian Americans have immigrated to the United States from different parts of Asia, including India, Pakistan, Bangladesh, Sri Lanka, the Philippines, China, Hong Kong, Cambodia, Vietnam, Laos, Thailand, Korea, and Japan. They are categorized by the Census Bureau under the broad classification of "Asian and Pacific Islanders in the United States." In 2000, Asian-born residents accounted for 26 percent (7.2 million) of the nation's total foreign-born population, with approximately half (about 45%) of them living in three metropolitan areas: Los Angeles, New York, and San Francisco.

Asian-American diets are based on rice and rice products, with less emphasis on the regular consumption of meat and dairy products, which differs from traditional American fare. *[AP/Wide World Photos. Reproduced by permission.]*

Food Habits

Two key elements draw the diverse cultures of the Asian region together: (1) the composition of meals, with an emphasis on vegetables and rice, with relatively little meat; and (2) cooking techniques. Eating is a vital part of the social matrix, and Asian-American cuisine includes a wide variety of meals, snacks, and desserts for social occasions. Asian food preparation techniques include stir-frying, barbecuing, deep-frying, boiling, and steaming. All in-

MERITS AND WEAKNESSES OF TRADITIONAL ASIAN DIETS

	Staple foods	Merits of diet	Weaknesses of diet	Common diseases
Cambodian	Rice Fish Tea	Low in fat Low in sugar	People often unable to obtain necessary food	Tuberculosis Polio
Chinese	Rice Vegetables Green Tea	Reduces risk for heart disease and certain cancers	Iodine deficiency Iron deficiency	Anemia
Filipino	Rice Vegetables Seafood Fruit	Reduces risk for heart disease and cancers	Protein deficiency Iron deficiency	Anemia Diarrhea Respiratory infections
Hmong	Rice Vegetables Meat Fish	Low in fat Low in sugar	Lack of fruit Calcium deficiency	
Asian Indian	Cereals Rice Vegetables	Low in fat Low in sugar	Protein deficiency Iron deficiency Vitamin A deficiency	Respiratory infections Intestinal infections Anemia Protein-energy malnutrition Diabetes
Laotian	Rice Vegetables Fish	Low in fat Low in sugar	Vitamin A deficiency Iron deficiency	Goiter Anemia
Vietnamese	Rice Fish Fruit	Low in fat Low in sugar	Iron deficiency	Anemia

nutrient: dietary substance necessary for health

diet: the total daily food intake, or the types of foods eaten

diversity: the variety of cultural traditions within a larger culture

socioeconomic status: level of income and social class

lactose intolerance: inability to digest lactose, or milk sugar

tofu: soybean curd, similar in consistency to cottage cheese

protein: complex molecule composed of amino acids that performs vital functions in the cell; necessary part of the diet

calcium: mineral essential for bones and teeth

gredients are carefully prepared (chopped, sliced, etc.) prior to starting the cooking process. The **nutrient** composition of the traditional Asian **diet** is very similar to the Mediterranean diet in that both are largely plant-based diets and meat is consumed only a few times a month (and often in very small amounts).

There exists great **diversity** in language, **socioeconomic status**, religion, age, education, social class, location, length of time in the United States, and country of origin among Asian Americans. Hence, caution needs to be taken not to generalize or imply that food habits are similar for all individuals of this group. For example, Chinese meals consist mainly of four food groups: grains, vegetables, fruit, and meat. Because of **lactose intolerance**, most Chinese do not consume large amounts of dairy products, substituting soymilk and **tofu** as sources of **protein** and **calcium**. Some Asian food, such as Thai food, is generally spicy, hot, and high in sodium. Hot peppers are used daily. The Japanese are very concerned about the visual appeal of food and the "separateness" of the foods and tastes. Garlic and hot pepper, commonly used among Asian Americans, are not common ingredients in the Japanese cuisine. Korean Americans eat kimchi with each meal. Kimchi is cabbage marinated in salt water, layered with peppers and spices in crockery, and left to ferment for a few days. South Asians (people from India, Pakistan, Bangladesh, and Sri Lanka) use spices (e.g., ginger, garlic, fenugreek, cumin, etc.) and condiments in their cuisine.

Most Asian Americans like to use fresh food in their cooking. Unlike the fast food society of the United States, they select live seafood, fresh meats, and seasonal fruits and vegetables from the local market to ensure freshness. Food preparation is meticulous, and consumption is ceremonious and deliberate. Most Asians living in America adhere to a traditional Asian diet interspersed with American foods, particularly breads and cereals. Dairy products are not consumed in large quantities, except for ice cream. Calcium is consumed through tofu and small fish (bones eaten). Fish, pork, and poultry are the main sources of protein. Significant amounts of nuts and dried beans are also eaten. Vegetables and fruits make up a large part of food intake. Rice is the mainstay of the diet and is commonly eaten at every meal.

The traditional Asian diet has received a lot of attention because many **chronic** diseases, such as **heart disease**, **diabetes**, and certain cancers, are not as common in Asia as in the United States and other Western nations. Researchers believe that the Asian plant-based diet provides protection against these chronic diseases. The diet is also believed to contribute to the long life spans commonly seen in Asia. To offer a healthful alternative to the 1992 U.S. Food Guide Pyramid, which lumped some animal and plant foods together in a single group, researchers developed an Asian Diet Pyramid, which emphasizes a wide base of rice, rice products, noodles, breads and grains, preferably whole grain and minimally **processed foods**, topped by another large band of fruits, vegetables, **legumes**, nuts, and seeds. Daily physical exercise, a small amount of vegetable oil, and a moderate consumption of plant-based beverages—including tea (especially black and green), sake, beer, and wine—are also recommended daily. Small daily servings of low-fat dairy products or fish are optional; sweets, eggs, and poultry are recommended no more than weekly; and red meat is recommended no more than monthly.

The Asian Diet Pyramid reflects the traditional, plant-based rural diets of Asia. Although there is an image of Asian Americans as a "model minority" who have overcome their "ethnic handicap" and are socioeconomically well off (Chen and Hawks), certain illnesses predominate in this group. For example, there is a particularly high rate of liver **cancer** among Asian Americans, while lung cancer is their leading cause of death. Vietnamese-American women's cervical cancer rate is five times that of Caucasian women. Asian Americans have among the highest rates of **tuberculosis** and **hepatitis** B in the United States. Asian Indian immigrants in the United States have an unusually high rate of coronary **artery** disease, and **parasitic** infections are particularly widespread among Southeast Asian refugees.

Studies indicate that the food habits of Asians become increasingly Westernized after they move to the United States or other Western countries (see Karim, Bloch, Falciglia, and Murthy). There is a general shift from vegetarianism to nonvegetarianism, and ethnic foods are consumed along with traditional ingredients found in American supermarkets. Consequently, diets of immigrants living in the United States have changed from being low in fat and rich in **fiber** to being high in **saturated fat** and animal protein and low in fiber. There is also an increased tendency to consume fast foods and **convenience foods**. These dietary changes, along with **sedentary** and stressful lifestyles, may increase their risk for chronic disease. SEE ALSO ASIANS, DIET OF.

Ranjita Misra

Bibliography

American Dietetic Association (2000). *Ethnic and Regional Food Practices: Indian and Pakistani Food Practices, Customs, and Holidays*, 2nd edition. Chicago: Author.

chronic: over a long period

heart disease: any disorder of the heart or its blood supply, including heart attack, atherosclerosis, and coronary artery disease

diabetes: inability to regulate level of sugar in the blood

processed food: food that has been cooked, milled, or otherwise manipulated to change its quality

legumes: beans, peas, and related plants

cancer: uncontrolled cell growth

tuberculosis: bacterial infection, usually of the lungs, caused by Mycobacterium tuberculosis

hepatitis: liver inflammation

artery: blood vessel that carries blood away from the heart toward the body tissues

parasitic: feeding off another organism

fiber: indigestible plant material that aids digestion by providing bulk

saturated fat: a fat with the maximum possible number of hydrogens; more difficult to break down that unsaturated fats

convenience food: food that requires very little preparation for eating

sedentary: not active

Chen, M. S., Jr., and Hawks, B. L. (1995). "A Debunking of the Myth of Healthy Asian Americans and Pacific Islanders." *American Journal of Health Promotion* 9:261–268.

Karim, N.; Bloch, D. S.; Falciglia, G.; and Murthy, L. (1986). "Modifications of Food Consumption Patterns Reported by People from India Living in Cincinnati, Ohio." *Ecology of Food and Nutrition* 19:11–18.

Internet Resources

Applesforhealth.com. "Chinese Diet Can Keep Heart Healthy." Available from <http://www.applesforhealth.com/chinesediet1.html>

Betancourt, Deidre (1995). "Cultural Diversity: Eating in America—Asian." Available from <http://www.ohioline.osu.edu>

Cornell University Science News (1995). "Asian Diet Pyramid Offers Alternative to U.S. Food Guide." Available from <http://www.news.cornell.edu/science/Dec95/st.asian.pyramid.html>

Lin, Kathy. "Chinese Food Cultural Profile." Harborview Medical Center/University of Washington. Available from <http://www.ethnomed.org>

National Library of Medicine. "Asian American Health." Available from <http://www.asianamericanhealth.nlm.nih.gov>

Asians, Diet of

With forty-seven countries, innumerable tribes, and thousands of distinct languages, Asia is home to more ethnic groups than any other part of the world. In addition, the geography and climate of Asia are as diverse as its nations and peoples. From the lush rice paddies of the Philippines to the crowded Tokyo metropolis to the rainforests of Indonesia, there is a staggering variety of fruit, food, and spices in this extraordinary part of the world. Asia can be divided into three regions: East Asia (including China, Taiwan, Japan, and Korea); Southeast Asia (including Malaysia, Singapore, and the Philippines); and South Asia (including India and Sri Lanka).

The Thread that Binds Asia: Rice

famine: extended period of food shortage

Though each Asian country and region has its distinct flavors and cooking styles, almost all share one food in common—rice. But rice is not eaten in the same manner in each country. As a staple food central to survival, especially during times of **famine**, rice has acquired an almost sacred status in Asian society, and it is served in many ways. It is cooked as a significant part of each meal of the day, incorporated as a main ingredient in confections such as candy and cakes, fermented to make wine (Japanese sake) or beer, or sometimes given as an offering to the gods to ensure a good harvest. Rice is a potent culinary and spiritual staple in Asia.

Asian Fruit

diet: the total daily food intake, or the types of foods eaten

The fruits of Asia are unlike those of any other part of the world. The tropical climate of South and Southeast Asia, and the mild climate of East Asia, create a hospitable environment for many different fruits to grow. Fruit is a significant part of the Asian **diet** and is usually eaten as a dessert with lunch or dinner. In East Asia, oranges, quince, dates, pears, strawberries, cherries, watermelon, peaches, and grapefruit are eaten widely. In South and Southeast Asia, there are unique fruits such as sweet mangoes (originally from India), which are eaten individually or made into ice cream or other confections, and green mangoes, which are used widely in Vietnam, the Philippines, and India, where they are made into chutneys or curries (which are used as a broth, stew, or dry seasoning).

Coconuts are popular in Southeast Asian cuisine. Coconut milk is used for curries in Thailand, Malaysia, Indonesia, South India, Myanmar, and the Philippines. It is also a delicious beverage, and is often drunk straight from the coconut with a straw. Coconut meat is added to desserts and salads. Other tropical fruits found in Asia include guava, papaya, pawpaw, starfruit (carambola), mangosteen, sour sop, jackfruit, longan, rambutan, durian, pineapple, and lychee.

Other Common Ingredients Used across Asia

Nuts are popular in Asia, eaten plain as snacks or mashed into porridge and sauces. In Malaysia and Indonesia, satays (peanut-based sauces) flavor chicken and beef dishes. The Chinese bake almond cookies and make rice cream with almonds or hazelnuts. Steamed cakes with almonds or macadamias are also common, and rice puddings with fruit, raisins, almonds, walnuts, or hazelnuts are popular desserts in India. Both East and Southeast Asia boast stir-fry dishes with peanuts, while India flavors its rice with lemon and peanuts.

East Asian Food

China. Different regions of China have distinct tastes in food. Shanghainese cooking is known for its spicy chili flavoring and trademark red-colored meats. The Cantonese and Chaozhao regions are known for cooked meats and vegetables; and in the Beijing, Mandarin, and Shandong regions steamed bread and noodles are used as **staples** instead of rice. The most prized food staples in China are rice and wheat, though yams, taros, and potatoes are eaten when rice and wheat are not available. Chinese vegetables are mostly imported from Central Asia, including cucumbers, coriander, peas, sesame, onions, grapes and pomegranates, tomatoes, maize, sweet potatoes, peanuts, mushrooms, and daikon (radish). Preserved foods are popular, including pickled foods, fermented vegetables, and smoked and salted meats. Other well-known seasonings that are used include salted black beans (douchi), sweet and salty sauce, garlic, oyster sauce, soy sauce, black fungus, chilies, hoisin sauce, ginger, sesame seeds, and sesame oil.

The Chinese cook most of their food by mincing the ingredients and sautéing them in a deep pan called a wok. Little **fat** is used to season the meals, but plenty of fresh flavorings are added, such as ginger, chilies, soy sauces, scallions, oyster sauce, and fagara (Szechuan pepper). In the cities, most people cook over a gas stovetop, while in the country they use a brick stove to cook several dishes at once, including the rice. Tea is the most common beverage, though sodas are also popular.

Japan. Sushi (slices of raw fish on rice), teriyaki meats, and tempura (batter-fried vegetables or shrimp) are not the only foods in the Japanese diet. Salted vegetables are part of everyday diets, as are soybean products such as **tofu**, soy sauce, miso (a soybean paste), and dashi (a stock whose base is dried fish and kelp). Meat and seafood are popular in Japanese cooking, and broths

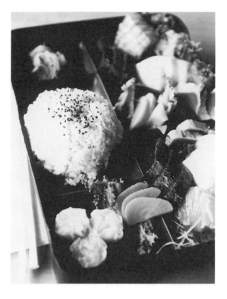

A healthy serving of rice is the centerpiece of this modern Japanese bento box. Though they differ in many ways, most Asian cultures share a dependence on rice. [Courtesy of Corinne Trang. Reproduced by permission.]

staples: essential foods in the diet

fat: type of food molecule rich in carbon and hydrogen, with high energy content

tofu: soybean curd, similar in consistency to cottage cheese

are also common. Ingredients for stock include dried sea tangle, dried bonito (a type of tuna), and brown mushrooms. Spices like pepper, wasabi (horse-radish), cloves, ginger, sesame, and garlic give special flavor to the food.

Japan centers its dishes on rice, with all other dishes thought of as side dishes. When rice stocks are low, millet or sweet potatoes are used. Different types of noodles are found in Japanese cuisine: soba (a buckwheat noodle) is popular in the west, and udon (a flour noodle) is popular in the east. Japanese rice wine (mirin or sake) is served both cold and warm. Green tea is especially popular.

Korea. Korea's cuisine is a blend of Chinese and Japanese, though with its own distinctive flavor. The Korean national dish is *bulgogi*, or "fire beef"—beef strips marinated in soy sauce, sesame oil, garlic, and chili. The mainstay of Korean food is kimchi (or gimchi), a side dish of pickled grated vegetables infused with ginger, garlic, and chili. Seafood is a major staple in Korea, in addition to pork, hens, deer, and wild boar. Popular vegetables include turnips, lotus roots, taro, leeks, lettuce, bamboo shoots, ferns, and mushrooms. Popular spices and nuts include pine nuts, hazelnuts, and ginseng, and chili peppers are used liberally.

herbal: related to or made from herbs

Noodles are usually made of wheat, buckwheat, soya, rice, or beans. Rice-cake soup, dumpling soup, five-grain rice, rice gruel, and sweet rice beverages are all popular. Green tea, scorched rice tea, **herbal** teas, and coffee are popular drinks. Other well-liked drinks are made from barley, corn rice, sesame seeds, ginseng, ginger, cinnamon, and citron.

Southeast Asia

Southeast Asia is located in the monsoon belt, where heavy rains fall for several months a year. Most Southeast Asian countries use plenty of spice and coconut in their dishes, except for Vietnam.

Vietnam. Vietnamese cuisine does not include large amounts of meat and fish; instead, rice is supplemented with vegetables and eggs. Similar to Chinese cooking, Vietnamese cooking uses little fat or oil for frying. Instead of using soy sauce for seasoning, *nuocmam* (fish sauce) is used as the main flavoring in almost every dish. *Pho* is a type of soup in which noodles, beef, chicken, or pork are added, and the soup is then garnished with basil, bean sprouts, and other seasonings. Fruits are an integral part of each meal—bananas, mangoes, papayas, oranges, coconuts, and pineapple are all popular. Vietnamese coffee is made with condensed milk to make the drink extra sweet and delicious. Hot green tea is very popular as well.

The Philippines. Philippine culture is a fusion of Malay origin and Spanish, Japanese, Chinese, Islamic, and American influence. In the Philippines, four meals a day are served: breakfast, lunch, *merienda* (snack), and dinner. *Pancit*, or noodles, is considered a *merienda* dish and is served with a sponge-cake called *puto* and a glutinous ricecake called *cuchinta*. Lunch is the heaviest meal and consists of rice, a vegetable, a meat, and sometimes fish as well. Vegetables include *kangkung* (a local spinach), broccoli, Chinese broccoli, bitter melon, mung bean, beansprouts, eggplant, and okra. However, vegetables are not considered as important to the diet as in East Asia. Meat is a major part of the diet, with pork being one of the more popular meats.

Beef and chicken are eaten often, and water buffalo are eaten in the provinces. The primary foods in the Philippines are rice, corn, coconuts, sugarcane, bananas, coffee, mangoes, and pineapples.

Malaysia and Singapore. These two countries have Indian, Muslim, and Chinese heritages that are reflected in their spicy **cuisines**. Authentic Malay food is difficult to find, though a wide selection of Chinese, Indian, Indonesian, and occasionally Western food is almost always available. *Nonya* is a Malaysian dish that has Chinese ingredients with local spices. Satays (meat kebabs in spicy peanut sauce) are a Malaysian creation, and fiery curries, Chinese noodles, fried tofu in peanut sauce, tamarind fish curry, curry prawns, and curried meat in coconut marinade are typical dishes. *Laksa* is a creamy curry with either seafood or chicken simmered in coconut milk. Popular desserts include *endol* (sugar syrup, coconut milk, and green noodles) and *is kacang* (beans and jellies topped with shaved ice, syrups, and condensed milk).

cuisine: types of food and traditions of preparation

South Asia

India's influence can be seen in Pakistan, Sri Lanka, Afghanistan, and even Bali (Indonesia). Sri Lankan cuisine is a snapshot of Indian food. Its fiery curry dishes with rice, and hoppers (fried pancake) served with yogurt and honey, are reminiscent of India. Meat and seafood are popular staples, as is tea.

India is the only country in this region that uses milk and dairy products in its diet, mostly in the form of yogurt and cheese. Indian seasonings include turmeric, tamarind, saffron, cumin, coriander, cardamom, mustard, ginger, celery seed, aniseed, fenugreek, curry leaf, and coconut milk. Cashews, pistachios, and almonds are also often found in meat dishes, as well as in the variety of breads that are baked, fried, or roasted to accompany the meals. Indian meals are served with chutney, a spicy relish, or *raita*, a chilled yogurt to soothe the spiciness of the dish.

In the north of India, meat dishes are more common and are usually made with goat, sheep, or chicken. The meals emphasize breads, grain, and spices. Southern meals focus on rice, vegetables, and chilies. Vegetables include onions, yams, potatoes, tomatoes, pumpkin, banana flowers, cucumbers, radishes, and lotus roots. The sacred status of the cow in the agrarian society has disallowed beef to be eaten by those who practice Hinduism. The **protein** in these diets comes primarily from **legumes** or dairy products.

protein: complex molecule composed of amino acids that performs vital functions in the cell; necessary part of the diet

legumes: beans, peas, and related plants

Food Security in Asia

Food is not always readily available across Asia because of a complex web of social and political factors. Weather also plays a heavy role in food security, which is the idea that everyone has access to food at a reasonable cost. If a typhoon causes devastating flooding or severe droughts destroy crops, people suffer because there will be no food to harvest. Droughts can also destroy food supplies and deplete drinking water supplies.

Micronutrient Deficiency

Micronutrients are essential **vitamins** and **minerals** that the body does not naturally produce. A certain amount of these vitamins and minerals are

vitamin: necessary complex nutrient used to aid enzymes or other metabolic processes in the cell

mineral: an inorganic (non-carbon-containing) element, ion, or compound

nutritional deficiency: lack of adequate nutrients in the diet

immune system: the set of organs and cells, including white blood cells, that protect the body from infection

cataract: clouding of the lens of the eye

hormone: molecules produced by one set of cells that influence the function of another set of cells

hemoglobin: the iron-containing molecule in red blood cells that carries oxygen

calcium: mineral essential for bones and teeth

cardiovascular: related to the heart and circulatory system

diabetes: inability to regulate level of sugar in the blood

high blood pressure: elevation of the pressure in the bloodstream maintained by the heart

obesity: the condition of being overweight, according to established norms based on sex, age, and height

body mass index: weight in kilograms divided by square of the height in meters; a measure of body fat

required for human development, but in areas of famine or insufficient food, populations are at high risk of micronutrient deficiencies. In areas of famine, or where insufficient varieties of foods are available, certain populations (such as pregnant women, infants, and growing children) are often at high risk for **nutritional deficiencies**.

Vitamin A. Vitamin A is necessary to develop a strong **immune system** and proper eyesight. Vitamin A deficiency (VAD) not only causes blindness and visual impairment (e.g., **cataract**), but also growth retardation and susceptibility to infections. When VAD is not detected early, it may make a child more prone to illness and even death. In Asia alone, it is estimated that 125 million children under five years of age are currently at risk, and 1.3 million are reported to be vitamin A deficient.

Iodine Deficiency Disorder (IDD). Iodine is essential for pregnant women, infants, and young children because it regulates the production of **hormones** necessary for children's development. Providing the recommended daily amount of iodine to mothers and children helps prevent brain damage, stunted growth, and goiters (ball-shaped tumors on the neck) in children. Some children with IDD are unable to move normally, speak, or hear. Asia has an estimated 200 million people at risk of IDDs.

Iron Deficiency and Anemia. Iron deficiency is the most common micronutrient deficiency in the world. The consequences of iron deficiency include impaired cognitive development. Iron deficiency is the most common cause of anemia (low levels of red blood cells or **hemoglobin**) in Asia, with over 600 million people affected. Young children, adolescent girls, and women are the most severely affected. Southeast Asia has the largest proportion of anemia—about 600 million are at risk for iron deficiency in this region.

Lactose Intolerance. Historically, milk and dairy products have not been used in East and Southeast Asia. As a result, the hereditary ability to digest lactose is most common in Asia and parts of Africa. Milk and dairy products are a major source of **calcium**, and people who avoid them because of lactose intolerance may compromise their nutritional status and bone strength. Low-lactose milk products have been developed to reduce the symptoms of lactose intolerance (diarrhea, abdominal bloating and gas, and stomach cramps).

The Nutritional Transition and Its Health Effects

With people living longer, and with low birth weight at an all-time low, Asian health should be improving. But with increased Westernization of the Asian diet, elevated tobacco use (generally among Asian men), and lifestyle changes (such as decreased physical activity), there has been a marked rise in **cardiovascular** disease (CVD), **diabetes** mellitus, hypertension (**high blood pressure**), and certain cancers. **Obesity** is also a growing health problem in Asia, and is strongly associated with hypertension (along with **body mass index** and age). Despite the low obesity levels in the Asia Pacific region, rates of obesity-related diseases such as diabetes and CVD are on the rise. High blood pressure is also a growing problem in Asia. In India, Indonesia, and Thailand alone, nearly 10 to 15 percent of adults have high

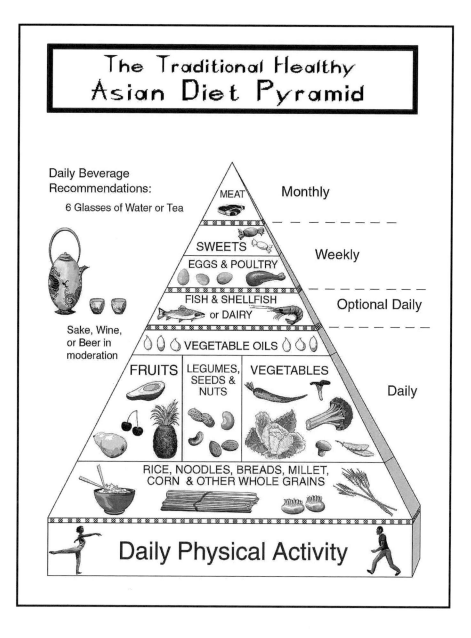

The Traditional Healthy Asian Diet Pyramid

Daily Beverage Recommendations:

6 Glasses of Water or Tea

Sake, Wine, or Beer in moderation

MEAT — Monthly

SWEETS — Weekly

EGGS & POULTRY

FISH & SHELLFISH or DAIRY — Optional Daily

VEGETABLE OILS

FRUITS | LEGUMES, SEEDS & NUTS | VEGETABLES — Daily

RICE, NOODLES, BREADS, MILLET, CORN & OTHER WHOLE GRAINS

Daily Physical Activity

The plant-based Asian diet, with its heavy reliance on rice, is reflected in the Asian food pyramid. The Asian diet does not include much meat or dairy and is low in total fat. [2000 Oldways Preservation & Exchange Trust. Reproduced by permission.]

blood pressure. Hypertension is dangerous because it increases a person's risk of developing CVD or having a **stroke**.

Changes in the dietary intake patterns of Asian countries have been called the nutritional transition, meaning a shift away from the traditional Asian diets to a more varied diet higher in sugars, fats, and **processed foods**. This new eating trend includes fewer **carbohydrates** and **fiber** and is higher in fat and meat. Together with a shift towards physical inactivity, obesity among the Asian population has risen. The nutritional and health effects of these new foods contribute to higher mortality rates due to CVD in many Asian countries.

Conclusion

Asian food and the diets of Asians are often believed to be the model of healthful eating. Rice and fruit figure prominently in each country's typical meal. However, as diets have diversified, **chronic** diseases, such as **heart disease**,

stroke: loss of blood supply to part of the brain, due to a blocked or burst artery in the brain

processed food: food that has been cooked, milled, or otherwise manipulated to change its quality

carbohydrate: food molecule made of carbon, hydrogen, and oxygen, including sugars and starches

fiber: indigestible plant material which aids digestion by providing bulk

chronic: over a long period

heart disease: any disorder of the heart or its blood supply, including heart attack, atherosclerosis, and coronary artery disease

nutrition: the maintenance of health through proper eating, or the study of same

have begun to affect Asians in a new and different way. Further, as weather patterns change over time and natural disasters occur, Asia, a largely agricultural society, is not always guaranteed a good crop. Asian food and **nutrition** is deeply rooted in the availability of food in each country. International organizations such as the United Nations Food and Agricultural Organization and Oxfam International continue to work on programs that ensure that continents like Asia will not suffer food shortages in the future. SEE ALSO ASIAN AMERICANS, DIETS OF; DIETARY TRENDS, INTERNATIONAL.

M. Cristina F. Garces

Bibliography

Achaya, K. T. (1994). *Indian Food: A Historical Companion*. Delhi, India: Oxford University Press.

Fiple, Kenneth F., and Ornelas, Kriemhil Coneè, eds. (2000). *The Cambridge World History of Food*, Volumes 1 and 2. Cambridge, UK: Cambridge University Press.

Gill, T. P. (2001). "Cardiovascular Risk in the Asia-Pacific Region from a Nutrition and Metabolic Point of View: Abdominal Obesity." *Asia Pacific Journal of Clinical Nutrition* 10(2):85–89.

Groff, James L.; Gropper, Sarren S.; and Hunt, Sara M., eds. (1995). *Advanced Nutrition and Human Metabolism*, 2nd edition. St. Paul, MN: West Publishing.

Hubert, Annie (1997). "Choices of Food and Cuisine in the Concept of Social Space among the Yao of Thailand." In *The Anthropology of Food and Nutrition*, Vol. 2: *Food Preferences and Taste Continuity and Change*, ed. Helen MacBeth. Oxford, UK: Berghahn.

Khor, Geok Lin (1997). "Nutrition and Cardiovascular Disease: An Asia-Pacific Perspective." *Asia Pacific Journal of Clinical Nutrition* 6(2):122–142.

Kotler, Neil G., ed. (1992). *Frontiers of Nutrition and Food Security in Asia, Africa, and Latin America*. Washington, DC: Smithsonian Institution Press.

McKeigue, P. M.; Shah, B.; and Marmot, M. G. (1991). "Relation of Central Obesity and Insulin Resistance with High Diabetes Prevalence and Cardiovascular Risk in South Asians." *Lancet* 337:382–386.

Mason, John; Mannar, Venkatesh; and Mock, Nancy (1999). "Controlling Micronutrient Deficiencies in Asia." *Asian Development Review* 17(2).

Popkin, Barry M.; Horton, Sue; and Kim, Soowon (2001). "The Nutritional Transition and Diet-Related Chronic Diseases in Asia: Implications for Prevention." Discussion Paper No. 105. International Food Policy Research Institute.

Underwood, B. A. (1999). "Perspectives from Micronutrient/Malnutrition Elimination Eradication Programmes." *Morbidity and Mortality Weekly Report* 48(SU01):37–42.

Internet Resources

Betancourt, Deidre. "Cultural Diversity: Eating in America: Vietnamese." Ohio State University Extension Fact Sheet. Available from <http://www.ohioline.osu.edu>

BBC News (12 July 2000). "144 Million Asian Children Stunted." Available from <http://news.bbc.co.uk>

British Nutrition Foundation (1999). "Adverse Reactions to Food" Available from <http://www.nutrition.org.uk>

Food and Agriculture Organization of the United Nations. "Staple Foods: What Do People Eat?" Available from <http://www.fao.org>

International Council for Control of Iodine Deficiency Disorders (2000). "About Iodine Deficiency Disorder: IDD Problem Statement." Available from <http://www.tulane.edu/~icec/>

United Nations Development Fund. "The Philippines at a Glance." Available from <http://www.undp.org>

World Health Organization (2001). "The South-East Asia Nutrition Research-cum-Action Network." Available from <http://www.who.int>

World Health Organization. "Vitamin A." Available from <http://www.who.int>

World Health Organization, South East Asia Regional Office (2001). "South-East Asia Progress Towards Health For All (1977-2000)." Available from <http://www.whosea.org/progress/index/htm>

Atherosclerosis

Macrovascular disease, or **atherosclerosis**, is the cause of more than half of all mortality in developed countries and the leading cause of death in the United States. It is a progressive disease of the large- and medium-sized **arteries**. The name is derived from the Greek *athero* meaning "gruel" or "paste" and *sclerosis* meaning "hardening." Thus, atherosclerosis is the hardening of the arteries due to the accumulation of this paste (commonly called plaque).

Any vessel in the body may be affected; however, the aorta, coronary, carotid, and iliac arteries are most frequently affected. When the coronary arteries are involved, it results in coronary artery disease (CAD). Hardening of the arteries is due to the build up of plaque and mineral deposits. As a result, the supply of blood to the heart is reduced, which can lead to chest pain or a myocardial infarction (**heart attack**). Hardening of the arteries causes an increase in resistance to blood flow and, therefore, an increase in **blood pressure**.

Everyone gets atherosclerosis. It is said that if every person lived to be 100 years old, each would eventually die of atherosclerosis. The process begins early in life. Therefore, physicians should obtain risk-factor profiles and a family history for children. Surgical procedures such as **angioplasty** and cardiac bypass may restore **cardiovascular** function. However, prevention is the key. Smoking, high blood **cholesterol**, **high blood pressure**, a high-fat **diet**, and lack of physical activity are the most serious risk factors for atherosclerosis and other cardiovascular diseases. Controlling one of these risk factors can help control the others. For example, regular exercise can help control cholesterol, blood pressure, weight, and **stress** levels. Smoking is the most preventable risk factor. For some, a low-dose aspirin taken daily is recommended for adults over age forty to thin the blood.

For optimal health, health professionals recommend a change to a healthful diet and lifestyle for those at risk, including daily physical activity; smoking cessation; a low-fat, low-cholesterol diet; reducing sodium intake; and managing stress. SEE ALSO ARTERIOSCLEROSIS; CARDIOVASCULAR DISEASES.

Delores C. S. James

Internet Resource

American Heart Association. "Common Cardiovascular Diseases." Available from <http://www.americanheart.org/stroke>

atherosclerosis: build-up of deposits within the blood vessels

artery: blood vessel that carries blood away from the heart toward the body tissues

heart attack: loss of blood supply to part of the heart, resulting in death of heart muscle

blood pressure: measure of the pressure exerted by the blood against the walls of the blood vessels

angioplasty: reopening of clogged blood vessels

cardiovascular: related to the heart and circulatory system

cholesterol: multi-ringed molecule found in animal cell membranes; a type of lipid

high blood pressure: elevation of the pressure in the bloodstream maintained by the heart

diet: the total daily food intake, or the types of foods eaten

stress: heightened state of nervousness or unease

Baby Bottle Tooth Decay

B

Baby bottle tooth decay occurs in young children when their teeth or gums are exposed to infant formula, milk, juice, or other sweet drinks for long

carbohydrate: food molecule made of carbon, hydrogen, and oxygen, including sugars and starches

bacteria: single-celled organisms without nuclei, some of which are infectious

plaque: material forming deposits on the surface of the teeth, which may promote bacterial growth and decay

caries: cavities in the teeth

periods of time. This often happens when infants or toddlers fall asleep while sucking on a bottle. Breastfed infants are usually not at risk, unless they feed for extended periods. The **carbohydrates** in the drink (lactose in milk, or fructose in fruit drinks) mix with the normal **bacteria** in the mouth. This bacteria is found in the **plaque** on teeth and gums. When plaque mixes with carbohydrates, acids are formed that dissolve tooth enamel, causing tooth decay and dental **caries**. To prevent baby bottle tooth decay, a child should not be put in bed with a bottle; and the bottle should be taken away as soon as mealtime is over. Further, only formula or water should be put in a bottle; juices and sweet drinks should be offered in a cup. SEE ALSO INFANT NUTRITION; ORAL HEALTH.

Heidi J. Silver

Bibliography

American Dietetic Association (1996). "Oral Health and Nutrition: Position of the American Dietetic Association." *Journal of the American Dietetic Association* 96:184–189.

Johnsen, D. and Nowjack-Raymer, R. (1989). "Baby Bottle Tooth Decay (BBTD): Issues, Assessment, and an Opportunity for the Nutritionist." *Journal of the American Dietetic Association* 89:1112–1116.

Internet Resource

American Academy of Pediatrics. Baby Bottle Tooth Decay. Available from <http://medem.com>

Battle Creek Sanitarium, Early Health Spa

The Western Health Reform Institute, which opened in 1866, was originally a residence belonging to Benjamin Graves, a judge of the Michigan Superior Court. Set on eight acres of land, this farm house gave no hint of what it was to become, but already there were ideas and propositions for the building that would lead to a worldwide reputation.

Upon its opening, in 1866, the Western Health Reform Institute was heralded far and wide through the Seventh-day Adventist journal *Review and Herald.* Dr. H. S. Lay, the first physician in charge, and James and Ellen White, early founders of the Seventh-day Adventist Church, were instrumental in founding this health institution. Taking in visitors and teaching simple principles, such as advocating the use of "Graham" bread and counseling eight hours of sleep at night, the institution struggled to live up to its grand name until 1876, when John Harvey Kellogg became medical director. In 1877, Kellogg changed the name to Battle Creek Sanitarium.

Ellen Gould White had come to Battle Creek, Michigan, in 1855 with her family. White was an advocate of healthful living, and she and her husband encouraged young John Harvey Kellogg to study medicine and eventually return to Battle Creek as medical director and surgeon.

The sanitarium, in its heyday during the 1880s, was the most famous health institution in the country, a reputation it held until World War II. The sanitarium was also instrumental in spawning the health food industry and lent strong support to the concept of vegetarianism.

Cereals put Battle Creek on the map. In November 1855, there were 3,000 inhabitants in all of Battle Creek, yet there were soon over forty cereal man-

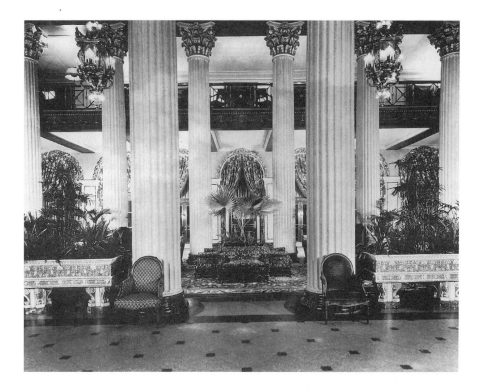

In the late nineteenth and early twentieth centuries, the Battle Creek Sanitarium was an incubator for nutritional health movements, including vegetarianism and temperance. Early sanitarium members developed such dietary innovations as breakfast cereal and graham crackers. *[AP/Wide World Photos. Reproduced by permission.]*

ufacturers in the city, and **entrepreneurs** and famous personalities would soon find their way to Battle Creek. Both Kellogg's brother Will and C. W. Post were to find great success and spawn businesses worth millions of dollars—all from the humble principles found in eating cereal breakfasts and promoting health foods for their **protein**, their **calories**, their **minerals** and **vitamins**, and, most of all, their bran. Famous personalities that visited the Battle Creek Sanitarium included J. C. Penney in 1929 and Professor Ivan Pavlov of Leningrad, Russia, who, at the age of eighty, visited in the summer of 1929.

The Great Depression interrupted the growth and expansion of this successful enterprise. On February 18, 1902, a fire burned two main buildings to the ground, and Kellogg immediately began an ambitious rebuilding project. He said at the time that "buildings may burn, but principles survive." The expansion cost $4 million and was done in 1928. But by 1930, with a capacity for 1,400, there were only 300 patients in residence. In 1930, at the age of seventy-eight, Kellogg retired to Florida to start another sanitarium, which ran at full capacity (100 beds) for the remaining thirteen years of his life.

The Battle Creek Sanitarium represented a haven to those who made pilgrimages to its abundant facilities. It afforded indoor exercise facilities, a steam-heated environment, and all the amenities of a first-class hotel, including Edison electric lights and polite attendants. In 1927, its golden anniversary year, the Battle Creek Sanitarium treated more than 7,000 patients. It eventually became the Percy Jones Army Hospital, which treated casualties of World War II and the Korean War. SEE ALSO KELLOGG, JOHN HARVEY; WHITE, ELLEN G.

Louise E. Schneider

entrepreneur: founder of a new business

protein: complex molecule composed of amino acids that performs vital functions in the cell; necessary part of the diet

calorie: unit of food energy

mineral: an inorganic (non-carbon-containing) element, ion or compound

vitamin: necessary complex nutrient used to aid enzymes or other metabolic processes in the cell

Bibliography

Sabate, Joan (2001). *Vegetarian Nutrition.* Boca Raton, FL: CRC.

Schwartz, Richard W. (1970). *John Harvey Kellogg.* Nashville, TN: Southern Publishing Association.

Whorton, James C. (1987). "Traditions of Folk Medicine." *Journal of the Medical Association* 257:1632–1640.

Beikost

The German word *beikost* translates as "foods other than milk or formula." It refers to the first strained foods that are given to a young infant as a supplement to breast milk or formula. Beikost is introduced between four and six months of age, when an infant develops the appropriate oral motor skills and can indicate disinterest by leaning back and turning away. The first foods introduced vary by country, but are generally soft mashed foods that are easily digested. If solid foods are added before four months, there is a risk of overfeeding or negative physical reactions such as diarrhea. SEE ALSO INFANT NUTRITION.

Sheah Rarback

Beriberi

water-soluble: able to be dissolved in water

energy: technically, the ability to perform work; the content of a substance that allows it to be useful as a fuel

legumes: beans, peas, and related plants

vitamin: necessary complex nutrient used to aid enzymes or other metabolic processes in the cell

mineral: an inorganic (non-carbon-containing) element, ion, or compound

clinical: related to hospitals, clinics, and patient care

nervous system: the brain, spinal cord, and nerves that extend throughout the body

Thiamin, or vitamin B_1, is a **water-soluble** vitamin that plays a role in **energy** production (through the synthesis of adenosine triphosphate [ATP]) and nerve conduction. (ATP is the major source of energy that the human body utilizes to do work.) Thiamin is found in abundance in foods such as lean pork, **legumes**, and yeast. In contrast, polished (white) rice, white flour, refined sugars, fats, and oils are foods lacking this vitamin. People at risk for thiamin deficiency include those who consume large quantities of alcohol and those who live in impoverished conditions, for such people are deficient in substantial amounts of **vitamins** and **minerals**.

Beriberi is a **clinical** manifestation of thiamin deficiency. Symptoms include **nervous system** abnormalities (e.g., leg cramps, muscle weakness), limb swelling, elevated pulse, and heart failure. Wernicke-Korsakoff syndrome is a related condition (with symptoms such as a jerky gait, disorientation, and impaired short-term memory) that occurs among alcoholics. SEE ALSO NUTRITIONAL DEFICIENCY; VITAMINS, WATER-SOLUBLE.

Kheng Lim

Bibliography

Morgan, Sarah L., and Weinsier, Roland L. (1998). *Fundamentals of Clinical Nutrition,* 2nd edition. St. Louis, MO: Mosby.

Kane, Agnes B., and Kumar, Vinay (1999). "Environmental and Nutritional Pathology." In *Robbins Pathologic Basis of Disease,* 6th edition. Philadelphia: W. B. Saunders.

Beta-Carotene

carotenoid: plant-derived molecules used as pigments

Beta-carotene is the most active of the deeply colored pigments called **carotenoids**. After consumption, beta-carotene converts to retinol, a readily usable form of vitamin A. Beta-carotene's beneficial effects include protecting the skin from sunlight damage, fighting early **cancer** cells, boosting immunity, and preventing **cataract** formation. It also stops the creation of **free radicals** (oxidants), which are DNA-damaging molecular fragments in the body.

Food sources of beta-carotene include carrots, spinach, kale, and broccoli, as well as animal sources such as liver, whole eggs, and whole milk. Since beta-carotene is fat-soluble, most fat-free milk has been **fortified** with vitamin A to replace what is lost when the fat is removed.

Vitamin A is stored in the body, and an excess amount can lead to **acute** symptoms, such as vomiting and muscle weakness, as well as **chronic** problems such as liver abnormalities, birth defects, and **osteoporosis**. In addition, beta-carotene supplements have been found in some studies to actually increase the risk of cancer in smokers. (Excess beta-carotene is not stored in the body, however.) Because of these dangers, the Institute of Medicine recommends that beta-carotene supplements are not to be used by the general public. The institute does advocate the use of such supplements for populations with inadequate vitamin A intake. SEE ALSO ANTIOXIDANTS; CAROTENOIDS; VITAMINS, FAT-SOLUBLE.

Chandak Ghosh

cancer: uncontrolled cell growth

cataract: clouding of the lens of the eye

free radical: highly reactive molecular fragment, which can damage cells

fortified: altered by addition of vitamins or minerals

acute: rapid-onset and short-lived

chronic: over a long period

osteoporosis: weakening of the bone structure

Bibliography

Margen, Sheldon, and the Editors of UC Berkeley Wellness Letter (2002). *Wellness Foods A to Z: An Indispensable Guide for Health-Conscious Food Lovers.* New York: Rebus.

Internet Resources

National Institutes of Health (NIH) Clinical Center. "Vitamin A and Carotenoids." Available from <http://www.cc.nih.gov>

Wellness Guide to Dietary Supplements. "Beta-Carotene." Available from <http://www.berkeleywellness.com>

Bezoars

Bezoars are balls of undigested materials, **insoluble fiber**, and undissolved medicines that resist the action of digestive **enzymes** in the stomach. Bezoars are the result of a lack of stomach hydrochloric acid secretion, without which medicine like sulfa **drugs**, **iron**, and antacid tablets may not dissolve. They may also be caused by poor stomach emptying.

Bezoars in humans cause the feeling of fullness, pain, **nausea**, and vomiting, and they reduce or prevent stomach emptying. Treatment may include avoidance of fibrous foods such as apples, berries, Brussels sprouts, beans, and sauerkraut, as well as changes in any medication being taken. Bezoars may also form in animals' stomachs. In ancient Persian medicine, bezoars were used as an antidote to poison. SEE ALSO CRAVINGS; PICA.

Simin B. Vaghefi

insoluble: not able to be dissolved in

fiber: indigestible plant material that aids digestion by providing bulk

enzyme: protein responsible for carrying out reactions in a cell

drugs: substances whose administration causes a significant change in the body's function

iron: nutrient needed for red blood cell formation

nausea: unpleasant sensation in the gut that precedes vomiting

Binge Eating

Binge eating disorder (BED), also known as compulsive overeating, has been designated as a psychiatric disorder requiring further study by the

binge: uncontrolled indulgence

eating disorder: behavioral disorder involving excess consumption, avoidance of consumption, self-induced vomiting, or other food-related aberrant behavior

American Psychiatric Association. Like bulimics, individuals suffering from binge eating disorder indulge in regular episodes of gorging, but unlike bulimics, they do not purge afterward. Binges are accompanied by a similar sense of guilt, embarrassment, and loss of self-control seen among bulimics. Because of the tremendous number of **calories** consumed, many people with BED are **overweight** or **obese**, and as a result they are more prone to complications such as **high blood pressure**, **diabetes**, high **cholesterol**, and **heart disease**.

A clinical diagnosis of BED requires bingeing at least two times a week for a period of six months or longer. SEE ALSO ADDICTION, FOOD; BULIMIA NERVOSA; EATING DISORDERS; EATING DISTURBANCES; YO-YO DIETING.

Karen Ansel

calorie: unit of food energy

overweight: weight above the accepted norm based on height, sex, and age

obese: above accepted standards of weight for sex, height, and age

high blood pressure: elevation of the pressure in the bloodstream maintained by the heart

diabetes: inability to regulate level of sugar in the blood

cholesterol: multi-ringed molecule found in animal cell membranes; a type of lipid

heart disease: any disorder of the heart or its blood supply, including heart attack, atherosclerosis, and coronary artery disease

Bibliography

American Dietetic Association (1998). *Nutrition Intervention in the Treatment of Anorexia Nervosa, Bulimia Nervosa, and Eating Disorder Not Otherwise Specified (ED-NOS)*. Chicago.

American Psychiatric Association (2000). *Diagnostic and Statistical Manual of Mental Disorders*, 4th edition. Washington, DC.

Escott-Stump, Sylvia, and Mahan, L. Kathleen (1996). *Krause's Food, Nutrition, and Diet Therapy*, 9th edition. Philadelphia: W. B. Saunders.

Bioavailability

bioavailability: availability to living organisms, based on chemical form

A nutrient's **bioavailability** is the proportion of the nutrient that, when ingested, actually gets absorbed by the body. The remaining amount cannot be metabolized and is removed as waste. The ability to absorb nutrients varies by gender, disease state, and physiologic condition (e.g., pregnancy, aging). The bioavailability of a nutrient can also increase or decrease if other substances are present. For example, **calcium** and magnesium lose much of their effectiveness if taken with fatty foods. The **intestines** themselves may also regulate the amount of a mineral that enters the bloodstream. For these reasons, taking high-potency vitamin supplements does not guarantee that all of the included nutrients will enter one's system. SEE ALSO NUTRIENTS.

Chandak Ghosh

calcium: mineral essential for bones and teeth

intestines: the two long tubes that carry out the bulk of the processes of digestion

Bibliography

"Nutrients Are Team Players." *University of California Wellness Letter* 20(7):5.

Internet Resource

British Nutrition Foundation. "Minerals." Available from <http://www.nutrition.org.uk>

Biotechnology

genetic: inherited or related to the genes

microorganisms: bacteria and protists; single-celled organisms

The term *biotechnology* refers to the use of scientific techniques, including **genetic** engineering, to improve or modify plants, animals, and **microorganisms**. In its most basic forms, biotechnology has been in use for millennia. For example, Middle Easterners who domesticated and bred deer, antelope, and sheep as early as 18,000 B.C.E.; Egyptians who made wine in

4000 B.C.E.; and Louis Pasteur, who developed **pasteurization** in 1861, all used biotechnology. In recent years, however, food biotechnology has become synonymous with the terms *genetically engineered foods* and *genetically modified organism* (GMO).

Traditional biotechnology uses techniques such as **crossbreeding**, **fermentation**, and **enzymatic** treatments to produce desired changes in plants, animals, and foods. Crossbreeding plants or animals involves the selective passage of desirable **genes** from one generation to another. *Microbial* fermentation is used in making wine and other alcoholic beverages, yogurt, and many cheeses and breads. Using **enzymes** as **food additives** is another traditional form of biotechnology. For example, papain, an enzyme obtained from papaya fruit, is used to tenderize meat and clarify beverages.

Genetic Engineering

The **DNA** contained in genes determines inherited characteristics. Modifying DNA to remove, add, or alter genetic information is called genetic modification or genetic engineering. In the early 1980s, scientists developed recombinant DNA techniques that allowed them to extract DNA from one species and insert it into another. Refinements in these techniques have allowed identification of specific genes within DNA—and the transfer of that particular gene sequence of DNA into another species. For example, the genes responsible for producing **insulin** in humans have been isolated and inserted into **bacteria**. The insulin that is then produced by these bacteria, which is identical to human insulin, is then isolated and given to people who have **diabetes**. Similarly, the genes that produce chymosin, an enzyme that is involved in cheese manufacturing, have also been inserted into bacteria. Now, instead of having to extract chymosin from the stomachs of cows, it is made by bacteria. This type of application of genetic engineering has not been very controversial. However, applications involving the use of plants have been more controversial.

Among the first commercial applications of genetically engineered foods was a tomato in which the gene that produces the enzyme responsible for softening was turned off. The tomato could then be allowed to ripen on the vine without getting too soft to be packed and shipped. As of 2002, over forty food crops had been modified using recombinant DNA technology, including pesticide-resistant soybeans, virus-resistant squash, frost-resistant strawberries, corn and potatoes containing a natural pesticide, and rice containing beta-carotene. Consumer negativity toward biotechnology is increasing, not only in the United States, but also in the United Kingdom, Japan, Germany, and France, despite increased consumer knowledge of biotechnology. The principle objections to biotechnology and foods produced using genetic modification are: concern about possible harm to human health (such as allergic responses to a "foreign gene"), possible negative impact to the environment, a general unease about the "unnatural" status of biotechnology, and religious concerns about modification.

Biotechnology in Animals

The most controversial applications of biotechnology involve the use of animals and the transfer of genes from animals to plants. The first animal-based application of biotechnology was the approval of the use of bacterially

pasteurization: heating to destroy bacteria and other microorganisms, after Louis Pasteur

crossbreeding: breeding between two different varieties of an organism

fermentation: reaction performed by yeast or bacteria to make alcohol

enzymatic: related to use of enzymes, proteins that cause chemical reactions to occur

gene: DNA sequence that codes for proteins, and thus controls inheritance

enzyme: protein responsible for carrying out reactions in a cell

food additive: substance added to foods to improve nutrition, taste, appearance, or shelf-life

DNA: deoxyribonucleic acid; the molecule that makes up genes, and is therefore responsible for heredity

insulin: hormone released by the pancreas to regulate level of sugar in the blood

bacteria: single-celled organisms without nuclei, some of which are infectious

diabetes: inability to regulate level of sugar in the blood

Scientists inserted daffodil genes and other genetic material into ordinary rice to make this *golden rice.* The result is a strain of rice that provides vitamin A, a nutrient missing from the diets of many people who depend on rice as a food staple. *[AP/Wide World Photos. Reproduced by permission.]*

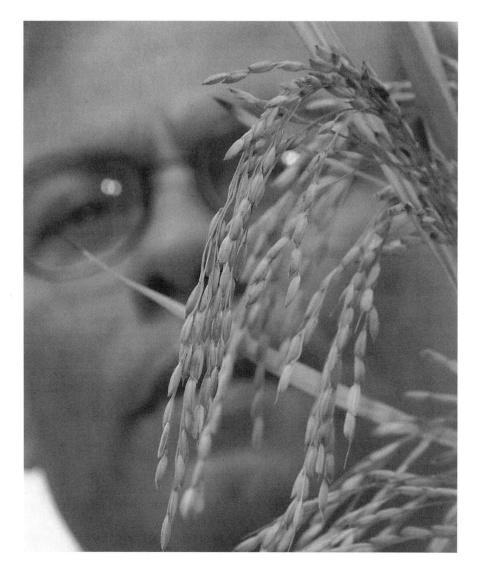

hormone: molecules produced by one set of cells that influence the function of another set of cells

cloning: creation of an exact genetic copy of an organism

protein: complex molecule composed of amino acids that performs vital functions in the cell; necessary part of the diet

allergen: a substance that provokes an allergic reaction

allergy: immune system reaction against substances that are otherwise harmless

produced bovine somatotropin (bST) in dairy cows. Bovine somatotropin, a naturally occurring **hormone**, increases milk production. This application has not been commercially successful, however, primarily because of its expense. The **cloning** of animals is another potential application of biotechnology. Most experts believe that animal applications of biotechnology will occur slowly because of the social and ethical concerns of consumers.

Concerns about Food Production

Some concerns about the use of biotechnology for food production include possible allergic reactions to the transferred **protein**. For example, if a gene from Brazil nuts that produces an **allergen** were transferred to soybeans, an individual who is allergic to Brazil nuts might now also be allergic to soybeans. As a result, companies in the United States that develop genetically engineered foods must demonstrate to the U.S. Food and Drug Administration (FDA) that they did not transfer proteins that could result in food **allergies**. When, in fact, a company attempted to transfer a gene from Brazil nuts to soybeans, the company's tests revealed that they had transferred a gene for an allergen, and work on the project was halted. In 2000 a brand

Biotechnology and Global Health

The World Health Organization estimates that more than 8 million lives could be saved by 2010 by combating infectious diseases and malnutrition through developments in biotechnology. A study conducted by the Joint Centre for Bioethics at the University of Toronto identified biotechnologies with the greatest potential to improve global health, including the following:

- Hand-held devices to test for infectious diseases including HIV and malaria. Researchers in Latin America have already made breakthroughs with such devices in combating dengue fever.

- Genetically engineered vaccines that are cheaper, safer, and more effective in fighting HIV/AIDS, malaria, tuberculosis, cholera, hepatitis, and other ailments. Edible vaccines could be incorporated into potatoes and other foods.

- Drug delivery alternatives to needle injections, such as inhalable or powdered drugs.

- Genetically modified bacteria and plants to clean up contaminated air, water, and soil.

- Vaccines and microbicides to help prevent sexually transmitted diseases in women.

- Computerized tools to mine genetic data for indications of how to prevent and cure diseases.

- Genetically modified foods with greater nutritional value.

—*Paula Kepos*

of taco shells was discovered to contain a variety of genetically engineered corn that had been approved by the FDA for use in animal feed, but not for human consumption. Although several antibiotechnology groups used this situation as an example of potential allergenicity stemming from the use of biotechnology, in this case the protein produced by the genetically modified gene was not an allergen. This incident also demonstrated the difficulties in keeping track of a genetically modified food that looks identical to the unmodified food. Other concerns about the use of recombinant DNA technology include potential losses of **biodiversity** and negative impacts on other aspects of the environment.

biodiversity: richness of species within an area

Safety and Labeling

In the United States, the FDA has ruled that foods produced though biotechnology require the same approval process as all other food, and that there is no inherent health risk in the use of biotechnology to develop plant food products. Therefore, no label is required simply to identify foods as products of biotechnology. Manufacturers bear the burden of proof for the safety of the food. To assist them with this, the FDA developed a decision-tree approach that allows food processors to anticipate safety concerns and know when to consult the FDA for guidance. The decision tree focuses on **toxicants** that are characteristic of each species involved; the potential for transferring food allergens from one food source to another; the concentration and **bioavailability** of **nutrients** in the food; and the safety and nutritional value of newly introduced proteins.

toxicant: harmful substance

bioavailability: availability to living organisms, based on chemical form

nutrient: dietary substance necessary for health

Labeling of genetically modified foods has sparked additional debate. Labels are required on food produced through biotechnology to inform consumers of any potential health or safety risk. For example, a label is required if a potential allergen is introduced into a food product. A label is also required if a food is transformed so that its nutrient content no longer resembles the original food. For example, so-called golden rice has been genetically engineered to have a higher concentration of beta-carotene than regular rice, and thus it must be included on the label. In response to consumer demands, regulators in England have instituted mandatory labeling laws for all packaged foods and menus containing genetically modified ingredients. Similar but less restrictive laws have been instituted in Japan. In Canada, the policy on labeling has remained similar to that of the United States.

Some consumer advocates maintain that not requiring a label on all genetically modified foods violates consumers' right to make informed food choices, and many producers of certain foods, such as foods containing soy protein, now include the term "non-GMO" on the label to indicate that the product does not contain genetically modified ingredients.

The application of recombinant DNA technology to foods, commonly called biotechnology, may be viewed as an extension of traditional cross-breeding and fermentation techniques. The technology enables scientists to transfer genetic material from one species to another, and may produce food crops and animals that are different than those obtained using traditional techniques. The FDA has established procedures for approval of food products manufactured using recombinant DNA technology that require food producers to demonstrate the safety of their products. The American Dietetic Association, the American Medical Association, and the World Health Organization have each adopted statements that techniques of biotechnology may have the potential to improve the food supply. These organizations and others acknowledge that long-term health and environmental impacts of the technology are not known, and they encourage continual monitoring of potential impacts. SEE ALSO ADDITIVES AND PRESERVATIVES; FOOD SAFETY; GENETICALLY MODIFIED FOODS.

M. Elizabeth Kunkel
Barbara H. D. Luccia

Bibliography

Altman, Arie, ed. (1998). *Agricultural Biotechnology.* New York: Marcel Dekker.

Johnson-Green, Perry (2002). *Introduction to Food Biotechnology.* Boca Raton, FL: CRC Press.

Serageldin, Ismail (1999). "Biotechnology and Food Security in the 21st Century." *Science* 285:387–389.

adipose tissue: tissue containing fat deposits

stroke: loss of blood supply to part of the brain, due to a blocked or burst artery in the brain

diabetes: inability to regulate level of sugar in the blood

cholesterol: multi-ringed molecule found in animal cell membranes; a type of lipid

triglyceride: a type of fat

obesity: the condition of being overweight, according to established norms based on sex, age, and height

Body Fat Distribution

Adipose tissue accumulation is referred to as body fat distribution. For individuals with *android* (apple-shaped) distribution, fat is centered around the abdominal area. This leads to an increased risk for coronary artery disease, **stroke**, **diabetes**, and high **cholesterol** and **triglyceride** levels. It is also an indicator for **obesity**. *Gynoid* (pear-shaped) distribution is associated with body fat that accumulates around the hip and thigh region.

Specific body fat distribution is often determined by measuring the waist-to-hip ratio, which is the circumference of the waist divided by the circumference of the hips. Android fat distribution is defined as a ratio greater than 1.0 for men and 0.8 for women. SEE ALSO ANTHROPOMETRIC MEASUREMENTS; BODY IMAGE; OBESITY; WAIST-TO-HIP RATIO; WEIGHT MANAGEMENT.

Diane L. Golzynski

Body Image

The term *body image* refers to the view that a person has of his or her own body size and proportion. Body-image distortion occurs when a person's view of their body is significantly different from reality.

Many factors impact the perception of one's body image, including the mass media, peer groups, ethnic groups, and family values. There is no such thing as an "ideal" or "perfect" body, and different cultures have different standards and norms for appropriate body size and shape. Even within a particular culture, societal standards shift periodically. For example, in the United States, the value of being thin has been the predominant stereotype for women since the model Twiggy arrived on the scene in the 1960s. The average fashion model (at the beginning of the twenty-first century) is almost six feet tall and weighs 130 pounds, whereas the average American woman is five feet, four inches tall and weighs 140 pounds. This disparity in height and weight may lead to problems with self-esteem when a woman finds herself not meeting the cultural ideal of body size and shape. The interesting factor is that women tend to feel **overweight**, not "under height" when comparing themselves to fashion models.

overweight: weight above the accepted norm based on height, sex, and age

Another example of body-image distortion can be seen among the contestants in the Miss America Beauty Pageant, the Miss Universe Pageant, and the Miss World Pageant. No winner of these pageants has ever been "overweight," and the winners have gotten progressively thinner over the years. Magazines and other media convey the image that being thin equates to being happy and successful, while cases of weight discrimination have been identified and argued in the courts. Fortunately, more emphasis is now being placed on health at any size, and on women becoming more muscular and fit, rather than simply thin. With increases in **obesity** statistics, however, some people may feel even more pressure to lose weight due to body-image distortion.

obesity: the condition of being overweight, according to established norms based on sex, age, and height

There are normal and predictable periods in life when body-image distortion occurs. One of these is **puberty**, when rapid changes in body size, body shape, and secondary sex characteristics take place. During this time, females tend to gain fat in the breasts, hips, buttocks, and thighs, developing a more pear-shaped body. Adolescent females may view their bodies as being heavier than they actually are, especially when compared to fashion models or celebrities. Adolescent males tend to gain height and muscle mass during puberty, and they may view their bodies as smaller than they actually are when compared to bodybuilders or professional athletes.

puberty: time of onset of sexual maturity

Body-image distortion also occurs when eating disorders develop. Most experts agree that the development of eating disorders is multifactorial and includes sociocultural, **psychological**, hereditary, and brain chemistry effects. Society plays a role in their development since eating disorders occur

psychological: related to thoughts, feelings, and personal experiences

Dissatisfaction with one's body can appear in adolescence and could lead to eating disorders. About 1 percent of teenage girls in the U.S. develop anorexia nervosa and up to 10 percent of those may die as a result. *[Photograph by Ariel Skelley. Corbis. Reproduced by permission.]*

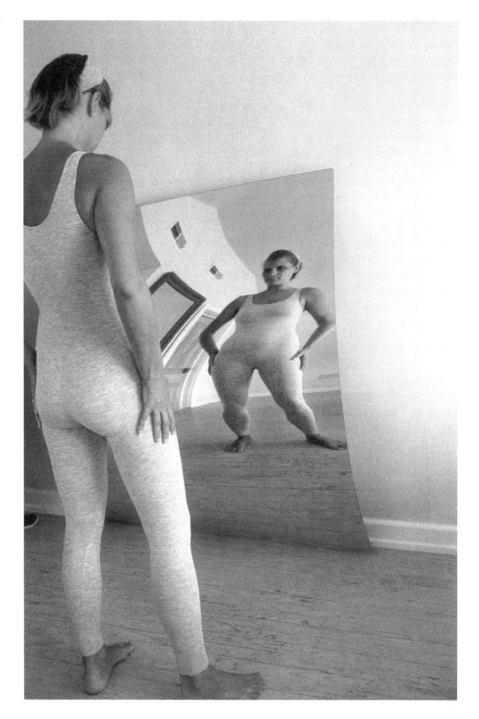

incidence: number of new cases reported each year

anorexia nervosa: refusal to maintain body weight at or above what is considered normal for height and age

bulimia: uncontrolled episodes of eating (bingeing) usually followed by self-induced vomiting (purging)

dysmorphia: the belief that one's body is different (fatter, thinner, etc.) than it really is

only in developed nations where food is prevalent and the **incidence** of these diseases increases with wealth. People diagnosed with eating disorders often see their body accurately only at the end of treatment—or not at all. No matter what their eventual weight is, the females with **anorexia** or **bulimia** may see themselves as overweight or fat, and males with muscle **dysmorphia** see themselves as underweight and scrawny. In anorexia, even when severe weight loss has occurred, patients may view their emaciated bodies as overweight. The diagnostic criteria for anorexia includes a "disturbance in the way in which one's body weight or shape is experienced; undue influence of body weight or shape on self-evaluation, or denial of the seriousness of current low body weight" (American Psychiatric Association). The diagnostic criteria for bulimia nervosa includes self-evaluation that is "unduly influenced by body shape and weight" (American Psychiatric Association). Body size or shape dissatisfaction appears to be one of the best predictors of dieting behavior. Another characteristic associated with body-image dissatisfaction, dieting, and **binge** eating is low self-esteem.

binge: uncontrolled indulgence

The earlier the treatment or intervention in eating disorders occurs, the better the prognosis is. With early diagnosis and treatment, body-image distortion may be minimal and can return to normal. The goals of body-image treatment are to correct distortions in body image and create a more positive body image. The longer the **eating disorder** has occurred, the more persistent the body-image distortion tends to be. Some female patients may never view their bodies as anything but overweight, and they may even view normal-weight women as fat. In males, the opposite is true: normal-weight men are viewed as scrawny, and only bodybuilders with significantly higher lean body mass than usual are considered ideal. Cognitive-behavioral therapy is commonly used as a major form of treatment for eating disorders and is often provided with a nondiet approach to improve self-esteem as bingeing or purging behaviors are reduced. SEE ALSO DIETING; EATING DISORDERS; EATING DISTURBANCES; WEIGHT MANAGEMENT.

eating disorder: behavioral disorder involving excess consumption, avoidance of consumption, self-induced vomiting, or other food-related aberrant behavior

Catherine Christie

Bibliography

American Psychiatric Association (2000). *Diagnostic and Statistical Manual*, 4th edition. Washington, DC: Author.

Eldredge, K.; Wilson, G. T.; and Whaley, A. (1990). "Failure, Self-Evaluation and Feeling Fat in Women." *International Journal of Eating Disorders* 9:37–50.

Rosen, J. C.; Gross, J.; and Vara, L. (1987). "Psychological Adjustment of Adolescents Attempting to Lose or Gain Weight." *Journal of Consulting and Clinical Psychology* 55:742–747.

Rubenstein, S., and Cabellero, B. (2000). "Is Miss America an Undernourished Role Model?" *Journal of the American Medical Association* 283:1569.

Body Mass Index

Body weight is used as an indicator of an individual's health. It is usually compared to tables that list "ideal" or "desirable" weight ranges for specific heights. Some of these tables use values gathered from research studies, while some include the heights and weights of individuals who have bought life insurance (e.g., the Metropolitan Height and Weight Tables). An individual's weight can be described as a percentage of the ideal or desirable weight listed, and can also be categorized as healthy, underweight, **overweight**, or **obese**. An additional method of comparing an individual to a population group is with the **body mass index**.

overweight: weight above the accepted norm based on height, sex, and age

obese: above accepted standards of weight for sex, height, and age

Body mass index (BMI) is an estimate of body composition that correlates an individual's weight and height to lean body mass. The BMI is thus an index of weight adjusted for stature. Body mass index is figured by dividing weight in kilograms by height in meters squared and multiplying by 100. It can also be figured by dividing weight in pounds by height in inches squared and multiplying by 705. High values can indicate excessive fat stores, while low values can indicate reduced fat stores. In this way, the BMI

body mass index: weight in kilograms divided by square of the height in meters; a measure of body fat

BMI, or body mass index, is a number that correlates a person's height and weight. It is a useful tool for diagnosing obesity or malnutrition; however, such diagnosis should take into account a person's age, gender, fitness, and ethnicity. *[Ed Bock/Corbis. Reproduced by permission.]*

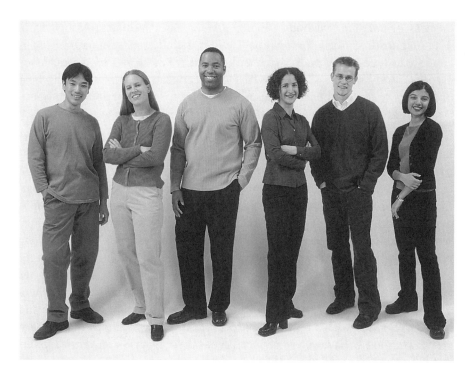

obesity: the condition of being overweight, according to established norms based on sex, age, and height

malnutrition: chronic lack of sufficient nutrients to maintain health

hydration: degree of water in the body

is a diagnostic tool for both **obesity** and protein-energy **malnutrition**. The BMI has also been associated with mortality, with lower values generally correlating with longer life.

However, when evaluating the BMI, several characteristics of an individual need to be known. An individual's age, gender, ethnicity, and level of fitness must be considered when using BMI to determine health risk. Also, the significance of the BMI is affected by disease state and **hydration** status. As with most assessment tools, the BMI is most effective when used in conjunction with other measurements.

Tables are available to identify the significance of the BMI. Calculations based on values for ideal body weight suggest the BMI for normal men and women should be in the range of 19 to 27 kg/m^2. This range corresponds to the 25th to 75th percentile values recorded from adults followed in the 1971–1974 National Health and Nutrition Examination Survey (NHANES). Tables also list levels of protein-energy malnutrition and obesity. These values were determined by research in which height, weight, and age were associated with functional measurements and health outcomes.

A BMI between 13 and 15 corresponds to 48 to 55 percent of desirable body weight for a given height and describes the lowest body weight that can sustain life. Body weight at this level consists of less than 5 percent fat. The maximum survival body weight is about 500 kg, which corresponds to a BMI of about 150.

Research with children indicates annual increases in BMI are usually due to increases in lean mass rather than fat tissue. Not until late adolescence does fat mass begin to affect the BMI—and adult values begin to be achieved.

There is a strong correlation between BMI and total fat mass, though individual variation in body type or height can cause misclassification. Un-

---

BODY MASS INDEX

Body mass index equation

$$BMI = \frac{weight\ (kg)}{height\ (m)\ (squared)} \times 100 \quad OR \quad \frac{pounds}{inches\ (squared)} \times 705$$

Significance of BMI values for adults

Condition Indicated	Men	Women
Protein-calorie malnutrition	< 17	< 17
Underweight	< 20	< 19
Acceptable weight	20.7 − 27.8	19.1 − 27.3
Intervention indicated	> 26.4	>25.8
Obese	> 27.8	> 27.3
Severely obese	> 31.1	> 32.2
Morbidly obese	> 45.4	> 44

Normal BMI Values for Infants and Children

Infants (at birth)	13	
1 year	18	
6 years	15	

fortunately, the same BMI value can correlate with a range of body-fat percentage. For example, athletes usually have large skeletal muscles (which weigh more than fat) and therefore a high BMI, but they are not obese. Shorter individuals can also be identified as obese, since their BMIs are usually high. An older individual may have a higher body-fat percentage than a younger individual, but have the same BMI. Adult females can have a BMI of 20, which correlates to a body-fat percentage of 13 to 32 percent, while adult males can have a BMI of 27 and a body-fat percentage of 10 to 31 percent.

Findings from the third NHANES (1988–1994) describe misidentification of the elderly when self-reported height, rather than measured height, is used in the BMI equation. Height decreases over an individual's lifetime due to vertebral compression, loss of muscle tone, and postural slump. An individual may, therefore, report a height that is no longer accurate, and the resulting value will be lower than the value that actually describes the individual, possibly leading to the wrong intervention.

Research has shown that both high BMIs and low BMIs can indicate increased **morbidity** and mortality. A low BMI, usually an indication of protein-energy malnutrition or the effects of **wasting** or a disease process, is a significant predictor of mortality among young and old hospitalized patients. A high BMI has been shown to be predictive of mortality only among young hospitalized patients, usually an effect of **cardiovascular** disease and obesity. Risk of mortality is only slightly elevated at the highest BMI for elderly hospitalized patients.

Because ethnicity has been shown to require adjustments to the levels of concern for the BMI, care must be taken when comparing different population groups. For example, Asian populations may require a lower BMI to describe health risk, while Pacific populations, specifically Hawaiian, may require a higher threshold to indicate that an individual is at risk. This variation can be explained by body type.

BMI and waist circumference have been used to evaluate health risks associated with overweight and obesity. Because both are easy measures to

morbidity: illness or accident

wasting: loss of body tissue often as a result of cancer or other disease

cardiovascular: related to the heart and circulatory system

do, standardization of both are encouraged for widespread use as a reference. Additionally, the two measurements have been used in an algorithm with a cardiovascular risk index to determine which individuals would benefit most from weight loss.

BMI is an easy measurement to make—only requiring a tape measure, scale, and, perhaps, a calculator. However, for individuals who have trouble standing up straight for an accurate height measurement—either from disease process, weakness, or kyphosis (abnormal backward curvature of the spine)—BMI may not be an easy or accurate assessment tool to use. Comparisons between BMI and mid-upper arm circumference (MUAC) measurements show that they identify the same level of malnutrition in individuals. MUAC is also easily measured (it requires only a tape measure), and it is a good indicator of change in body weight and muscle mass. Standardization of these two assessment tools for reference would benefit the science of nutrition assessment. SEE ALSO AGING AND NUTRITION; BODY FAT DISTRIBUTION; DIET; MALNUTRITION; NUTRITION ASSESSMENT; OBESITY; OVERWEIGHT; UNDERWEIGHT; WAIST-TO-HIP RATIO.

Carole S. Mackey

Bibliography

Collins, Steve (1996). "Using Middle Upper Arm Circumference to Assess Severe Adult Malnutrition During Famine." *Journal of the American Medical Association* 276(5):391–395.

Kiernan, M. (2000). "Identifying Patients for Weight-Loss Treatment: An Empirical Evaluation of the NHLBI Obesity Education Initiative Expert Panel Treatment Recommendations." *Archives of Internal Medicine* 160:2169–2176.

Kuczmarski, Marie Fanelli (2001). "Effects of Age on Validity of Self-Reported Height, Weight, and Body Mass Index: Findings from the Third National Health and Nutrition Survey, 1988–1994." *Journal of the American Dietetic Association* 101(1):28–34.

Landi, F. (2000). "Body Mass Index and Mortality Among Hospitalized Patients." *Archives of Internal Medicine* 160:2641–2644.

Maskarinec, G. (2000). "Dietary Patterns Are Associated with Body Mass Index in Multiethnic Women." *Journal of Nutrition* 130:3068–3072.

Maynard, L. M. (2001). "Childhood Body Composition in Relation to Body Mass Index." *Pediatrics* 107:344–350.

Pike, Ruth, and Brown, Myrtle L. (1984). *Nutrition, An Integrated Approach.* New York: John Wiley.

Seidel, J. C. (2001). "Report from a CDC Prevention Workshop on Use of Adult Anthropometry for Public Health and Primary Health Care." *American Journal of Clinical Nutrition* 73:123–126.

Shills, Maurice E.; Olson, James A.; and Shike, Moshe. (1994). *Modern Nutrition in Health and Disease*, 8th edition. Philadelphia: Lea & Febiger.

White, Jane V. (1999). "The Utility of Body Mass Index in Predicting Health Risk." *Consultant Dietitian* 24(2).

Breastfeeding

Before 1900, most mothers breastfed their infants. Breastfeeding rates declined sharply worldwide after 1920, when evaporated cow's milk and infant formula became widely available. These were promoted as being more convenient for mothers and more nutritious than human milk. Breastfeeding rates began rising again in the late 1950s and early 1960s.

BENEFITS OF BREASTFEEDING

Benefits for Infant	Benefits for Mother
• Perfect food for infant	• Promotes faster shrinking of the uterus
• Guarantees safe, fresh milk	• Promotes less postpartum bleeding
• Enhances immune system	• Promotes faster return to pre-pregnancy weight
• Protects against infectious and noninfectious diseases	• Eliminates the need for preparing and mixing formula
• Protects against food allergies and intolerances	• Saves money not spent on formula
• Decreases risk of diarrhea and respiratory infections	• Decreases risk of breast and ovarian cancer
• Promotes correct development of jaw, teeth, and speech patterns	• Increases bonding with infant
• Decreases risk of childhood obesity	• Enhances self-esteem in the maternal role
• Increases cognitive function	• Delays the menstrual cycle
• Increases bonding with mother	

Breastfeeding, or lactation, is, in fact, the ideal method of feeding and nurturing infants. Most health organizations recommend infants be exclusively breastfed during the first four to six months of life, but ideally through the first year. Premature infants also benefit from their mothers' milk. In developing countries, breastfeeding up to age two, with appropriate supplementary solid foods, maintains good nutritional status and prevents diarrhea.

Benefits of Breastfeeding

Human milk contains the right balance of **nutrients** for human growth and development. It is low in total **protein** and high in **carbohydrates**, making it more digestible and less stressful on the immature kidneys. In addition, each mammal produces milk that is nutritionally and immunologically tailored for its young. In rare cases, such as **galactosemia** and **phenylketonuria**, some infants cannot **metabolize** human milk or other milk products. A significant benefit of human milk is that it contains many **immunologic** agents that protect the infant against **bacteria**, **viruses**, and **parasites**. Breastfeeding also provides many benefits for the mother.

Breastfeeding Trends

Despite the many benefits of breastfeeding, only 64 percent of mothers in the United States initiate breastfeeding, with 29 percent still breastfeeding six months after birth. The U.S. goals for 2000 were to increase to 75 percent the proportion of women who initiate breastfeeding, and to increase to 50 percent the proportion of women who breastfeed for five to six months. In the United States, ethnic minorities are less likely to breastfeed than their white counterparts.

Based on a 2001 report by the World Health Organization (WHO), 35 percent of infants worldwide are exclusively breastfed (no other food or drink, not even water) for the first four months of life. Rates are very low in a number of African countries, especially Nigeria, Central African Republic, and Niger. Some countries, such as Benin, Mali, Zambia, and Zimbabwe have had small increases, due mainly to breastfeeding campaigns, baby-friendly hospitals, and the commitment of trained breastfeeding counselors. In Southeast Asia, the exclusive breastfeeding rate, though low, has increased. Breastfeeding rates are also low in many European countries, especially France, Italy, Netherlands, Spain, Switzerland, and the United Kingdom. Sweden, however, has a rate of 98 percent, the highest level in the world.

nutrient: dietary substance necessary for health

protein: complex molecule composed of amino acids that performs vital functions in the cell; necessary part of the diet

carbohydrate: food molecule made of carbon, hydrogen, and oxygen, including sugars and starches

galactosemia: inherited disorder preventing digestion of milk sugar, galactose

phenylketonuria: inherited disease marked by the inability to process the amino acid phenylalanine, causing mental retardation

metabolize: processing of a nutrient

immunologic: related to the immune system, which protects the body from infection

bacteria: single-celled organisms without nuclei, some of which are infectious

virus: noncellular infectious agent that requires a host cell to reproduce

parasite: organism that feeds off of other organisms

An increase in breastfeeding could save the lives of millions of children a year worldwide. However, the aggressive marketing campaigns by infant formula companies and the promotion of infant formula by health professionals combine to discourage breastfeeding. Other factors that determine whether a woman will breastfeed include:

- The father's preference for a specific feeding method
- Whether the mother was breastfed as an infant
- Social support
- Whether relatives and/or friends breastfeed
- Whether the mother gets help with household chores
- The mother's need to work
- Hospital policies

Physiology of Breastfeeding

hormone: molecules produced by one set of cells that influence the function of another set of cells

During pregnancy, the body increases its production of a **hormone** called prolactin, which stimulates the breast to make milk. Suckling by the infant stimulates the release of prolactin. The size of the breasts is not a factor in milk production. Oxytocin, another hormone, allows the breast tissue to "let down" or release milk from the milk ducts to the nipples.

Colostrum, the first milk produced, has all the nutrients a newborn infant needs. It also contains many substances to protect against infections. The body produces colostrum for several days until the "mature milk" comes in. Mature milk adjusts to the baby's needs for the rest of the time the infant is breastfed.

Nutritional Needs of the Mother

calorie: unit of food energy

Recommended Dietary Allowances: nutrient intake recommended to promote health

nutritional requirements: the set of substances needed in the diet to maintain health

folate: one of the B vitamins, also called folic acid

iron: nutrient needed for red blood cell formation

niacin: one of the B vitamins, required for energy production in the cell

zinc: mineral necessary for many enzyme processes

diet: the total daily food intake, or the types of foods eaten

drugs: substances whose administration causes a significant change in the body's function

wean: cease breast-feeding

malnourished: lack of adequate nutrients in the diet

Milk production requires about 800 **calories** a day. The **Recommended Dietary Allowances** for calories during breastfeeding is 500 more calories a day than is required by a nonpregnant woman. **Nutritional requirements** do not change significantly from pregnancy, with the exception of decreases in **folate** and **iron**, and increases in vitamin A, vitamin C, **niacin**, and **zinc**. The **diet** can be the same as during pregnancy, plus an additional glass of milk. Women who are on medication should check with their physicians, since most **drugs** are absorbed in breast milk.

Weaning

The decision to **wean** should be based on the desires and needs of the mother and child. Weaning should be gradual. Women returning to work can pump and store their milk for later use. Solid foods should be given based on the age and developmental stage of the child. In some countries, many toddlers become **malnourished** because they are given too many high carbohydrate foods, such as cassava, potatoes, and other root vegetables, too early. These foods are filling, but they are low in protein and other nutrients essential for growth and development.

Breast Implants and Breast Reduction

Many women with breast implants breastfeed successfully, though it is not known whether the health of the infant is affected by breast implants.

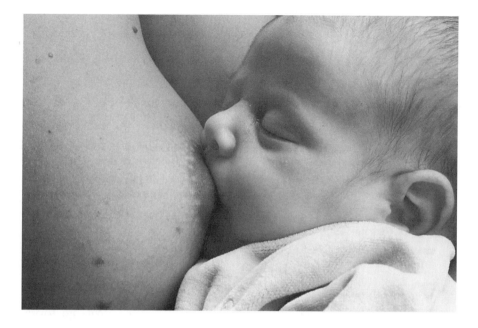

Human milk contains nutrients and antibodies that keep babies healthy. Although it is considered the ideal feeding method for infants, 36 percent of mothers in the United States do not breastfeed at all. *[Photograph by Jim Trois. Photo Researchers, Inc. Reproduced by permission.]*

Women who have had a breast reduction may not be able to breastfeed, since the surgical procedure removes glandular tissue and realigns the nipple.

Who Should Not Breastfeed?

Women with HIV/AIDS, **hepatitis**, **cancer**, and other conditions where the **immune system** may be compromised should not breastfeed. A case-by-case assessment should be made with women exposed to certain environmental **toxins** and those who use illicit drugs.

hepatitis: liver inflammation

cancer: uncontrolled cell growth

immune system: the set of organs and cells, including white blood cells, that protect the body from infection

toxins: poisons

Policies and Recommendations

A woman's ability to breastfeed for the optimal recommended time depends on the support she receives from her family, health care providers, and the workplace. Health care institutions should adopt policies and initiatives that include:

- A written breastfeeding policy
- A breastfeeding education program
- Rooming-in of mother and child
- Breastfeeding on demand
- Limited use of pacifiers, water, and formula

With the increased number of women in the workforce, employers can do a lot to support and encourage breastfeeding, such as providing adequate breaks; flexible hours; **job sharing**; part-time work; refrigerators for storage of breast milk; and on-site child care.

job sharing: splitting a single job among two or more people

A public health campaign can greatly increase the initiation and duration of breastfeeding. These campaigns should target all social groups, including men, future parents, grandparents, health care providers, and employers. In addition, culturally appropriate programs and materials should be available. Breastfeeding saves lives and money, and it benefits all of society. SEE ALSO BEIKOST; INFANT NUTRITION; MASTITIS; PREGNANCY.

Delores C. S. James

Bibliography

James, Delores C.; Jackson, Robert T.; and Probart, Claudia K. (1994). "Factors Affecting Breastfeeding Prevalence and Duration among International Students." *Journal of the American Dietetic Association* 94(2):194–196.

Worthington-Roberts, Bonnie S., and Rodwell-Williams, Sue (1993). *Nutrition in Pregnancy and Lactation*, 6th edition. Madison, WI: Brown & Benchmark.

U.S. Department of Health and Human Services, Office on Women's Health (2000). *HHS Blueprint for Action on Breastfeeding.* Washington, DC: U.S. Government Printing Office.

Internet Resources

American Academy of Pediatrics. "A Woman's Guide to Breastfeeding." Available from <http://www.aap.org/>

Ryan, A. S. (1997). "The Resurgence of Breastfeeding in the United States." *Pediatrics* (online). Available from <http://www.pediatrics.org>

UNICEF. "Breastfeeding and Complementary Feeding." Available from <http://www.childinfo.org/>

World Health Organization. "Global Databank on Breastfeeding." Available from <http://www.who.int/nut>

Brillat-Savarin, Jean Anthelme

French politician and writer
1755–1826

Jean Anthelme Brillat-Savarin was a French lawyer and politician. He served as mayor of Belley, the city where he was born, but his opposition to the Jacobins during the French Revolution made it necessary for him to flee to Switzerland in 1792. He then made his way to New York, where he taught language and played violin in the John Street Theater Orchestra to support himself.

After two years in New York, Brillat-Savarin spent time in Connecticut familiarizing himself with American culture and food. He took advantage of the opportunity to ask Thomas Jefferson how to prepare a wild turkey. Approximately four years after his exile, Brillat-Savarin was able to return to France after being reinstated as an honorable person. Soon after, he began serving as a judge of the Supreme Court of Appeal in Paris, a post he held for the rest of his life.

Brillat-Savarin embraced Parisian society and intellectual life, but he is best known for his culinary expertise and his twenty aphorisms on food, one of which was, "Tell me what you eat, and I will tell you what you are." Even as a child he loved to be near the kitchen. While in Paris, he wrote *Physiology of Taste, or Meditations on Transcendental Gastronomy*, which he published anonymously. Chapters discussed, among other things, the aphrodisiac properties of certain foods, the nature of digestion, and the dangers of acids in the stomach. The book was a success, and the people of Paris were anxious to learn the identity of this very witty and elegant author. His colleagues were not as impressed as the public and looked down on him, not considering him to be an expert in a relevant field of study. He had pre-

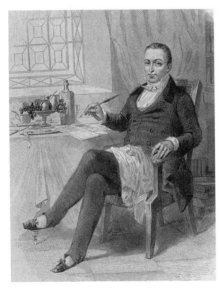

"The destiny of nations depends on the manner in which they are fed." Jean Anthelme Brillat-Savarin, whose culinary writings and passion for food distinguished him in Napoleonic France. [*Photograph by Gianni Dagli Orti. Corbis. Reproduced by permission.*]

viously written various treatises on dueling, economics, and history, but these were not very well known.

Brillat-Savarin contributed to the knowledge of digestion and **nutrition** through his essays on food and taste. He also shared his ideas on food preparation and its role in life and philosophy, and he provided discourses on **obesity** and its cure (and on thinness and its cure). In recognition of his achievements, various dishes, garnishes, and a cheese bear his name.

nutrition: the maintenance of health through proper eating, or the study of same

obesity: the condition of being overweight, according to established norms based on sex, age, and height

Brillat-Savarin's work reflects interactions with philosophers and physicians of his time. While he remained a bachelor all his life, he had many prominent guests sitting at his table for meals, and he often sat at the best tables of Paris. Among his guests were Napoleon's doctor, Jean-Nicolas Corvisart, the surgeon Guillaume Dupuytren, the pathologist Jean Cruveilhier, and other great minds. Cruveilhier was such an authority on the stomach that **gastric ulcers** are referred to as Cruveilhier's disease. Through such interactions, Brillat-Savarin undoubtedly gained knowledge about the chemistry of food and how it relates to the physiology of digestion. So passionate was Brillat-Savarin about food that many people identified him more often as a chef rather than a lawyer.

gastric: related to the stomach

ulcer: erosion in the lining of the stomach or intestine due to bacterial infection

Slande Celeste

Bibliography

Brillat-Savarin, Jean-Anthelme (1999). *The Physiology of Taste, or, Meditations on Transcendental Gastronomy*, tr. M. F. K. Fisher. Washington, DC: Counterpoint Press.

Modlin, I. M., and Lawton, G. P. (1996). "Observations on the Gastric Illuminati." *Perspectives in Biology and Medicine* 39(4):527–543.

Schnetzer, Amanda (1999). "The Gastronomic Servings of Brillat-Savarin." *Washington Times* July 11.

Internet Resources

Kansas State University Library. "Rare Books, The Cookery Exhibit: *Physiologie du Gout*." Available from <http://www.lib.ksu.edu/>

Vanderbilt Medical Center. "Culinary History." Available from <http://www.mc.vanderbilt.edu/biolib>

Bulimia Nervosa

Bulimia nervosa is an **eating disorder** characterized by frequent episodes of **binge** eating, which are followed by purging to prevent weight gain. During these incidents, unusually large portions of food are consumed in secret, followed by compensatory behaviors such as self-induced vomiting or diuretic and laxative abuse. Although the types of food chosen may vary, sweets and high-calorie foods are commonly favored. Bulimic episodes are typically accompanied by a sense of a loss of self-control and feelings of shame.

bulimia: uncontrolled episodes of eating (bingeing) usually followed by self-induced vomiting (purging)

eating disorder: behavioral disorder involving excess consumption, avoidance of consumption, self-induced vomiting, or other food-related aberrant behavior

binge: uncontrolled indulgence

A clinical diagnosis of bulimia nervosa requires that the behavior occur at least two times a week for a minimum of three months. SEE ALSO ADDICTION, FOOD; ANOREXIA NERVOSA; BINGE EATING; BODY IMAGE; EATING DISORDERS; EATING DISTURBANCES.

Karen Ansel

Bibliography

American Dietetic Association (1998). *Nutrition Intervention in the Treatment of Anorexia Nervosa, Bulimia Nervosa, and Eating Disorder Not Otherwise Specified (EDNOS)*. Chicago: Author.

American Psychiatric Association (2000). *Diagnostic and Statistical Manual of Mental Disorders*, 4th edition. Washington, DC: Author.

Escott-Stump, Sylvia, and Mahan, L. Kathleen (1996). *Krause's Food, Nutrition, & Diet Therapy*, 9th edition. Philadelphia: W. B. Saunders.

C Caffeine

Caffeine is a naturally occurring stimulant found in the leaves, seeds, or fruit of over sixty plants around the world. Caffeine exists in the coffee bean in Arabia, the tea leaf in China, the kola nut in West Africa, and the cocoa bean in Mexico. Because of its use throughout all societies, caffeine is the most widely used psychoactive substance in the world. The most common caffeine sources in North America and Europe are coffee and tea. Since about 1980, extensive research has been conducted on how caffeine affects health. Most experts agree that moderate use of caffeine (300 milligrams, or about three cups of coffee, per day) is not likely to cause health problems.

How Caffeine Affects the Body

Caffeine is best known for its stimulant, or "wake-up," effect. Once a person consumes caffeine, it is readily absorbed by the body and carried around in the bloodstream, where its level peaks about one hour after consumption. Caffeine mildly stimulates the nervous and **cardiovascular** systems. It affects the brain and results in elevated mood, decreased **fatigue**, and increased attentiveness, so a person can think more clearly and work harder. It also increases the heart rate, blood flow, respiratory rate, and **metabolic** rate for several hours. When taken before bedtime, caffeine can interfere with getting to sleep or staying asleep.

Exactly how caffeine will affect an individual, and for how long, depends on many factors, including the amount of caffeine ingested, whether one is male or female, one's height and weight, one's age, and whether one is pregnant or smokes. Caffeine is converted by the liver into substances that are excreted in the urine.

Some people are more sensitive to the effects of caffeine than others. With frequent use, **tolerance** to many of the effects of caffeine will develop. At doses of 600 milligrams (about six cups of coffee) or more daily, caffeine can cause nervousness, sweating, tenseness, upset stomach, **anxiety**, and insomnia. It can also prevent clear thinking and increase the side effects of certain medications. This level of caffeine intake represents a significant health risk.

Caffeine can be mildly addictive. Even when moderate amounts of caffeine are withdrawn for 18 to 24 hours, one may feel symptoms such as headache, fatigue, irritability, **depression**, and poor concentration. The symptoms peak within 24 to 48 hours and progressively decrease over the course of a week. To minimize withdrawal symptoms, experts recommend reducing caffeine intake gradually.

cardiovascular: related to the heart and circulatory system

fatigue: tiredness

metabolic: related to processing of nutrients and building of necessary molecules within the cell

tolerance: development of a need for increased amount of drug to obtain a given level of intoxication

anxiety: nervousness

depression: mood disorder characterized by apathy, restlessness, and negative thoughts

CAFFEINE IN FOODS AND BEVERAGES.

Food/Beverage	Caffeine (milligrams)
Coffee	
Espresso coffee, brewed, 8 fluid ounces	502
Coffee, brewed, 8 fluid ounces	85
Coffee, instant, 8 fluid ounces	62
Coffee, brewed, decaffeinated, 8 fluid ounces	3
Coffee, instant, decaffeinated, 8 fluid ounces	2
Tea	
Tea, brewed, 8 fluid ounces	47
Tea, herbal, brewed, 8 fluid ounces	0
Tea, instant, 8 fluid ounces	29
Tea, brewed, decaffeinated, 8 fluid ounces	3
Chocolate Beverages	
Hot chocolate, 8 fluid ounces	5
Chocolate milk, 8 fluid ounces	5
Soft Drinks	
Cola, 12 ounce can	37
Cola, with higher caffeine, 12 ounce can	100
Cola or pepper-type, diet, 12 ounce can	49
Cola or pepper-type, regular or diet, without caffeine, 12 ounce can	0
Lemon-lime soda, regular or diet, 12 ounce can	0
Lemon-lime soda, with caffeine, 12 ounce can	55
Ginger ale, regular or diet, 12 ounce can	0
Root beer, regular or diet, 12 ounce can	0
Chocolate	
Milk chocolate bar, 1.55 ounces	9
M & M milk chocolate candies, 1.69 ounces	5
Dark chocolate, semisweet, 1 ounce	20

SOURCE: U.S. Department of Agriculture National Nutrient Database for Standard Reference, Release 16 July 2003.

Caffeine in Food and Drugs

Due to its stimulant properties, caffeine is used around the world in any of its many forms, such as coffee, tea, soft drinks, and chocolate. The accompanying table displays the amount of caffeine in foods. An eight-ounce cup of drip-brewed coffee has about 85 milligrams of caffeine, whereas the same amount of brewed tea contains about 47 milligrams. Twelve-ounce cans of soft drinks (soda) provide about 35 to 45 milligrams of caffeine.

The caffeine content of coffee and tea depends on the variety of the coffee bean or tea leaf, the particle size, the brewing method, and the length of brewing or steeping time. Brewed coffee has more caffeine than instant coffee, and espresso has more caffeine than brewed coffee. Espresso is made by forcing hot pressurized water through finely ground, dark-roast beans. Because it is brewed with less water, it contains more caffeine than regular coffee per fluid ounce.

In soft drinks, caffeine is both a natural and an added ingredient. About 5 percent of the caffeine in colas and pepper-flavored soft drinks is obtained naturally from cola nuts; the remaining 95 percent is added. Caffeine-free drinks contain virtually no caffeine and make up a small part of the soft-drink market.

Numerous prescription and nonprescription drugs also contain caffeine. Caffeine increases the ability of aspirin and other painkillers to do their job, and it is often used in headache and pain-relief remedies as well as in cold products and alertness or stay-awake tablets. When caffeine is an ingredient, it must be listed on the product label.

Though it has mildly addictive properties, caffeine taken in moderation is not considered to be a health risk, and may improve athletic performance. *[AP/Wide World Photos. Reproduced by permission.]*

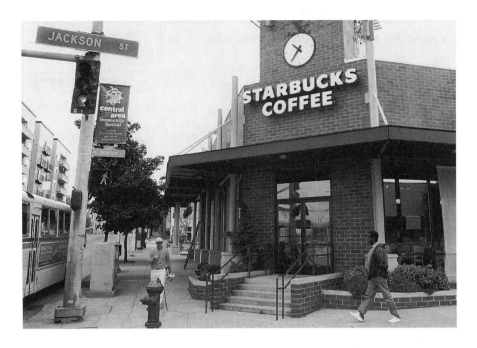

Caffeine and Health

Current research on how caffeine affects a variety of health issues is summarized below. Keep in mind that most experts agree that moderate use of caffeine is not likely to cause any health problems.

- Studies have looked at the effects of caffeine on heart health. Moderate caffeine consumption does not appear to adversely affect cardiovascular health.

calcium: mineral essential for bones and teeth

osteoporosis: weakening of the bone structure

- Caffeine appears to increase the excretion of **calcium**, a mineral needed for healthy bones. Calcium is particularly important to prevent **osteoporosis**, a bone disease characterized by loss of bone strength and seen especially in older women (although men get it too). Moderate caffeine intake does not seem to cause a problem with calcium, as long as one is consuming the recommended amount (adult men and women should be taking between 1,000 and 1,200 milligrams of calcium, depending on age and gender).

cancer: uncontrolled cell growth

- In the past there have been concerns that the caffeine in coffee may cause **cancer**. Research has shown that caffeine in coffee does not cause breast or intestinal cancer. However, not enough research has been done to determine if caffeine in coffee is involved in urinary bladder or pancreatic cancer. Taken in moderation, it is unlikely that caffeine will cause cancer.

- Evidence suggests that, at levels over 500 milligrams per day, caffeine may delay conception. Moderate caffeine consumption does not appear to be of concern to women trying to get pregnant. Moderate consumption is also important for a healthy pregnancy. Excessive caffeine intake has been associated with **miscarriages** and low birth weight babies.

miscarriage: loss of a pregnancy

- Because children have developing nervous systems, it is important to moderate their caffeine consumption. For children, major sources of caffeine include soft drinks and chocolate.

- Caffeine may be useful as part of a weight control program because it increases the rate at which the body burns **calories** for three or more hours after being consumed.

- Caffeine's ability to improve physical performance is well known among well-trained athletes. Through a mechanism that is not completely understood, caffeine seems to increase endurance and speed in some situations. Excessive use of caffeine is restricted in international competitions.

Karen Eich Drummond

Bibliography

Heaney, R. P. (2002). "Effects of Caffeine on Bone and the Calcium Economy." *Food and Chemical Toxicology* 40:1263–1270.

Juhn, M. S. (2002). "Ergogenic Aids in Aerobic Activity." *Current Sports Medicine Reports* 1:233–238.

Kaiser, Lucia Lynn, and Allen, Lindsay. (2002). "Position of the American Dietetic Association: Nutrition and Lifestyle for a Healthy Pregnancy Outcome." *Journal of the American Dietetic Association* 102:1479–1490.

Nawrot, P.; Jordan, S.; Eastwood, J.; Rotstein, J.; Hugenholtz, A.; and Feeley, M. (2003). "Effects of Caffeine on Human Health." *Food Additives and Contaminants* 20:1–30.

Sizer, Frances, and Whitney, Eleanor. (2003). *Nutrition: Concepts and Controversies.* Belmont, CA: Wadsworth/Thomson Learning.

Smith, A. (2002). "Effects of Caffeine on Human Behavior." *Food and Chemical Toxicology* 40:1243–1255.

Weinberg, Bennett Alan, and Bealer, Bonnie K. (2002). *The World of Caffeine: The Science and Culture of the World's Most Popular Drug.* London: Taylor & Francis.

Internet Resource

Spriet, Lawrence L., and Graham, Terry. "Caffeine and Exercise Performance." American College of Sports Medicine. Available from <http://mplus.nlm.nih.gov/medlineplus>

Calcium

Calcium is one of the most important elements in the **diet** because it is a structural component of bones, teeth, and soft tissues and is essential in many of the body's **metabolic** processes. It accounts for 1 to 2 percent of adult body weight, 99 percent of which is stored in bones and teeth. On the cellular level, calcium is used to regulate the permeability and electrical properties of **biological** membranes (such as cell walls), which in turn control muscle and nerve functions, glandular secretions, and blood vessel dilation and contraction. Calcium is also essential for proper **blood clotting**.

Because of its biological importance, calcium levels are carefully controlled in various compartments of the body. The three major regulators of blood calcium are parathyroid **hormone** (PTH), **vitamin D**, and calcitonin. PTH is normally released by the four parathyroid glands in the neck in response to low calcium levels in the bloodstream (hypocalcemia). PTH acts in three main ways: (1) It causes the **gastrointestinal** tract to increase calcium **absorption** from food, (2) it causes the bones to release some of their

calorie: unit of food energy

calcium: mineral essential for bones and teeth

diet: the total daily food intake, or the types of foods eaten

metabolic: related to processing of nutrients and building of necessary molecules within the cell

biological: related to living organisms

blood clotting: the process by which blood forms a solid mass to prevent uncontrolled bleeding

hormone: molecules produced by one set of cells that influence the function of another set of cells

vitamin D: nutrient needed for calcium uptake and therefore proper bone formation

gastrointestinal: related to the stomach and intestines

absorption: uptake by the digestive tract

rickets: disorder caused by vitamin D deficiency, marked by soft and misshapen bones and organ swelling

osteomalacia: softening of the bones

protein: complex molecule composed of amino acids that performs vital functions in the cell; necessary part of the diet

constipation: difficulty passing feces

kidney stones: deposits of solid material in kidney

intravenous: into the veins

nausea: unpleasant sensation in the gut that precedes vomiting

elemental: made from predigested nutrients

calcium stores, and (3) it causes the kidneys to excrete more phosphorous, which indirectly raises calcium levels.

Vitamin D works together with PTH on the bone and kidney and is necessary for intestinal absorption of calcium. Vitamin D can either be obtained from the diet or produced in the skin when it is exposed to sunlight. Insufficient vitamin D from these sources can result in **rickets** in children and **osteomalacia** in adults, conditions that result in bone deformities. Calcitonin, a hormone released by the thyroid, parathyroid, and thymus glands, lowers blood levels by promoting the deposition of calcium into bone.

Most dietary calcium is absorbed in the small intestine and transported in the bloodstream bound to albumin, a simple **protein**. Because of this method of transport, levels of albumin can also influence blood calcium measurements. Calcium is deposited in bone with phosphorous in a crystalline form of calcium phosphate.

Deficiency and Toxicity

Because bone stores of calcium can be used to maintain adequate blood calcium levels, short-term dietary deficiency of calcium generally does not result in significantly low blood calcium levels. But, over the long term, dietary deficiency eventually depletes bone stores, rendering the bones weak and prone to fracture. A low blood calcium level is more often the result of a disturbance in the body's calcium regulating mechanisms, such as insufficient PTH or vitamin D, rather than dietary deficiency. When calcium levels fall too low, nerve and muscle impairments can result. Skeletal muscles can spasm and the heart can beat abnormally—it can even cease functioning.

Toxicity from calcium is not common because the gastrointestinal tract normally limits the amount of calcium absorbed. Therefore, short-term intake of large amounts of calcium does not generally produce any ill effects aside from **constipation** and an increased risk of **kidney stones**. However, more severe toxicity can occur when excess calcium is ingested over long periods, or when calcium is combined with increased amounts of vitamin D, which increases calcium absorption. Calcium toxicity is also sometimes found after excessive **intravenous** administration of calcium. Toxicity is manifested by abnormal deposition of calcium in tissues and by elevated blood calcium levels (hypercalcemia). However, hypercalcemia is often due to other causes, such as abnormally high amounts of PTH. Usually, under these circumstances, bone density is lost and the resulting hypercalcemia can cause kidney stones and abdominal pain. Some cancers can also cause hypercalcemia, either by secreting abnormal proteins that act like PTH or by invading and killing bone cells causing them to release calcium. Very high levels of calcium can result in appetite loss, **nausea**, vomiting, abdominal pain, confusion, seizures, and even coma.

Requirements and Supplementation

Dietary calcium requirements depend in part upon whether the body is growing or making new bone or milk. Requirements are therefore greatest during childhood, adolescence, pregnancy, and breastfeeding. Recommended daily intake (of **elemental** calcium) varies accordingly: 400 mg for

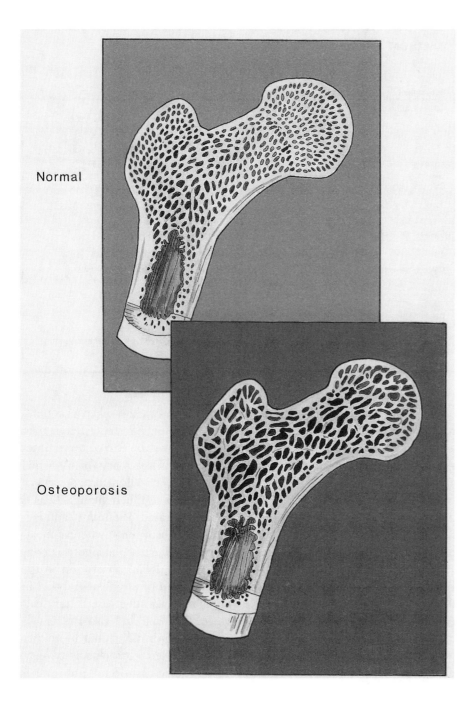

Normal

Osteoporosis

Calcium supplements can help prevent osteoporosis, which is a condition that occurs when bone breaks down more quickly than it is replaced. In this illustration, the bone above is normal, but the bone below is more porous and therefore more susceptible to fracture. [*Custom Medical Stock Photo, Inc. Reproduced by permission.*]

infants 0–6 months, 600 mg for infants 6–12 months, 800 mg for children 1–10 years, 1,200 mg for ages 11–24 years, and 800 mg for individuals over 24 years of age. Pregnant women require additional calcium (RDA 1,200 mg). Many experts believe that elderly persons should take as much as 1,500 mg to help prevent **osteoporosis**, a common condition in which bones become weak and fracture easily due to a loss of bone density. Dairy products, meats, and some seafood (sardines, oysters) are excellent sources of calcium. Spinach, beet greens, beans, and peanuts are among the best plant-derived sources.

Calcium absorption is affected by many factors, including age, the amount needed, and what foods are eaten at the same time. In general,

osteoporosis: weakening of the bone structure

85

CALCIUM SUPPLEMENTS

Supplement	Elemental calcium by weight	Comment
Calcium carbonate	40%	• Most commonly used • Less well absorbed in persons with decreased stomach acid (e.g., elderly or those on anti-acid medicines) • Natural preparations from oyster shell or bone meal may contain contaminants such as lead • Least expensive
Calcium citrate	21%	• Better absorbed, especially by those with decreased stomach acid • May protect against kidney stones • More expensive.
Calcium phosphate	38% or 31%	• Tricalcium or dicalcium phosphate • Used more in Europe • Absorption similar to calcium carbonate
Calcium gluconate	9%	• Used intravenously for severe hypocalcemia • Well absorbed orally, but low content of elemental calcium • Very expensive
Calcium glubionate	6.5%	• Available as syrup for children • Low content elemental calcium.
Calcium lactate	13%	• Well absorbed, but low content elemental calcium.

SOURCE: Gregory, Philip J. (2000) "Calcium Salts." *Prescriber's Letter.* Document #160313.

growth spurts: periods of rapid growth

fat: type of food molecule rich in carbon and hydrogen, with high energy content

intestines: the two long tubes that carry out the bulk of the processes of digestion

fiber: indigestible plant material which aids digestion by providing bulk

pH: level of acidity, with low numbers indicating high acidity

acidity: measure of the tendency of a molecule to lose hydrogen ions, thus behaving as an acid

hypertension: high blood pressure

cancer: uncontrolled cell growth

cardiovascular: related to the heart and circulatory system

obesity: the condition of being overweight, according to established norms based on sex, age, and height

stroke: loss of blood supply to part of the brain, due to a blocked or burst artery in the brain

calcium from food sources is better absorbed than calcium taken as supplements. Children absorb a higher percentage of their ingested calcium than adults because their needs during **growth spurts** may be two or three times greater per body weight than adults. Vitamin D is necessary for intestinal absorption, making Vitamin D–fortified milk a very well-absorbed form of calcium. Older persons may not consume or make as much vitamin D as is optimal, so their calcium absorption may be decreased. Vitamin C and lactose (the sugar found in milk) enhance calcium absorption, whereas meals high in **fat** or protein may decrease absorption. Excess phosphorous consumption (as in carbonated sodas) can decrease calcium absorption in the **intestines**. High dietary **fiber** and phytate (a form of phytic acid found in dietary fiber and the husks of whole grains) may also decrease dietary calcium absorption in some areas of the world. Intestinal **pH** also affects calcium absorption—absorption is optimal with normal stomach **acidity** generated at meal times. Thus, persons with reduced stomach acidity (e.g., elderly persons, or persons on acid-reducing medicines) do not absorb calcium as well as others do.

Calcium supplements are widely used in the treatment and prevention of osteoporosis. Supplements are also recommended, or are being investigated, for a number of conditions, including **hypertension**, colon **cancer**, **cardiovascular** disease, premenstrual syndrome, **obesity**, **stroke**, and pre-eclampsia (a complication of pregnancy). There are several forms of calcium salts used as supplements. They vary in their content of elemental calcium, the amount effectively absorbed by the body, and cost. Whatever the specific form, the supplement should be taken with meals to maximize absorption.

Calcium is one of the most important macronutrients for the body's growth and function. Sufficient amounts are important in preventing many diseases. Calcium levels are tightly controlled by a complex interaction of hormones and **vitamins**. Dietary requirements vary throughout life and are greatest during periods of growth and pregnancy. However, recent reports suggest that many people do not get sufficient amounts of calcium in their diet. Various calcium supplements are available when dietary intake is inadequate. SEE ALSO MINERALS; OSTEOMALACIA; OSTEOPOROSIS; RICKETS.

Donna Staton
Marcus Harding

vitamin: necessary complex nutrient used to aid enzymes or other metabolic processes in the cell

Bibliography

Berkow, Robert, ed. (1997). *The Merck Manual of Medical Information, Home Edition.* Whitehouse Station, NJ: Merck & Co.

National Research Council (1989). *Recommended Dietary Allowances*, 10th edition. Washington, DC: National Academy Press.

Olendorf, Donna; Jeryan, Christine; and Boyden, Karen, eds. (1999). *The Gale Encyclopedia of Medicine.* Farmington Hills, MI: Gale Research.

Internet Resources

Food and Nutrition Board (1999). *Dietary Reference Intakes for Calcium, Phosphorous, Magnesium, Vitamin D, and Fluoride.* Washington, DC: National Academy Press. Available from <http://www.nap.edu>

Gregory, Philip J. (2000) "Calcium Salts." *Prescriber's Letter* Document #160313. Available from <http://www.prescribersletter.com>

Calorie

Technically, a **calorie** is the amount of heat needed to raise the temperature of 1 kilogram (kg) of water 1 degree Celsius. One calorie is 1/1000 of a kilocalorie (a kcalorie or Calorie). The kcalorie is the unit by which food, and the amount of **energy** a person takes in is measured. To maintain one's weight, energy intake should equal energy expenditure. If energy intake is negative (if a person consumes fewer kilocalories than he or she needs or expends) then weight loss will occur. If energy intake is positive (if a person consumes more kilocalories than he or she needs and expends), weight gain will occur.

Judith C. Rodriguez

calorie: unit of food energy

energy: technically, the ability to perform work; the content of a substance that allows it to be useful as a fuel

Cancer

Cancer is a disease characterized by the uncontrolled growth and spread of abnormal cells. Around the world, over 10 million cancer cases occur annually. Half of all men and one-third of all women in the United States will develop some form of cancer during their lifetime. It is one of the most feared diseases, primarily because half of those diagnosed with cancer in the United States will die from it. Cancer is a leading cause of death around the world, causing over 6 million deaths a year. The exact causes of most types of cancer are still not known, and there is not yet a cure for cancer. However, it is now known that the risk of developing many types of cancer can be reduced by adopting certain lifestyle changes, such as quitting smoking and eating a better **diet**.

cancer: uncontrolled cell growth

diet: the total daily food intake, or the types of foods eaten

Prevalence

Cancer is, in general, more common in industrialized nations, but there has been a growth in cancer rates in developing countries, particularly as these nations adopt the diet and lifestyle habits of industrialized countries. Over one million people in the United States get cancer each year. Anyone can get cancer at any age; however, about 80 percent of all cancers occur in people over the age of fifty-five.

Cancer can affect any site in the body. About one hundred human cancers are recognized. The four most common cancers in the United States are: lung, colon/rectum, breast, and **prostate**. Together, these cancers account for over 50 percent of total cancer cases in the United States each year.

There is a marked variation among countries in **incidence** of different cancers. Most of the variation in cancer risk among populations, and among individuals, is due to environmental factors, such as cigarette smoking and certain dietary patterns, that can affect one's risk of developing cancer. For example, individuals living in Australia have the highest worldwide lifetime risk of skin cancer, at over 20 percent, due to the high level of exposure to the sun of people in Australia. People in India have twenty-five times the average risk of developing oral cancer sometime during their lives due to the popularity of chewing tobacco in that country. In fact, India has the world's highest incidence of oral cancer, with 75,000 to 80,000 new cases a year. The population of Japan has the highest rates of stomach cancer in the world due to the high consumption of raw fish by the Japanese.

Types of Cancer

Cancers are classified according to the types of cells in which they develop. Most human cancers are *carcinomas*, which arise from the **epithelial cells** that form the superficial layer of the skin and some internal organs. *Leukemias* affect the blood and blood-forming organs such as **bone marrow**, the **lymphatic system**, and the spleen. *Lymphomas* affect the **immune system**. *Sarcoma* is a general term for any cancer arising from muscle cells or connective tissues.

Growth and Spread of Cancer

Cancer develops when cells in a particular part of the body begin to grow out of control. Normal body cells grow, divide, and die in an orderly way. Cancer cells, however, continue to grow and divide without dying. Instead, they outlive normal cells and continue to form new abnormal cancer cells. As most cancer cells continue to grow, they lump together and form an extra mass of tissue. This mass is called a **malignant** tumor.

As a malignant tumor grows, it damages nearby tissue. Some cancers, like leukemia, do not form tumors. Instead, these cancer cells involve the blood and blood-forming organs and circulate through other tissues, where they grow.

Cancer can begin in one part of the body and spread to others. The spread of a tumor to a new site is called *metastasis*. This process occurs as cancer cells break away from a tumor and travel through the bloodstream or the **lymph system** to other areas of the body. Once in a new location, cancer cells continue to grow out of control and form a new malignant tumor.

prostate: male gland surrounding the urethra that contributes fluid to the semen

incidence: number of new cases reported each year

epithelial cell: sheet of cells lining organs throughout the body

bone marrow: dividing cells within the long bones that make the blood

lymphatic system: group of ducts and nodes through which fluid and white blood cells circulate to fight infection

immune system: the set of organs and cells, including white blood cells, that protect the body from infection

malignant: spreading to surrounding tissues; cancerous

lymph system: system of vessels and glands in the body that circulates and cleans extracellular fluid

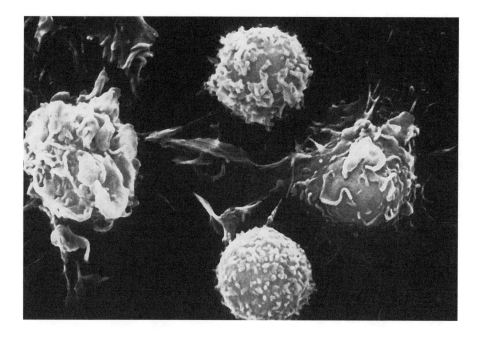

An image showing the division of cancer cells (left and right) and two healthy white blood cells (above and below). In normal cells, cell division is balanced by cell death, but cancerous cells continue to divide and accumulate, damaging nearby tissues. *[Nibsc/Photo Researchers, Inc. Reproduced by permission.]*

Causes of Cancer

The exact cause of cancer is not known. Most cancers result from permanent damage to **genes** or from mutations, which occur either due to internal factors, such as **hormones**, immune conditions, **metabolism**, and the digestion of **nutrients** within cells, or by exposure to environmental or external factors. A chemical or other environmental agent that produces cancer is called a *carcinogen.*

Overall, environmental factors, defined broadly to include tobacco use, diet, **infectious diseases**, chemicals, and radiation, are believed to cause between 75 and 80 percent of all cancer cases in the United States. Tobacco use, including cigarettes, cigars, chewing tobacco, and snuff, can cause cancers of the lung, mouth, throat, larynx, bladder, kidney, esophagus, and pancreas. Smoking alone causes one-third of all cancer deaths in the United States. Heavy consumption of alcohol has also been shown to increase the risk of developing cancer of the mouth, pharynx, larynx, esophagus, liver, and breast.

Overweight and **obesity** are associated with increased risk of cancers of the breast, colon, endometrium, esophagus, kidney, and gallbladder. The following chemicals have been found to cause cancer: coal tars and their derivatives, such as benzene; some hydrocarbons; aniline, a substance used to make dyes; and asbestos. Radiation from a variety of sources, including the ultraviolet light from the sun, is known to lead to skin cancer.

Several infectious agents have also been implicated in cancer. Evidence suggests that **chronic** viral infections are associated with up to one-fifth of all cancers. These include hepatitis B virus (HBV), which can lead to cancer of the liver; the Epstein-Barr virus, a type of herpes virus that causes infectious mononucleosis and has been associated with Hodgkin's disease, non-Hodgkin's lymphomas, and nasopharyngeal cancer; the human immunodeficiency virus (HIV), which is associated with an increased risk of developing several cancers, especially Kaposi's sarcoma and non-Hodgkin's

gene: DNA sequence that codes for proteins, and thus controls inheritance

hormone: molecules produced by one set of cells that influence the function of another set of cells

metabolism: the sum total of reactions in a cell or an organism

nutrient: dietary substance necessary for health

infectious diseases: diseases caused by viruses, bacteria, fungi, or protozoa, which replicate inside the body

overweight: weight above the accepted norm based on height, sex, and age

obesity: the condition of being overweight, according to established norms based on sex, age, and height

chronic: over a long period

Tobacco use is a major cause of lung, lip, mouth, larynx, and throat cancer, and is a contributing cause of many other cancers. In India, where this photo was taken, the prevalence of tobacco use among students approaches 60 percent in some states. [© AFP/Corbis. Reproduced by permission.]

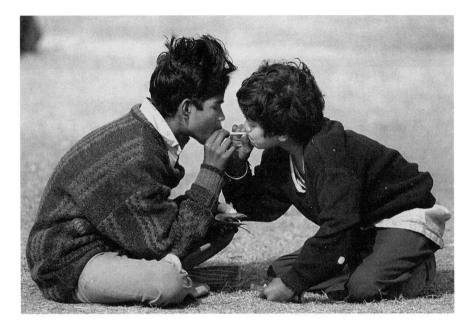

virus: noncellular infectious agent that requires a host cell to reproduce

DNA: deoxyribonucleic acid; the molecule that makes up genes, and is therefore responsible for heredity

lymph node: pocket within the lymph system in which white blood cells reside

genetic: inherited or related to the genes

When cells in some area of the body divide without control, these cells accumulate and form lumps. A *tumor,* or *neoplasm,* is an abnormal lump or mass of tissue that may compress, invade, and destroy normal tissue. Tumors may be benign or malignant. Cancer is a malignant neoplasm, though not all tumors are malignant. A noncancerous growth is called a benign tumor. Benign tumors do not metastasize and, with very rare exceptions, are not life threatening.

lymphoma; and human papilloma **viruses** (HPV), which have been proven to cause cervical cancer and have also been associated with cancers of the vagina, vulva, penis, and colon. The bacterium *Helicobacter pylori* has been linked to stomach cancer.

About 5 to 10 percent of cancers are hereditary, in that a faulty gene or damaged **DNA** that has been inherited predisposes a person to be at a very high risk of developing a particular cancer. Two genes, BRCA1 and BRCA2, have been found to cause some breast cancers. Other genes have been discovered that are associated with some cancers that run in families, such as cancers of the colon, rectum, kidney, ovary, esophagus, **lymph nodes**, skin melanoma, and pancreas.

Carcinogenesis Process

All cancers involve the malfunction of genes that control cell growth and division. The process by which cancers develop is called *carcinogenesis.* This process usually starts when chemicals or radiation damage DNA, the **genetic** structure inside cells. Viruses induce carcinogenesis by introducing new DNA sequences. Most of the time, when DNA becomes damaged the body is able to repair it. In cancer cells, however, the damaged DNA is not repaired. While normal cells with damaged DNA die, cancer cells with damaged DNA continue to multiply.

There is a long time lag between exposure to a carcinogen and the occurrence of cancer. While cellular mutations cause cancer to develop, it is not exactly clear how this happens. Carcinogenesis is a multistep process, in which as many as ten distinct mutations may have to accumulate in a cell before it becomes cancerous. The fact that so many mutations are needed for a cancer to develop indicates that cell growth is normally controlled through many sets of checks and balances.

The cell cycle is regulated by a large number of cellular genes that are expressed, or exhibited, at different stages of the cycle. The genes code for, or determine, **growth factors**, growth-factor receptors, and **proteins** that control gene functions and cell survival. Damaged DNA can lead to cancer because the cell cycle is distorted by the alteration and activation of *oncogenes*, genes that stimulate cell growth, or by the inactivation of *tumor suppressor genes*, which ordinarily suppress cell growth. Activated oncogenes drive abnormal, unregulated cell proliferation and lead to tumor formation. Mutations of the tumor suppressor gene p53 are found in about 50 percent of human cancers.

In experimental animals, three stages of chemical carcinogenesis have been identified. These are: (1) initiation, where DNA is irreversibly altered; (2) promotion, which is the multiplication of altered cells; and (3) progression, which involves chromosomal changes, high growth rate, invasiveness, and potential to metastasize.

Prevention

All cancers caused by cigarette smoking and heavy use of alcohol could be prevented completely. Approximately 30 percent of all cancers worldwide are due to tobacco use. Many of the skin cancers could be prevented by protection from sunlight. Certain cancers that are related to infectious exposures, such as HBV, HPV, HIV, and *Helicobacter* could be prevented through **behavioral** changes, **vaccines**, or **antibiotics**. Research shows that about 30 to 40 percent of all cancers worldwide are due to dietary factors and lack of physical activity, including obesity, and could therefore have been prevented. By making changes in regard to diet, exercise, healthy weight maintenance, and tobacco use, the incidence of cancer around the world could be reduced by 60 to 70 percent.

The Relationship between Diet, Physical Activity, and Cancer

While the exact mechanisms by which diet is related to cancer have not been completely understood, research has shown that food plays a role in cancer prevention. For example, populations whose diet includes at least five servings of fruits and vegetables a day have lower rates of some of the most common cancers. Fruits and vegetables contain many **antioxidants** and **phytochemicals**, such as vitamins A, C, and E, and beta-carotene, which have been shown to prevent cancer. It is not completely clear, however, whether it is individual phytochemicals, or a combination of them, or the **fiber** in fruits and vegetables that result in reduced risk of cancer.

Studies have shown the risk of prostate cancer drops for men who eat tomato products, possibly because of the phytochemical lycopene. In addition, it has been shown that colon cancer declines among those who drink green tea, which contains antioxidants and phytochemicals, and who regularly eat soy products and foods rich in selenium, an antioxidant.

Those who eat a diet low in **fat**, especially animal fat, also have lower cancer rates, but again it is not clear whether it is the **calories**, the amount and distribution of body fat, or the likelihood that a low-fat diet is high in fiber, fruits, and vegetables that is protective against cancer. High-fiber diets are thought to reduce the risk of colon cancer because the fiber helps move food through the lower digestive tract, possibly reducing the contact of any **carcinogens** with the **bowel** lining.

growth factor: protein that stimulates growth of surrounding cells

protein: complex molecule composed of amino acids that performs vital functions in the cell; necessary part of the diet

behavioral: related to behavior, in contrast to medical or other types of interventions

vaccine: medicine that promotes immune system resistance by stimulating pre-existing cells to become active

antibiotic: substance that kills or prevents the growth of microorganisms

antioxidant: substance that prevents oxidation, a damaging reaction with oxygen

phytochemical: chemical produced by plants

fiber: indigestible plant material that aids digestion by providing bulk

fat: type of food molecule rich in carbon and hydrogen, with high energy content

calorie: unit of food energy

carcinogen: cancer-causing substance

bowel: intestines and rectum

Scientific evidence indicates that physical activity may reduce the risk of certain cancers. This effect may be due to the fact that physical activity is associated with the maintenance of a healthy body weight. Other mechanisms by which physical activity may help to prevent certain cancers may involve both direct and indirect effects. For colon cancer, physical activity accelerates the movement of food through the intestine, thereby reducing the length of time that the bowel lining is exposed to potential carcinogens. For breast cancer, vigorous physical activity may decrease the exposure of breast tissue to circulating **estrogen**, a hormone that has been implicated in breast cancer. Physical activity may also affect cancers of the colon, breast, and other sites by improving **energy** metabolism and reducing circulating concentrations of **insulin** and related growth factors.

Because of these factors, recommendations of the American Cancer Society to reduce the risk of cancer include: consumption of a mostly plant-based diet, including five or more servings of fruits and vegetables each day; consumption of whole grains in preference to processed or refined grains and sugar; limited consumption of high-fat foods, particularly from animal sources; physical activity; and limited consumption of alcohol.

Nutrition for People with Cancer

People with cancer often have increased nutritional needs. As such, it is important for them to consume a variety of foods that provide the nutrients needed to maintain health while fighting cancer. These nutrients include: protein, **carbohydrates**, fat, water, vitamins, and **minerals**. Nutrition suggestions for people with cancer often emphasize eating high-calorie, high-protein foods. Protein helps to ensure growth, repair body tissue, and maintain a healthy immune system. Therefore, people with cancer often need more protein than usual.

Great progress has been made in the fight against cancer, and cancer detection and treatments have improved significantly. However, there is a disparity in cancer death rates between developed and developing countries. Between 80 and 90 percent of cancer patients in developing countries have late-stage and often incurable cancer at the time of diagnosis.

A growing body of evidence shows that simple changes in diet and lifestyle can help prevent many cancers. Further research into the exact mechanisms by which certain diets may help prevent cancer is ongoing. SEE ALSO ANTIOXIDANTS; FUNCTIONAL FOODS; PHYTOCHEMICALS.

Gita C. Gidwani

estrogen: hormone that helps control female development and menstruation

energy: technically, the ability to perform work; the content of a substance that allows it to be useful as a fuel

insulin: hormone released by the pancreas to regulate level of sugar in the blood

carbohydrate: food molecule made of carbon, hydrogen, and oxygen, including sugars and starches

mineral: an inorganic (non-carbon-containing) element, ion, or compound

Bibliography

American Institute for Cancer Research (1997). *Food, Nutrition, and the Prevention of Cancer: A Global Perspective.* Washington, DC: Author.

Cooper, Geoffrey M. (1992). *Elements of Human Cancer.* Boston: Jones and Bartlett.

Tortora, Gerald J., and Grabowski, Sandra Reynolds (2003). *Principles of Anatomy and Physiology*, 10th edition. New York: Wiley.

Internet Resources

American Cancer Society. "Cancer Facts and Figures, 2002." Available from <http://www.cancer.org/downloads>

National Cancer Institute (2000). "Cancer Facts: Questions and Answers About Cancer." Available from <http://www.nci.nih.gov>

Carbohydrates

Carbohydrates are one of three macronutrients that provide the body with **energy** (**protein** and fats being the other two). The chemical compounds in carbohydrates are found in both simple and complex forms, and in order for the body to use carbohydrates for energy, food must undergo digestion, **absorption**, and **glycolysis**. It is recommended that 55 to 60 percent of caloric intake come from carbohydrates.

Chemical Structure

Carbohydrates are a main source of energy for the body and are made of carbon, hydrogen, and **oxygen**. Chlorophyll in plants absorbs light energy from the sun. This energy is used in the process of photosynthesis, which allows green plants to take in carbon dioxide and release oxygen and allows for the production of carbohydrates. This process converts the sun's light energy into a form of chemical energy useful to humans. Plants transform carbon dioxide (CO_2) from the air, water (H_2O) from the ground, and energy from the sun into oxygen (O_2) and carbohydrates ($C_6H_{12}O_6$) (6 CO_2 + 6 H_2O + energy = $C_6H_{12}O_6$ + 6 O_2). Most carbohydrates have a ratio of 1:2:1 of carbon, hydrogen, and oxygen, respectively.

Humans and other animals obtain carbohydrates by eating foods that contain them. In order to use the energy contained in the carbohydrates, humans must **metabolize**, or break down, the structure of the molecule in a process that is opposite that of photosynthesis. It starts with the carbohydrate and oxygen and produces carbon dioxide, water, and energy. The body utilizes the energy and water and rids itself of the carbon dioxide.

Simple Carbohydrates

Simple carbohydrates, or simple sugars, are composed of *monosaccharide* or *disaccharide* units. Common monosaccharides (carbohydrates composed of single sugar units) include **glucose**, fructose, and galactose. Glucose is the most common type of sugar and the primary form of sugar that is stored in the body for energy. It sometimes is referred to as blood sugar or dextrose and is of particular importance to individuals who have **diabetes** or **hypoglycemia**. Fructose, the primary sugar found in fruits, also is found in honey and high-fructose corn syrup (in soft drinks) and is a major source of sugar in the **diet** of Americans. Galactose is less likely than glucose or fructose to be found in nature. Instead, it often combines with glucose to form the disaccharide lactose, often referred to as milk sugar. Both fructose and galactose are metabolized to glucose for use by the body.

Oligosaccharides are carbohydrates made of two to ten monosaccharides. Those composed of two sugars are specifically referred to as disaccharides, or double sugars. They contain two monosaccharides bound by either an alpha bond or a beta bond. Alpha bonds are digestible by the human body, whereas beta bonds are more difficult for the body to break down.

There are three particularly important disaccharides: **sucrose**, maltose, and lactose. Sucrose is formed when glucose and fructose are held together by an alpha bond. It is found in sugar cane or sugar beets and is refined to make granulated table sugar. Varying the degree of purification alters the

carbohydrate: food molecule made of carbon, hydrogen, and oxygen, including sugars and starches

energy: technically, the ability to perform work; the content of a substance that allows it to be useful as a fuel

protein: complex molecule composed of amino acids that performs vital functions in the cell; necessary part of the diet

absorption: uptake by the digestive tract

glycolysis: cellular reaction that begins the breakdown of sugars

oxygen: O_2, atmospheric gas required by all animals

metabolize: processing of a nutrient

glucose: a simple sugar; the most commonly used fuel in cells

diabetes: inability to regulate level of sugar in the blood

hypoglycemia: low blood sugar level

diet: the total daily food intake, or the types of foods eaten

sucrose: table sugar

SUGAR COMPARISON

Sugar	Carbohydrate	Monosaccharide or disaccharide	Additional information
Beet sugar (cane sugar)	Sucrose	Disaccharide (fructose and glucose)	Similar to white and powdered sugar, but varied degree of purification
Brown sugar	Sucrose	Disaccharide (fructose and glucose)	Similar to white and powdered sugar, but varied degree of purification
Corn syrup	Glucose	Monosaccharide	
Fruit sugar	Fructose	Monosaccharide	Very sweet
High-fructose corn syrup	Fructose	Monosaccharide	Very sweet and inexpensive. Added to soft drinks and canned or frozen fruits
Honey	Fructose and glucose	Monosaccharides	
Malt sugar	Maltose	Disaccharide (glucose and glucose)	Formed by the hydrolysis of starch, but sweeter than starch
Maple syrup	Sucrose	Disaccharide (fructose and glucose)	
Milk sugar	Lactose	Disaccharide (glucose and galactose)	Made in mammary glands of most lactating animals
Powdered sugar	Sucrose	Disaccharide (fructose and glucose)	Similar to white and brown sugar, but varied degree of purification
White sugar	Sucrose	Disaccharide (fructose and glucose)	Similar to brown and powdered sugar, but varied degree of purification

SOURCE: Mahan and Escott-Stump, 2000; Northwestern University; Sizer and Whitney, 1997; and Wardlaw and Kessel, 2002.

enzyme: protein responsible for carrying out reactions in a cell

nutrition: the maintenance of health through proper eating, or the study of same

glycogen: storage form of sugar

fiber: indigestible plant material that aids digestion by providing bulk

final product, but white, brown, and powdered sugars all are forms of sucrose. Maltose, or malt sugar, is composed of two glucose units linked by an alpha bond. It is produced from the chemical decomposition of starch, which occurs during the germination of seeds and the production of alcohol. Lactose is a combination of glucose and galactose. Because it contains a beta bond, it is hard for some individuals to digest in large quantities. Effective digestion requires sufficient amounts of the **enzyme** lactase.

Complex Carbohydrates

Complex carbohydrates, or *polysaccharides*, are composed of simple sugar units in long chains called polymers. Three polysaccharides are of particular importance in human **nutrition**: starch, **glycogen**, and dietary **fiber**.

Starch and glycogen are digestible forms of complex carbohydrates made of strands of glucose units linked by alpha bonds. Starch, often contained in seeds, is the form in which plants store energy, and there are two types: amylose and amylopectin. Starch represents the main type of digestible complex carbohydrate. Humans use an enzyme to break down the bonds linking glucose units, thereby releasing the sugar to be absorbed into the bloodstream. At that point, the body can distribute glucose to areas that need energy, or it can store the glucose in the form of glycogen.

Glycogen is the polysaccharide used to store energy in animals, including humans. Like starch, glycogen is made up of chains of glucose linked by alpha bonds; but glycogen chains are more highly branched than starch. It is this highly branched structure that allows the bonds to be more quickly broken down by enzymes in the body. The primary storage sites for glycogen in the human body are the liver and the muscles.

Another type of complex carbohydrate is dietary fiber. In general, dietary fiber is considered to be polysaccharides that have not been digested at the point of entry into the large intestine. Fiber contains sugars linked by bonds that cannot be broken down by human enzymes, and are there-

Pastas and whole-grain breads contain complex carbohydrates, which are long strands of glucose molecules. Nutritionists recommend that 55–60 percent of calories come from carbohydrates, and especially complex carbohydrates. *[Photograph by James Noble. Corbis. Reproduced by permission.]*

fore labeled as indigestible. Because of this, most fibers do not provide energy for the body. Fiber is derived from plant sources and contains polysaccharides such as **cellulose**, hemicellulose, pectin, gums, mucilages, and lignins.

The indigestible fibers cellulose, hemicellulose, and lignin make up the structural part of plants and are classified as **insoluble** fiber because they usually do not dissolve in water. Cellulose is a nonstarch carbohydrate polymer made of a straight chain of glucose **molecules** linked by beta bonds and can be found in whole-wheat flour, bran, and vegetables. Hemicellulose is a nonstarch carbohydrate polymer made of glucose, galactose, xylose, and other monosaccharides; it can be found in bran and whole grains. Lignin, a noncarbohydrate polymer containing alcohols and acids, is a woody fiber found in wheat bran and the seeds of fruits and vegetables.

In contrast, pectins, mucilages, and gums are classified as soluble fibers because they dissolve or swell in water. They are not broken down by human enzymes, but instead can be metabolized (or fermented) by **bacteria**

cellulose: carbohydrate made by plants; indigestible by humans

insoluble: not able to be dissolved in water

molecule: combination of atoms that form stable particles

bacteria: single-celled organisms without nuclei, some of which are infectious

95

legumes: beans, peas, and related plants

present in the large intestine. Pectin is a fiber made of galacturonic acid and other monosaccharides. Because it absorbs water and forms a gel, it is often used in jams and jellies. Sources of pectin include citrus fruits, apples, strawberries, and carrots. Mucilages and gums are similar in structure. Mucilages are dietary fibers that contain galactose, manose, and other monosaccharides; and gums are dietary fibers that contain galactose, glucuronic acid, and other monosaccharides. Sources of gums include oats, **legumes**, guar, and barley.

Digestion and Absorption

Carbohydrates must be digested and absorbed in order to transform them into energy that can be used by the body. Food preparation often aids in the digestion process. When starches are heated, they swell and become easier for the body to break down. In the mouth, the enzyme amylase, which is contained in saliva, mixes with food products and breaks some starches into smaller units. However, once the carbohydrates reach the acidic environment of the stomach, the amylase is inactivated. After the carbohydrates have passed through the stomach and into the small intestine, key digestive enzymes are secreted from the pancreas and the small intestine where most digestion and absorption occurs. Pancreatic amylase breaks starch into disaccharides and small polysaccharides, and enzymes from the cells of the small-intestinal wall break any remaining disaccharides into their monosaccharide components. Dietary fiber is not digested by the small intestine; instead, it passes to the colon unchanged.

Sugars such as galactose, glucose, and fructose that are found naturally in foods or are produced by the breakdown of polysaccharides enter into absorptive intestinal cells. After absorption, they are transported to the liver where galactose and fructose are converted to glucose and released into the bloodstream. The glucose may be sent directly to organs that need energy, it may be transformed into glycogen (in a process called glycogenesis) for storage in the liver or muscles, or it may be converted to and stored as fat.

Glycolysis

The molecular bonds in food products do not yield high amounts of energy when broken down. Therefore, the energy contained in food is released within cells and stored in the form of adenosine triphosphate (ATP), a high-energy compound created by cellular energy-production systems. Carbohydrates are metabolized and used to produce ATP molecules through a process called glycolysis.

enzymatic: related to use of enzymes, proteins that cause chemical reactions to occur

cytoplasm: contents of a cell minus the nucleus

lactic acid: breakdown product of sugar in the muscles in the absence of oxygen

Krebs Cycle: cellular reaction that breaks down numerous nutrients and provides building blocks for other molecules

Glycolysis breaks down glucose or glycogen into pyruvic acid through **enzymatic** reactions within the **cytoplasm** of the cells. The process results in the formation of three molecules of ATP (two, if the starting product was glucose). Without the presence of oxygen, pyruvic acid is changed to **lactic acid**, and the energy-production process ends. However, in the presence of oxygen, larger amounts of ATP can be produced. In that situation, pyruvic acid is transformed into a chemical compound called *acetyle coenzyme A*, a compound that begins a complex series of reactions in the **Krebs Cycle** and the electron transport system. The end result is a net gain of up to thirty-nine molecules of ATP from one molecule of glycogen (thirty-eight molecules of ATP if glucose was used). Thus, through certain systems, glucose can be used very efficiently in the production of energy for the body.

Recommended Intake

At times, carbohydrates have been incorrectly labeled as "fattening." Evidence actually supports the consumption of more, rather than less, starchy foods. Carbohydrates have four **calories** per gram, while dietary fats contribute nine per gram, so diets high in complex carbohydrates are likely to provide fewer calories than diets high in fat. Recommendations are for 55 to 60 percent of total calories to come from carbohydrates (approximately 275 to 300 grams for a 2,000-calorie diet). The majority of carbohydrate calories should come from complex rather than simple carbohydrates. Of total caloric intake, approximately 45 to 50 percent of calories should be from complex carbohydrates, and 10 percent or less from simple carbohydrates.

calorie: unit of food energy

It is important to consume a minimum amount of carbohydrates to prevent **ketosis**, a condition resulting from the breakdown of fat for energy in the absence of carbohydrates. In this situation, products of fat breakdown, called ketone bodies, build up in the blood and alter normal **pH** balance. This can be particularly harmful to a fetus. To avoid ketosis, daily carbohydrate intake should include a minimum of 50 to 100 grams. In terms of dietary fiber, a minimum intake of 20 to 35 grams per day is recommended.

ketosis: build-up of ketone bodies in the blood, due to fat breakdown

pH: level of acidity, with low numbers indicating high acidity

---

Low-Carb Diets

Low-carbohydrate diets, such as the Atkins and South Beach diets, are based on the proposition that it's not fat that makes you fat. Allowing dieters to eat steak, butter, eggs, bacon, and other high-fat foods, these diets instead outlaw starches and refined carbohydrates on the theory that they are metabolized so quickly that they lead to hunger and overeating. This theory, which was first popularized in the nineteenth century, came under scathing criticism from the medical establishment during the early 1970s when Dr. Robert Atkins published the phenomenally popular low-carb diet bearing his name. According to the American Medical Association (AMA), the Atkins diet was a "bizarre regimen" that advocated "an unlimited intake of saturated fats and cholesterol-rich foods" and therefore presented a considerable risk of heart disease. Most doctors recommended instead a diet low in fat and high in carbohydrates, with plenty of grains, fruits, and vegetables and limited red meat or dairy products. This became the received wisdom during the 1980s, at the same time that the U.S.

waistline began to expand precipitously. As dieters found that weight loss was difficult to maintain on a low-fat diet, low-carb diets regained popularity—with as many as 30 million people trying a low-carb diet in 2003. Several small-scale studies began to suggest that a low-carb diet may indeed be effective and may not have the deleterious effects its detractors have claimed; other research found that any benefits of a low-carb diet are short-lived, and that the negative effects will take decades to become evident. The National Institutes of Health has pledged $2.5 million for a five-year study of the Atkins diet with 360 subjects. While the results of this and other large-scale studies are awaited, many researchers stress that the key issue in maintaining a healthy weight is the number of calories consumed, not the type of calories. The National Academy of Sciences recommends that adults obtain 45 to 65 percent of their calories from carbohydrates, 20 to 35 percent from fat, and 10 to 35 percent from protein.

—*Paula Kepos*

Exchange System

The exchange system is composed of lists that describe carbohydrate, fat, and protein content, as well as caloric content, for designated portions of specific foods. This system takes into account the presence of more than one type of nutrient in any given food. Exchange lists are especially useful for individuals who require careful diet planning, such as those who monitor intake of calories or certain nutrients. It is particularly useful for diabetics, for whom carbohydrate intake must be carefully controlled, and was originally developed for planning diabetic diets.

Diabetes, Carbohydrate-Modified Diets, and Carbohydrate Counting

Diabetes is a condition that alters the way the body handles carbohydrates. In terms of diet modifications, diabetics can control blood sugar levels by appropriately managing the carbohydrates, proteins, and fats in their meals. The amount of carbohydrates, not necessarily the source, is the primary issue. Blood glucose levels after a meal can be related to the process of food preparation, the amount of food eaten, fat intake, sugar absorption, and the combination of foods in the meal or snack.

insulin: hormone released by the pancreas to regulate level of sugar in the blood

One method of monitoring carbohydrate levels—carbohydrate counting—assigns a certain number of carbohydrate grams or exchanges to specific foods. Calculations are used to determine **insulin** need, resulting in better control of blood glucose levels with a larger variety of foods. Overall, diabetic diets can include moderate amounts of sugar, as long as they are carefully monitored. SEE ALSO DIABETES MELLITUS; FATS; NUTRIENTS; PROTEIN; WEIGHT LOSS DIETS.

Catherine N. Rasberry

Bibliography

Bounds, Laura E.; Agnor, Dottiedee; Darnell, Gayden S.; and Shea, Kirstin Brekken (2003). *Health and Fitness: A Guide to a Healthy Lifestyle*, 2nd edition. Dubuque, IA: Kendall/Hunt.

Duyff, Roberta Larson (2002). *American Dietetic Association: Complete Food and Nutrition Guide*, 2nd edition. Hoboken, NJ: John Wiley.

Mahan, L. Kathleen, and Escott-Stump, Sylvia (2000). *Krause's Food, Nutrition, and Diet Therapy*, 10th edition. Philadelphia: W. B. Saunders.

Robbins, Gwen; Powers, Debbie; and Burgess, Sharon (2002). *A Wellness Way of Life*, 5th edition. New York: McGraw-Hill.

Sizer, Frances, and Whitney, Eleanor (1997). *Nutrition: Concepts and Controversies*, 7th edition. Belmont, CA: Wadsworth Publishing.

Wardlaw, Gordon M., and Kessel, Margaret (2002). *Perspectives in Nutrition*, 5th edition. New York: McGraw-Hill.

Wilmore, Jack H., and Costill, David L. (1999). *Physiology of Sport and Exercise*, 2nd edition. Champaign, IL: Human Kinetics.

Internet Resources

American Diabetes Association. <http://www.diabetes.org>

American Dietetic Association. <http://www.eatright.org>

Carpi, Anthony. "Carbohydrates." Visionlearning. Available from <http://www.visionlearning.com>

Kennedy, Ron. "Carbohydrates in Nutrition." Doctor's Medical Library. Available from <http://www.medical-library.net/sites>

Northwestern University, Department of Preventive Medicine. "Nutrition Fact Sheets: Carbohydrates." Available from <http://www.feinberg.northwestern.edu/nutrition>

Cardiovascular Disease

The **cardiovascular** system comprises the heart, veins, **arteries**, and capillaries, which carry blood back and forth from the heart to the lungs (pulmonary circulation) and from the heart to the rest of the body (systemic circulation). The heart works on electrical impulses and produces them constantly, unless **stress**, fear, or danger is involved, in which case the impulses will increase dramatically. The body's largest artery is the aorta and the largest vein is the vena cava. Veins are thinner than arteries, which resemble rubber bands in that they expand more easily (depending on the amount of blood passing through them). Smaller blood vessels, or capillaries, channel **oxygen** and blood to tissues. The process is a cycle in which the capillaries deliver oxygen-rich blood to the body and pick up oxygen-poor blood, which is then taken into the veins and finally to the heart to be "rejuvenated" or cleansed.

Cardiovascular disease (CVD), and the resulting complications, is the main cause of death for both males and females in the United States and other technologically advanced countries of the world. It usually is in the top five causes of death in lesser-developed countries. Diseases of the cardiovascular system include those that compromise the pumping ability of the heart, cause failure of the valves, or result in narrowing or hardening of the arteries. In addition, **toxins** and infectious agents may damage the heart and blood vessels. Injury or failure of the cardiovascular system, especially the heart, also will affect the peripheral tissues that depend on the delivery of **nutrients** and the removal of wastes through the blood vascular system. CVD is a family of diseases that includes **hypertension, atherosclerosis, coronary heart disease**, and **stroke**.

Hypertension (High Blood Pressure)

Blood pressure is a measure of the force of blood against the walls of arteries. It is recorded as two numbers: the systolic pressure over the diastolic pressure. Systolic pressure is the pressure as the heart beats, while diastolic pressure measures the pressure when the heart relaxes between beats.

Blood pressure is normally measured at the brachial artery with a sphygmomanometer (pressure cuff) in millimeters of mercury (mm Hg) and given as systolic over diastolic pressure. Normal blood pressure is less than 120 mm Hg systolic and less than 80 mm Hg diastolic—usually expressed as "120 over 80." However, normal for an individual varies with the height, weight, fitness level, age, and health of a person. Blood pressure is normally maintained within narrow limits, but it can drop during sleep or increase during exercise. Hypertension (HTN), or high blood pressure, occurs when the force of blood passing through blood vessels is above normal. The increase in pressure forces the blood to hit the blood vessel walls. HTN is called "the silent killer" because many people do not know they have the condition. Consistently high blood pressure increases the risk for a stroke or a **heart attack**.

cardiovascular: related to the heart and circulatory system

artery: blood vessel that carries blood away from the heart toward the body tissues

stress: heightened state of nervousness or unease

oxygen: O_2, atmospheric gas required by all animals

toxins: poison

nutrient: dietary substance necessary for health

hypertension: high blood pressure

atherosclerosis: build-up of deposits within the blood vessels

coronary heart disease: disease of the coronary arteries, the blood vessels surrounding the heart

stroke: loss of blood supply to part of the brain, due to a blocked or burst artery in the brain

blood pressure: measure of the pressure exerted by the blood against the walls of the blood vessels

heart attack: loss of blood supply to part of the heart, resulting in death of heart muscle

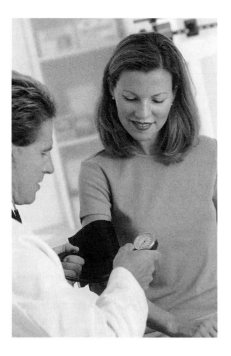

The sphygmomanometer around this woman's arm is inflated until it collapses her brachial artery, and then gradually deflated. Blood rushing into the vessel makes Korotkoff sounds that are used to time the measurements of systolic and diastolic pressure. *[Photograph by Michael Keller. Corbis. Reproduced by permission.]*

diet: the total daily food intake, or the types of foods eaten

obesity: the condition of being overweight, according to established norms based on sex, age, and height

plaque: material forming deposits on the surface of the teeth, which may promote bacterial growth and decay

lipid: fats, waxes and steroids; important components of cell membranes

cholesterol: multi-ringed molecule found in animal cell membranes; a type of lipid

triglyceride: a type of fat

trans-fatty acids: type of fat thought to increase the risk of heart disease

diabetes: inability to regulate level of sugar in the blood

It may be caused by poor **diet**, **obesity**, smoking, stress, and inactivity. The Dietary Approach to Stop Hypertension (DASH) project recommends a diet that is low in sodium and high in fruits, vegetables, and low-fat dairy products. Other approaches to controlling HTN include weight loss, smoking cessation, increased physical activity, and stress management.

Atherosclerosis

Atherosclerosis, or hardening of the arteries, is the cause of more than half of all mortality in developed countries and the leading cause of death in the United States. When the coronary arteries are involved, it results in coronary artery disease (CAD). The hardening of the arteries is due to the build up of fatty deposits called **plaque**, and mineral deposits. As a result, the supply of blood to the heart muscle (myocardium) is reduced and can lead to ischema (deficiency of blood) to the heart, causing chest pain or a myocardial infarction (heart attack). The hardening of the arteries causes an increase in resistance to blood flow, and therefore an increase in blood pressure. Any vessel in the body may be affected by atherosclerosis; however, the aorta and the coronary, carotid, and iliac arteries are most frequently affected. The process begins early in life. Therefore, physicians should obtain risk-factor profiles and a family history for children.

Coronary Artery Disease

Coronary artery disease (CAD) refers to any of the conditions that affect the coronary arteries and reduces blood flow and nutrients to the heart. It is the leading cause of death worldwide for both men and women. Atherosclerosis is the primary cause of CAD. Controlled risk factors associated with CAD include hypertension, cigarette smoking, elevated blood **lipids** (e.g., **cholesterol**, **triglyceride**), a high-fat diet (especially saturated fats and **trans-fatty acids**), physical inactivity, obesity, **diabetes**, and stress. Lifestyle changes can assist in prevention of CAD. Uncontrolled risk factors include a family history of CAD, gender (higher in males), and increasing age.

Stroke

Stroke, or a cerebrovascular accident (CVA), occurs when the brain does not receive sufficient oxygen-rich blood through blood vessels or when a blood vessel bursts. A stroke may result from blockage of the blood vessels due to a blood clot (ischemic) or from ruptures of the blood vessels (hemorrhagic bursts). Uncontrolled hypertension is a major risk factor for strokes.

Preventing CVD

The symptoms of CVD develop over many years and often do not manifest themselves until old age. Autopsies of young servicemen indicate significant accumulation of plaque and hardening of the arteries (atherosclerosis). Thus, primary prevention for CVD must begin in early childhood. Preventing premature CVD (before age 60) is crucial. Heart attacks between the ages of forty and sixty are primarily due to lifestyle factors.

Smoking, high blood cholesterol, high blood pressure, and lack of physical activity are the most serious risk factors for CVD and heart attack. Controlling one of these risk factors can help control others. For example, regular

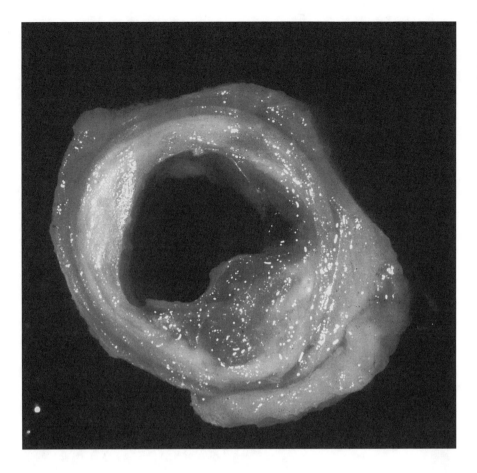

This cross section of a coronary artery shows plaque buildup, possibly indicating coronary artery disease—the most common cause of death worldwide. Risk factors for the disease include poor diet, cigarette smoking, and stress, among others. *[B&B Photos/Custom Medical Stock Photo. Reproduced by permission.]*

exercise can help control cholesterol, blood pressure, weight, and stress levels. Smoking is the most preventable risk factor. Smokers have twice the risk for heart attack that nonsmokers have. Tobacco use alters the blood chemistry and increases **blood clotting**. Nearly one-fifth of all deaths are due to tobacco use, and a smoker lives an average of seven to eight fewer years than a nonsmoker.

The worldwide increase in obesity and type 2 diabetes (in both children and adults) point to a high-fat, high-calorie diet and a **sedentary** lifestyle. Poverty increases the risk for poor dietary habits and poor access to healthful foods. Many of the world's urban poor have more access to highly **processed foods, convenience foods**, and fast foods than to fresh fruits and vegetables. But even in the most wealthy and technologically advanced countries, the affluent are choosing to eat more fast foods and processed foods that are high in fat, cholesterol, and sodium. For optimal health, health professionals recommend:

- Maintaining a healthy weight, with a **body mass index** (BMI) of 18.5–24.9.
- Limiting dietary fat to 30 percent or less of total calories—10 percent **saturated fat**, 10 percent **polyunsaturated** fat, and 10 percent mononunsaturated fats. Consumers should be aware that ounce for ounce, all sources of fat have approximately the same amounts of calories.
- Limiting saturated fats to 10 percent of calories. Saturated fats come primarily from animal sources (e.g., high-fat dairy and meats), but also are found in coconut and palm oil.

blood clotting: the process by which blood forms a solid mass to prevent uncontrolled bleeding

sedentary: not active

processed food: food that has been cooked, milled, or otherwise manipulated to change its quality

convenience food: food that requires very little preparation for eating

body mass index: weight in kilograms divided by square of the height in meters; a measure of body fat

saturated fat: a fat with the maximum possible number of hydrogens; more difficult to break down than unsaturated fats

polyunsaturated: having multiple double bonds within the chemical structure, thus increasing the body's ability to metabolize it

This scan of the cardiovascular system shows the heart and lungs, with major blood vessels radiating from them. Cardiovascular diseases, which affect the pumping of the heart and the circulation of blood, are the leading cause of death in developed nations. *[Photograph by Howard Sochurek. Corbis. Reproduced by permission.]*

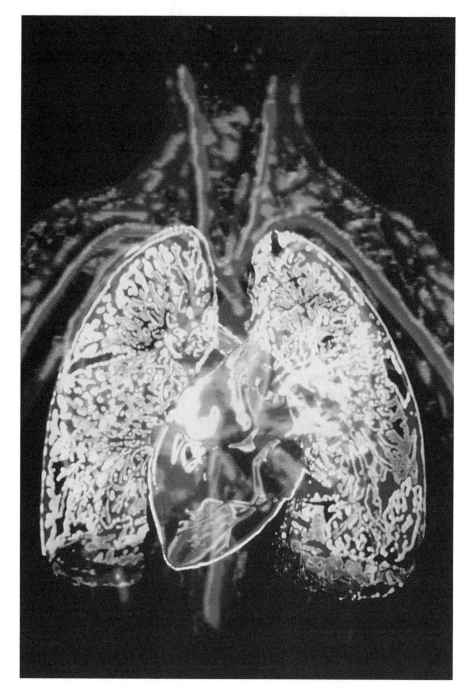

heart disease: any disorder of the heart or its blood supply, including heart attack, atherosclerosis, and coronary artery disease

fatty acids: molecules rich in carbon and hydrogen; a component of fats

- Limiting polyunsaturated fats to 10 percent of calories. Polyunsaturated fats come primarily from vegetable oils (e.g., corn oil, safflower oil).

- Limiting monounsaturated fats to 10 percent of calories. Monounsaturated fats may have a protective role in **heart disease**. Excellent sources of monounsaturated fats include olive oils, nuts, avocado, and canola oil.

- Increasing intake of omega-3 **fatty acids**. Two to four grams daily of omega-3 fatty acids may lower risk for CVD by reducing blood clotting, making platelets less sticky, and lowering triglycerides. Patients should inform their physician if they are using omega-3 supplements, since they may increase the risk of bleeding. Excellent sources of omega-3 include fatty fish (such as salmon and sardines), fish oils, and flax seed.

- Limiting sodium intake to 2,400 milligrams per day.

- Increasing potassium intake to at least 3,500 milligrams per day.

- Eating at least five servings a day of fruits and vegetables.

- Eating a plant-based diet consisting primarily of whole grains, fruits, and vegetables is also recommended.

- Eating at least 25 grams of **fiber** daily.

- Eating 25 grams of soy **protein** daily.

fiber: indigestible plant material that aids digestion by providing bulk

protein: complex molecule composed of amino acids that performs vital functions in the cell; necessary part of the diet

In addition to diet modification, research is increasingly focused on the role of physical activity in preventing CVD. People who are not physically active have twice the risk of heart disease as those who are active. More than half of U.S. adults do not achieve recommended levels of physical activity. Studies indicate a correlation between the amount of television viewing, playing videos, and other sedentary activities and increased rates of childhood obesity. In general, the more sedentary the activities, the more high-fat and sugary foods are consumed. At least thirty minutes of moderate physical activity, five times a week, is recommended. Moderate physical activity slows down the narrowing of the blood vessels, due to contraction of the smooth muscles in the vessel walls. It also increases coronary blood flow, strengthens the heart muscles, and reduces stress.

Worldwide, HTN is linked to about 50 percent of CVDs and approximately 75 million "lost healthy life years" each year. Thus, controlling HTN may greatly reduce the risk of disability and death from CVD. Secondary prevention involves treating the signs and symptoms of CVD. These strategies include management of hypertension, cholesterol, and other blood lipids. Dietary and lifestyle modification are tried first. However, medication may also be prescribed, depending on other clinical factors. Compliance with a medication regimen is extremely important, as is the monitoring of blood pressure and blood lipids. Recommended total **serum** cholesterol should not exceed 200 milligrams per deciliter (mg/dl); low-density **lipoproteins** (LDLs or "bad cholesterol") should not exceed 100 mg/dl, and high-density lipoproteins (HDLs or "good cholesterol") should not be lower than 40 mg/dl.

serum: noncellular portion of the blood

lipoprotein: blood protein that carries fats

Conclusion

Surgical intervention may restore cardiovascular function. Vessels may be opened by **angioplasty** or repaired by the use of grafts or stents, heart valves can be repaired or replaced with artificial valves, and pacemakers or **drugs** may aid heart function. A heart transplant may be an individual's last resort. Many large-scale international studies have focused on preventing cardiovascular disease through smoking cessation, healthful eating, physical activity, hypertension and cholesterol control, health education, and media campaigns. These include the Stanford Three City, the Stanford Five City Projects, the Framingham Heart Study, the Bogalusa Heart Study, the Multiple Risk Factor Intervention Trial (MRFIT), Active Australia, the Whickham Study (based on the Framingham model), and the North Karelia Study (Finland). Small, gradual changes in diet and exercise and smoking cessation are

angioplasty: reopening of clogged blood vessels

drugs: substances whose administration causes a significant change in the body's function

the best way to produce long-term effects. SEE ALSO ARTERIOSCLEROSIS; ATHEROSCLEROSIS; HEART DISEASE.

Teresa Lyles

Bibliography

Bauman, A.; Bellow, B.; Owen, N.; and Vita, P. (2001). "Impact of an Australian Mass Media Campaign Targeting Physical Activity in 1998." *American Journal of Preventive Medicine* 21:41–47.

Bijnen, F. C.; Caspersen, C. J.; Feskens, E. J.; Saris, W. H.; Mosterd, W. L.; and Kromhout, D. (1998). "Physical Activity and 10-Year Mortality from Cardiovascular Diseases and All Causes." *Archives of Internal Medicine* 158(14):1499–1505.

Elward, K., and Larson, E. K. (1992). "Benefits of Exercise for Older Adults: A Review of Existing Evidence and Current Recommendations for the General Population." *Journal of Clinical Gerontology Medicine* 8(1):35–50.

Fortman, S. P., and Varady, A. N. (2000). "Effects of a Community-Wide Health Education Program on Cardiovascular Disease Morbidity and Mortality: The Stanford Five-City Project." *American Journal of Epidemiology* 152:316–323.

Fox, S. I. (1999). *Human Physiology*, 6th edition. Boston: McGraw-Hill.

Insel, P. M., and Roth, W. T. (2004). "Cardiovascular Disease and Cancer." In *Core Concepts in Health*, 9th (brief) edition. Boston: McGraw-Hill.

Internet Resources

American Heart Association/American Stroke Association. "Heart Disease and Stroke Statistics—2003 Update." Available from <http://www.americanheart.org>

American Heart Association. "Common Cardiovascular Diseases." Available from <http://americanheart.org/stroke>

Bogalusa Heart Study (n.d.). Tulane Center for Cardiovascular Health. Available from <http://www.som.tulane.edu/cardiohealth>

HeartCenterOnline. "Coronary Artery." Available from <http://www.heartcenter online.com/myheartdr>

National Heart, Lung, and Blood Institute. "Framingham Heart Study: 50 Years of Research Success." Available from <http://www.nhlbi.nih.gov>

National Institutes of Health, National Cancer Institute. "Action Guide for Healthy Eating." Available from <http://www.5aday.nci.nih.gov/actionguide>

National Public Health Partnership of Australia. "Developing an Active Australia: A Framework for Action for Physical Activity and Health." Available from <http://www.health.gov.au/pubhlth>

World Health Organization. "Cardiovascular Death and Disability Can Be Reduced More than 50 Percent." Available from <http://www.who.int/mediacentre>

Careers in Dietetics

nutrition: the maintenance of health through proper eating, or the study of same

clinical: related to hospitals, clinics, and patient care

The science and profession of **nutrition** and dietetics is based on the application of foods and nutrition to promote health and treat disease. Most dietitians and nutritionists work in **clinical**, community, public health, or food service settings. Others work as consultants or researchers, in the food industry, in university, worksite, medical school, home health, or fitness center settings. Some persons work for world or regional health organizations. At least a bachelor's degree in dietetics, foods, and nutrition is needed to practice as a dietitian or a nutritionist. Dietetic technicians need an associate's degree.

Practice Roles

diet: the total daily food intake, or the types of foods eaten

Clinical dietitians, also known as medical nutrition therapists, usually work in a hospital setting as generalists or specialists and as part of a health care team. This person is responsible for using **diet** to treat disease and as part of the treatment plan. Clinical dietitians assess needs, manage the nutrition care of patients, and conduct individual or group counseling sessions. In almost all settings in the United States, a dietitian must be registered (R.D.) to practice medical nutrition therapy.

As generalists, clinical dietitians may rotate through, or work in a variety of the clinical settings, such as the medical and obstetrics areas. As specialists they have additional training. Some dietitians may also be Certified **Diabetes** Educators (CDE) or Certified in Nutrition Support (CNS).

diabetes: inability to regulate level of sugar in the blood

Community Nutritionist refers to persons that work in community programs that are funded by governmental organizations or private groups. The terms Public Health Nutritionist and Nutrition Educator usually refer to persons that are employed by governmental health agencies. These persons do one-to-one counseling, conduct assessments, design, implement, and evaluate programs. Some are involved in the screening, surveillance or monitoring of community programs.

Dietitians involved in food service work in hospitals, schools, and **long-term care facilities**. They have responsibilities related to the day-to-day preparation and delivery of foods, food acquisition, employee supervision, and fiscal matters. Advanced-level practitioners manage program budgets, design marketing strategies, promote programs, or initiate collaborative ventures, such as a joint program with a local clinic or health club.

long-term care facilities: hospitals or nursing homes in which patients remain for a long time for chronic care, rather than being treated and quickly discharged

As nutrition has gained popularity, so have the opportunities for innovative and entrepreneurial practice. Many nontraditional areas of practice are emerging, especially in the area of consultation. Nutritionists work in mass media, rehabilitation, sports, law, marketing, pharmaceuticals, and **wellness** settings. **Entrepreneurs** participate in a variety of creative activities, such as development of materials, creation or editing of newsletters or websites, or in the use of new technologies to promote nutrition.

wellness: related to health promotion

entrepreneur: founders of new businesses

For example, a consulting nutritionist may work at a long-term care facility on Mondays, see individual clients at a medical clinic on Tuesdays, spend Wednesdays and Thursdays writing articles for the local newspaper, and provide "brown-bag lunch" lectures to employees of a local company on Fridays.

Academic (Didactic) and Supervised Practice Training

In the United States, preparation for the dietetic profession is a formal process. The Commission on Accreditation of Dietetics Education (CADE) has two career paths for persons who wish to be eligible to take the national Registration Examination. In the more common path, students complete a baccalaureate degree and then a supervised practice experience (**internship**). In the second path, students complete a coordinated undergraduate program (CUP), in which they work on the baccalaureate degree requirements and the supervised practice simultaneously. In either path, the student must complete academic (didactic) and supervised practice (internship) training.

internship: training program

Didactic training emphasizes theoretical knowledge and is generally achieved by completing a baccalaureate-level degree from a CADE-accredited program in a college or university. The supervised practice component is an internship. The student rotates through a series of preplanned learning experiences in community, clinical, food-service, and selected specialty practice

Registered dietitians (RDs) use their expertise in food and nutrition to prevent disease and improve health through diet. RDs work at hospitals, at research institutions, for governments, and for private companies. *[© 1994 SIU Biomed Comm. Custom Medical Stock Photo, Inc. Reproduced by permission.]*

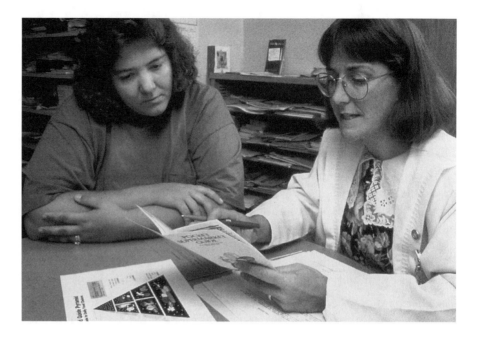

settings. Upon successful completion of these two elements of learning, the individual becomes eligible to take the national Registration Exam. Related professions include culinary careers (e.g., chefs) and the food sciences.

Knowledge and Skills

nutrient: dietary substance necessary for health

Nutritionists and dietitians have a basic knowledge of nutrition, **nutrient** needs throughout the life cycle, medical nutrition therapy, food service, food and consumer science, health education, and food habits and behavior. They have assessment, counseling, program design, marketing, and management skills. Some have advanced training in specialty areas such as pediatric nutrition, nutrition support, or diabetes education.

Registration and Licensure in the United States

health-promotion: related to advocacy for better health, preventive medicine, and other aspects of well-being

The terms *nutritionist* and *dietitian* are sometimes used interchangeably. In most cases a nutritionist, or nutrition educator, works in a community or **health-promotion** setting, while a dietitian works in a clinical setting. In international health and nutrition programs, the term *nutritionist* is generally used, and training, activities, and levels of responsibility can vary greatly. However, some U.S. states have licensure laws that define the requirements and scope of practice for a nutritionist. Persons who wish to practice in these states must meet the eligibility requirements to obtain a license.

Dietitians in the United States are credentialed by the profession's accrediting body, the Commission on Dietetic Registration (CDR) of the American Dietetic Association (ADA), as registered dietitians (RDs). Dietetic technicians, who assist in program service and delivery, are credentialed as dietetic technicians, registered (DTR). In some settings, such as long-term care facilities, DTRs may be responsible for day-to-day operations, with guidance from a consulting dietitian. SEE ALSO AMERICAN DIETETIC ASSOCIATION; DIETETIC TECHNICIAN, REGISTERED (DTR); DIETITIAN; NUTRITIONIST.

Judith C. Rodriguez

Bibliography

Barker, A. M.; Arensberg, M. B. F.; and Schiller, M. R. (1994). *Leadership in Dietetics*. Chicago: American Dietetic Association.

Boyle, Marie A., and Morris, Diane H. (1999). *Community Nutrition in Action*. New York: Wadsworth Publishing.

Chmelynski, Carol Ciprione. (2000). *Opportunities in Food Service Careers*. Chicago: VGM Career Horizons NTC/Contemporary Publishing.

Donovan, Mary D. (1998). *Opportunities in Culinary Careers*. Chicago: VGM Career Horizons NTC/Contemporary Publishing.

Ullrich, Helen D. (1992). *The SNE Story: 25 Years of Advancing Nutrition Education*. Berkeley, CA: Nutrition Communication Associates.

Internet Resources

American Dietetic Association. "Check It Out: Careers in Dietetics." Available from <http://www.eatright.org>

U.S. Department of Labor. "Occupational Outlook Handbook, Dietitians and Nutritionists." Available from <http://www.bls.gov>

Caribbean Islanders, Diet of

Travel advertisements for the Caribbean Islands portray long stretches of sun-drenched beaches and swaying palm trees, with people dancing to jazz, calypso, reggae, or meringue music. Indeed, the beauty, warmth, and lush landscapes had Christopher Columbus in awe in 1492 when he came upon these tropical islands, stretching approximately 2,600 miles between Florida and Venezuela.

European Settlement

The Arawaks and Caribs, the first natives of the islands, were not treated kindly, however, as the Spanish, French, Dutch, and British conquered the islands at different periods, all but wiping out the native populations. Today, only a few aboriginals remain in the Caribbean.

The European settlers soon realized that sugarcane was a profitable crop that could be exported to the European market. However, there was a shortage of European farmers, and slaves were brought from Africa to work on the sugar plantations. The slave trade started in 1698. European settlers fought to keep their territories and hoped for great wealth, while actively pursuing the sugar and slave trades.

Two things changed the situation on the islands. In 1756, missionaries from Germany (Moravian Protestants), came to the islands, though the landowners were opposed to their presence, fearing that any education of the slaves could lead to a revolution. At about the same time a German scientist by the name of Margraf discovered that sugar could be produced from beets, and many European countries began to produce their own sugar.

In 1772, after many revolts and uprisings, the Europeans began to free their slaves. The sugar plantations still needed laborers, however, and indentured workers were brought from China and India to work in the fields. Sugar cane, and its by-products, molasses and rum, brought great prosperity to the settlers. However, not wanting to depend solely on sugar, they began to grow yams, maize, cloves, nutmeg, cinnamon, coconuts, and pineapples on a very

The ancestors of many Caribbean islanders were brought as slaves to work on the sugarcane plantations. In the New World, their traditional African cuisines integrated new flavors both from their new environment and from the cuisines of various European colonial powers. *[Catherine Karnow/ Corbis. Reproduced by permission.]*

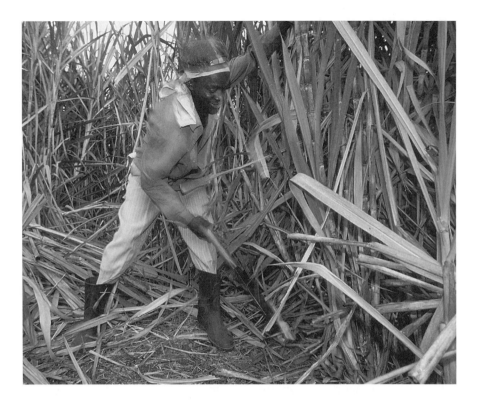

diet: the total daily food intake, or the types of foods eaten

large scale. Coffee also began to flourish. Many of the islands had wild pigs and cattle on them, and spiced, smoked meat became part of the **diet**. Today, jerk meat is a specialty.

Foods of the Islands

The foods of the Caribbean are marked by a wide variety of fruits, vegetables, meats, grains, and spices, all of which contribute to the area's unique cuisine. Foods of Creole, Chinese, African, Indian, Hispanic, and European origin blend harmoniously to produce mouth-watering dishes.

Fruits and Vegetables. There are many fruits and vegetables found in the various Caribbean Islands, and because many of them have been exported to North America and Europe, people have become familiar with them. This exotic array of fruits and vegetables in vibrant colors forms the heart of island cooking.

Chayote, also called Christophene or Cho-cho, is a firm pear-shaped squash used in soups and stews. The Chinese vegetable bokchoy (or pakchoy) has become widely used on the islands. Plantains, which resemble bananas, are roasted, sautéed, fried, and added to stews and soups. The breadfruit grows profusely, and is either boiled or baked, sliced, and eaten hot, or ground into flour. The breadfruit blossoms make a very good preserve.

tuber: swollen plant stem below the ground

Yucca, also known as cassava or manioc, is a slender **tuber** with bark-like skin and a very starchy flesh that must be cooked and served like a potato, or it can be made into cassava bread. Mangoes can be picked from the tree and eaten by peeling the skin and slicing the flesh off the large pit. They are used in salads, desserts, frozen drinks, and salsa. Papaya, which has a cantaloupe-like flavor, contains the **enzyme** papain, which aids in digestion. To be eaten, the black seeds must be removed and the flesh scooped out.

enzyme: protein responsible for carrying out reactions in a cell

The soursop is a large, oval, dark-green fruit with a thick skin that is soft to the touch when it ripens. The fruit has a creamy flesh with a sweet, tart flavor. Its rich custard-like flavor can be made into a sherbet, ice cream, or refreshing drink.

Spices and Condiments. The food of the Caribbean can be highly spiced. The Scotch bonnet, a colorful pepper with a hot aroma, is widely used in soups, salads, sauces, and marinades. Some other important spices are annatto, curry, pimento, cinnamon, and ginger. Annatto seeds are often steeped in oil and used to flavor soups, stews, and fish dishes. Curry powder is made from a variety of freshly grounded spices. Curry dishes and hot sauces, which are used regularly in cooking, were brought to the islands by Indian settlers.

Pimento, also known as allspice, is used in pickles, marinades, soups, and stews and is an important ingredient in jerking, a method of cooking meat and poultry over an open fire. To bring out the flavor of meat and chicken, they are marinated in a mixture of scallions, garlic, thyme, onion, lemon juice, and salt. The spices and the method of slow cooking over a fire give jerk meat its distinctive flavor.

Protein Sources. Although fish, conch (a pink shellfish), goat meat, pork, and beef are used throughout the Caribbean, **legumes** make up a fair percentage of the region's protein intake. Kidney and lima beans, chickpeas, lentils, black-eyed peas, and other legumes are used in soups, stews, and rice dishes. Accra fritters, made from soaked black-eyed peas that are mashed, seasoned with pepper, and then fried, is a dish of West African origin similar to the Middle Eastern falafel. Sancocho is a hearty Caribbean stew made with vegetables, tubers, and meats.

legumes: beans, peas, and related plants

Cooking Methods. A "cook-up" dish is one made with whatever ingredients an individual has on hand, and is an opportunity to be creative. Such a dish will often include rice, vegetables, and possibly meat. By adding coconut milk, this could turn into an enticing coconut-scented pilaf. Burning sugar to color stews is another technique used in island cooking. This process begins by heating oil, then adding sugar, and stirring until the sugar becomes an amber color.

The roti is a griddle-baked flour wrapping that is filled with curried meat, chicken, or potatoes. Coucou, or fungi, is a cornmeal mush that is served with meat, poultry, fish, or vegetable dishes.

Beverages and Desserts. A variety of fruit beverages are often served in the Caribbean. Beverages include green tea and "bush tea," served sweetened with sugar or honey, with or without milk. Bush tea is an infusion of tropical shrubs, grasses, and leaves that has a number of medicinal uses. People drink it as a remedy for gas, the common cold, **asthma, high blood pressure**, fever, and other ailments. Sweetened commercial drinks made from carrot, beet, guava, tamarind, and other fruits and vegetables are also popular.

asthma: respiratory disorder marked by wheezing, shortness of breath, and mucus production

high blood pressure: elevation of the pressure in the bloodstream maintained by the heart

A number of fermented drinks are also popular. *Garapina* is made from pineapple peelings, while *mauby* is made from the bark of the mauby tree. Grated ginger is used to produce ginger beer. *Horlicks* is a malted milk made with barley.

POPULAR DISHES OF SELECTED CARIBBEAN ISLANDS

Island	Special dishes
Antigua, Montserrat, Nevis	Fish soup, pepper pot soup (any available fish, meat, chicken, and vegetables cooked in fermented cassava juice); saltfish with avocado and eggplant
Barbados	Flying fish; jug-jug (mashed stew of pigeon peas, usually served at Christmas)
	Black pudding (a type of sausage made by combining cooked rice mixed with fresh pig's blood, seasoned with salt, pepper, and other condiments, and placed in thoroughly cleaned pieces of pig's intestine, and then tied on both ends and boiled in seasoned water)
Belize	Rice and chicken, tamales, conch fritters, refried beans and iswa (fresh corn tortillas)
Dominica	Tannia (coco, a starch tuber soup); mountain chicken (frog's legs)
Grenada	Callaloo (soup with green vegetables)
	Lambi souse (conch marinated in lime juice, hot pepper, onion); oil-down (a highly seasoned dish of coconut milk and salted fish)
Guyana	Mellagee (one-pot stew of pickled meat/fish and coconut milk with tubers and vegetables); rice treat (rice with shrimp, vegetables, and pineapple)
Jamaica	Saltfish and ackee (a fruit commonly used as a vegetable, boiled and then sautéed in oil); escoveitched fish (fried fish marinated in vinegar spices, seasoning); roasted breadfruit; asham or brown George (parched dried corn that is finely beaten in a mortar, sifted, and mixed with sugar)
St. Vincent and the Grenadines	Stewed shark
British Virgin Islands	Fish chowder, conch salad, saltfish and rice
Trinidad and Tobago	Pelau (rice with meat, fish, peas, vegetables); pakoras; kachouri; palouri (fried vegetable fritters)
Guadeloupe and Martinique	Mechoui (spit-roasted sheep); pate en pot (finely chopped sheep and lamb parts cooked into a thick, highly seasoned stew)

Fruit is eaten anytime of the day, but is not considered a dessert unless prepared in a fruit salad or some other form. Coconut and banana form the basis for many desserts. A sweet pudding that goes by many names (e.g., duckunoo, blue drawers, pain me, paimee, and konkee) is made from grated banana, plantain, or sweet potato, which is then sugared, spiced, and mixed with coconut milk or grated coconut, and then wrapped in banana leaves and boiled in spiced water. A prepared sweet pone (pudding) cake or pie is a popular dessert. Black fruitcake, made from dried fruits soaked in wine, is popular at Christmas time, and is also used for weddings and other celebrations.

Health Issues

chronic: over a long period

malnutrition: chronic lack of sufficient nutrients to maintain health

calorie: unit of food energy

In the Caribbean region, nutrition-related **chronic** diseases are common, threatening the well-being of the people of the islands. In the 1950s, the governments of the Caribbean were concerned about the **malnutrition** that permeated the region. They were able to increase the protein and **calorie** needs by making meat, fats, oils, and refined sugar more available. The health and nutrition initiatives introduced helped curbed the malnutrition, but new and related health and nutrition problems began to emerge.

The health administrators of the Caribbean region are concerned with the rise of iron-deficiency **anemia** in pregnant women and school-aged children due to inadequate iron intake and poor **absorption**. The increased **incidence** of **diabetes**, **hypertension**, **coronary heart disease**, **cancer**, and **obesity**, especially in the thirty-five-and-over age group, is thought to be directly linked to the existing lifestyle and dietary practices of the islanders.

The Caribbean Islands have seen a proliferation of **fast-food** restaurants, and the increased consumption of meals high in **fat**, sugar, and salt has contributed to the increase in chronic diseases. In addition, there has been a reduction in the amount of cereals, grains, fruits, vegetables, tubers, and legumes that are eaten. The popularity of fast foods among the young has led the government to focus on improving nutrition in the schools. Also contributing to the health problems is the dependency on costly imported **processed foods** that do the body harm. Overconsumption of imported foods high in fat and sodium has led to a deterioration of the health status of people throughout the region, with an increase in health problems such as obesity, diabetes, hypertension, **cardiovascular** disease, and cancer.

Innovative Programs

Due to insufficient resources and less than adequate planning, the school feeding programs on most of the islands exhibit many shortcomings. However, on the island of Dominica, where a self-help initiative involving the parents was introduced, the eating habits of school-aged children improved and the parents and communities adopted many of the program's menus and preparation methods. As a result, school attendance increased and the attention span of the children in class improved.

School nutrition programs need constant monitoring to improve the nutritional status of the children involved. Furthermore, a good nutrition promotion campaign must be designed to educate and promote a healthy lifestyle for the population at large.

The Caribbean region has the tremendous task of putting in place appropriate policies, plans, and programs to address the changing health and disease patterns of the region's people. This effort is made more difficult because of the socioeconomic, political, and cultural differences among the Caribbean countries. The various countries must not only examine the food availability and how it is consumed, but they must also assess and evaluate the quality of the food and the nutrition intake of those most at risk.

The Caribbean Food and Nutrition Institute (CFNI), established in 1967, aims to improve the food and nutrition status in member countries, which include Anguilla, Antigua, Bahamas, Barbados, Belize, the British Virgin Islands, Cayman Islands, Dominica, Grenada, Guyana, Jamaica, Montserrat, St. Christopher-Nevis, St. Lucia, St. Vincent, Suriname, Trinidad and Tobago, and Turks and Caicos Islands.

The governments of the Caribbean have come together under an initiative called Caribbean Cooperation in Health. They hope to work closely together through five types of activities: service, education training, providing information, coordination, and research. The food goals of each country must be analyzed, with care and attention paid to the agricultural policies and economic opportunities in each specific country.

anemia: low level of red blood cells in the blood

absorption: uptake by the digestive tract

incidence: number of new cases reported each year

diabetes: inability to regulate level of sugar in the blood

hypertension: high blood pressure

coronary heart disease: disease of the coronary arteries, the blood vessels surrounding the heart

cancer: uncontrolled cell growth

obesity: the condition of being overweight, according to established norms based on sex, age, and height

fast-food: food requiring minimal preparation before eating, or food delivered very quickly after ordering in a restaurant

fat: type of food molecule rich in carbon and hydrogen, with high energy content

processed food: food that has been cooked, milled, or otherwise manipulated to change its quality

cardiovascular: related to the heart and circulatory system

Forming Healthy Communities

Desiring a longer and richer quality of life, many governments of the Caribbean Islands have introduced programs to combat chronic diseases and promote a more physically active lifestyle. For example, in Grenada, a campaign to "grow what you eat and eat what you grow" demonstrates a move to increase consumption of local foods.

Adequate nutrition cannot be achieved without the consumption of sufficient foods containing a wide array of **nutrients**. Poor health status, whether as a result of insufficient food intake, overconsumption, or nutrition imbalance, threatens longevity and increases health care costs. The challenge is to improve the availability of nutritious foods and the eating habits of the varied population. SEE ALSO AFRICANS, DIETS OF; AFRICAN AMERICANS, DIET OF; DIETARY TRENDS, INTERNATIONAL; FAST FOODS.

Paulette Sinclair-Weir

nutrient: dietary substance necessary for health

Bibliography

"Assessing Dietary Trends in the Caribbean" (1998). *Cajanus, the Caribbean Food and Nutrition Quarterly* 31(4).

Campbell, Versada (1988). *Caribbean Foodways.* Kingston, Jamaica: Caribbean Food and Nutrition Institute.

"Food Consumption Issues and Trends" (2000). *Cajanus, the Caribbean Food and Nutrition Quarterly* 33(1).

"Food Marketing Trends" (2000). *Cajanus, the Caribbean Food and Nutrition Quarterly* 33(4).

Forrester, Clare (1999). "Selling Nutrition Behavior." *Cajanus, the Caribbean Food and Nutrition Quarterly* 32(1).

Kutler, Pamela Goyan, and Sucher, Kathryn P. (2000). *Food and Culture,* 3rd edition, New York: Thomson Learning.

McIntosh, E. Curtis (2000). "Food, Nutrition, and Health for National Development." *Cajanus, the Caribbean Food and Nutrition Quarterly* 33(4).

Prasad, P. V. Devi (1986). *Edible Fruits and Vegetables of the English-Speaking Caribbean.* Kingston, Jamaica: Caribbean Food and Nutrition Institute.

Sheridan, Richard B. (1974) *Sugar and Slavery.* Johns Hopkins University Press.

Stein-Barer, Thelma (1999). *You Eat What You Are: People, Culture, and Food Tradition,* 2nd edition. Toronto: Firefly.

Internet Resource

Pan American Health Organization. <http://www.paho.org>

carotenoid: plant-derived molecules used as pigments

antioxidant: substance that prevents oxidation, a damaging reaction with oxygen

cancer: uncontrolled cell growth

macular degeneration: death of cells of the macula, part of the eye's retina

heart disease: any disorder of the heart or its blood supply, including heart attack, atherosclerosis, and coronary artery disease

cholesterol: multi-ringed molecule found in animal cell membranes; a type of lipid

artery: blood vessel that carries blood away from the heart toward the body tissues

Carotenoids

Carotenoids are a group of red and yellow fat-soluble compounds that pigment different types of plants, such as flowers, citrus fruits, tomatoes, and carrots, as well as animals, such as salmon, flamingos, and goldfish. The ingestion of carotenoids is essential to human health, not only because some convert into Vitamin A, but also because they have **antioxidant** effects, which may combat such diverse problems as **cancer** and **macular degeneration**. Carotenoids also help prevent **heart disease** by inhibiting low-density lipoprotein (LDL) **cholesterol** (the "bad" cholesterol) from sticking to **artery** walls and creating plaques.

Up to one-third of the Vitamin A consumed by humans comes from the conversion of alpha-carotene and beta-carotene, the two most active of the over 600 carotenoids that have been identified. These two compounds combat early cancers, regulate the **immune system**, and maintain the integrity of the skin, lungs, liver, and urinary tract, among other organs. Food sources include eggs, liver, milk, spinach, and mangos.

Lycopene is a carotenoid that offers protection to the **prostate** and the **intestines**. It has also been associated with a decreased risk of lung cancer. Found in tomatoes, it remains intact despite the processing involved in making ketchup and tomato paste. The carotenoids lutein and zeaxanthin seem to aid in the prevention of **cataracts** and macular degeneration, and can be found in spinach and collard greens. SEE ALSO ANTIOXIDANTS; BETA-CAROTENE; VITAMINS, FAT-SOLUBLE.

Chandak Ghosh

immune system: the set of organs and cells, including white blood cells, that protect the body from infection

prostate: male gland surrounding the urethra that contributes fluid to the semen

intestines: the two long tubes that carry out the bulk of the processes of digestion

cataract: clouding of the lens of the eye

Bibliography

Margen, Sheldon, and Editors of U.C. Berkeley Wellness Letter (2002). *Wellness Foods A to Z: An Indispensable Guide for Health-Conscious Food Lovers.* New York: Rebus.

Internet Resources

National Institutes of Health Clinical Center. "Facts about Dietary Supplements: Vitamin A and Carotenoids." Available from <http://www.cc.nih.gov>

WebMD Health. "What Are Vitamins and Carotenoids and What Are the Adverse Effects of Deficiencies and Overdose?" Available from <http://www.my.webmd.com>

Central Americans and Mexicans, Diets of

The diets of peoples in Mexico and Central America (Guatemala, Nicaragua, Honduras, El Salvador, Belize, and Costa Rica) have several commonalities, though within the region great differences in methods of preparation and in local recipes exist. The basis of the traditional **diet** in this part of the world is corn (maize) and beans, with the addition of meat, animal products, local fruits, and vegetables. As in other parts of the world, the diet of people in this area has expanded to include more **processed foods**. In many parts of Mexico and Central America, access to a variety of foods remains limited, and **undernutrition**, particularly among children, is a major problem. Although access to an increased variety of foods can improve the adequacy of both **macronutrient** and **micronutrient** status, there is evidence that the use of processed foods is contributing to the rapidly increasing **prevalence** of **obesity** and diet-related **chronic** diseases such as **diabetes**.

Traditional Dietary Habits

The central staple in the region is maize, which is generally ground and treated with lime and then pressed into flat cakes called *tortillas*. In Mexico and Guatemala, these are flat and thin, while in other Central American countries tortillas are thicker. In El Salvador, for example, small, thick cakes of maize, filled with meat, cheese, or beans, are called *pupusas*. Maize is also used in a variety of other preparations, including tacos, tamales, and a thin gruel called **atole**. The complementary staple in the region is beans (*frijoles*), most commonly black or pinto beans. Rice is also widely used, particularly

diet: the total daily food intake, or the types of foods eaten

processed food: food that has been cooked, milled, or otherwise manipulated to change its quality

undernutrition: food intake too low to maintain adequate energy expenditure without weight loss

macronutrient: nutrient needed in large quantities

micronutrient: nutrient needed in very small quantities

prevalence: describing the number of cases in a population at any one time

obesity: the condition of being overweight, according to established norms based on sex, age, and height

chronic: over a long period

diabetes: inability to regulate level of sugar in the blood

atole: a porridge made of corn meal and milk

A Tzotzil mother makes tortillas with her daughters. The Tzotzil live in Chiapas, Mexico, near Guatemala. Central Americans traditionally have simple diets that depend on corn, beans, and local fruits and vegetables. *[© Corbis. Reproduced by permission.]*

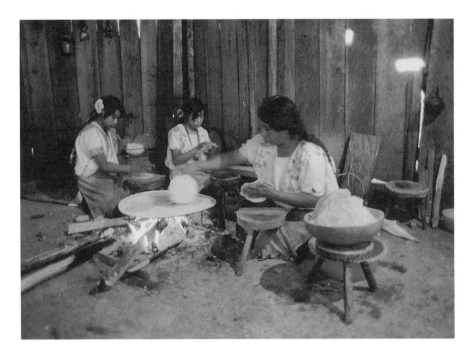

in the southernmost countries, such as El Salvador, Honduras, Nicaragua, and Costa Rica. Historically, major changes in the traditional diet occurred during colonial times, when the Spaniards and others introduced the region to wheat bread, dairy products, and sugar. Wheat is commonly consumed in the form of white rolls or sweet rolls, or, in the northern part of Mexico, as a flour-based tortilla. Noodles (*fideos*), served in soups or mixed with vegetables, have also become popular.

The consumption of meat and animal products, although popular, is often limited due to their cost. Beef, pork, chicken, fish, and eggs are all used. Traditional cheeses are prepared locally throughout the region as *queso del pais*, a mild, soft, white cheese, and milk is regularly used in *café con leche* and with cereal gruels.

Commonly Used Fruits and Vegetables

The region is a rich source of a variety of fruits and vegetables. Best known among these are the chile peppers, tomatoes, and tomatillos that are used in the salsas of Mexico. Avocado is also very popular in Mexican and Central American **cuisines**. Other commonly used vegetables include *calabaza* (pumpkin), carrots, plantains, onions, locally grown greens, and cacti. Fruits are seasonal but abundant in the rural areas and include guavas, papayas, mangoes, melons, pineapples, bananas, oranges, and limes, as well as less-known local fruits such as *nances*, *mamey*, and *tunas* (prickly pears from cacti). Traditional drinks (*frescos*, *chichas*, or *liquados*) are made with fruit, water, and sugar.

Methods of Cooking

The traditional preparation of maize involves boiling and soaking dried maize in a lime-water solution and then grinding it to form a soft dough called *masa*. Soaking in lime softens the maize and is an important source of **calcium** in the diet. The masa is shaped and cooked on a flat metal or

cuisine: types of food and traditions of preparation

calcium: mineral essential for bones and teeth

114

clay surface over an open fire. In some areas, lard or margarine, milk, cheese, and/or baking powder may be added to the tortilla during preparation. Beans are generally boiled with seasonings such as onion, garlic, and sometimes tomato or chile peppers. They are served either in a soupy liquid or are "re-fried" with lard or oil into a drier, and higher **fat**, preparation.

fat: type of food molecule rich in carbon and hydrogen, with high energy content

Meat, poultry, and fish are commonly prepared in local variations of thin soup (*caldo* or *sopa*), or thicker soups or stews (*cocido*) with vegetables. In Mexico and Guatemala, grilled meats are cut into pieces and eaten directly on corn tortillas as tacos.

These are often served with a variety of salsas based on tomato or tomatillo with onion, chile, coriander leaves (cilantro), and other local seasonings. Tamales are made with corn (or corn and rice) dough that is stuffed with chicken and vegetables. The tamales are steamed after being wrapped in banana leaves. Salvadorian *pupusas* are toasted tortillas filled with cheese, beans, or pork rind eaten with coleslaw and a special hot sauce.

Central American and Mexican Dishes

Beyond the basic **staples**, the cuisine of Mexico and Central America is rich with many regional variations. The tortilla-based Mexican preparations familiar in the United States are generally simpler in form in Mexico. *Tacos* are generally made with meat, chicken, or fish grilled or fried with seasoning and served on tortillas; *enchiladas* are filled tortillas dipped in a chile-based sauce and fried; and *tostadas* are fried tortillas topped with refried beans or meat, and sometimes with vegetables and cream. *Chiles rellenos* are made with the large and sweet chile *poblano* and filled with ground meat. Examples of specialty dishes include *mole*, a sauce made with chocolate, chile, and spices and served over chicken, beef, or enchiladas; and *ceviche*, raw marinated fish or seafood made along the coast throughout Central America and Mexico.

staples: essential foods in the diet

Nutritional Benefits

The staple diet of the region—corn and beans, supplemented with meat, dairy products, and local fruit and vegetables—is nutritionally complete and well suited to a healthful lifestyle. The proper combination of tortilla and beans provides an excellent complement of **amino acids**, thus supplying the necessary amount of complex **protein**. The process of liming the maize makes the calcium and the **niacin** in the tortilla more bioavailable, and this food is a major source of these **nutrients**. In addition, the traditional preparation of tortillas with a hand mill and grinding stones appears to add **iron** and **zinc** to the tortilla. Beans are excellent sources of **B vitamins**, magnesium, **folate**, and **fiber**. The tomato and chile-based salsas, along with several of the tropical fruits such as limes and oranges are important sources of vitamin C, and the variety of vegetables and yellow fruits such as papaya, melon, and mango provide excellent sources of **carotenoids**, which are precursors of vitamin A.

amino acid: building block of proteins, necessary dietary nutrient

protein: complex molecule composed of amino acids that performs vital functions in the cell; necessary part of the diet

niacin: one of the B vitamins, required for energy production in the cell

nutrient: dietary substance necessary for health

iron: nutrient needed for red blood cell formation

zinc: mineral necessary for many enzyme processes

B vitamins: a group of vitamins important in cell energy processes

folate: one of the B vitamins, also called folic acid

fiber: indigestible plant material which aids digestion by providing bulk

carotenoid: plant-derived molecules used as pigments

vitamin: necessary complex nutrient used to aid enzymes or other metabolic processes in the cell

Nutritional Limitations

Unfortunately, limited financial access to this variety of foods for many people in Central America and Mexico means that the diet often does not include sufficient levels of **vitamins** and **minerals**. For low-income groups,

mineral: an inorganic (non-carbon-containing) element, ion or compound

saturated fat: a fat with the maximum possible number of hydrogens; more difficult to break down than unsaturated fats

cholesterol: multi-ringed molecule found in animal cell membranes; a type of lipid

Americanized: having adopted more American habits or characteristics

nutrition: the maintenance of health through proper eating, or the study of same

globalization: development of worldwide economic system

diversity: the variety of cultural traditions within a larger culture

lack of access to animal products contributes to deficiencies in iron, zinc, vitamin A, and other nutrients. When animal products are included, there has been a tendency to choose high-fat products such as sausage and fried pork rinds (*chicharron*). The use of lard and a preference for fried foods also contributes to high intakes of **saturated fat** and **cholesterol** among subsets of the population.

Influence of Central American and Mexican Culture

As two cultures intermingle, foods and preparations from each tend to infiltrate the other. This is clearly the case near the U.S.-Mexican border, where Mexican immigrants and return immigrants have incorporated foods from U.S. diets into their traditional diets. The result has been a modified form of Mexican cuisine popularly known as "Tex-Mex." Beyond the border, this **Americanized** version of popular Mexican foods has spread throughout the United States through the popularity of Mexican restaurants. In the United States, tacos and tostadas tend to have less Mexican seasoning, but include lettuce and shredded processed cheese. Flour, rather than corn, tortillas are more widely used along the border. Many foods, such as soups and chiles, prepared along the border have become known for their spicy hotness, due to the Mexican-influenced use of chiles and chile powder.

Changes in Dietary Practices

Throughout the world, the diets of traditional cultures have experienced what has been called the "**nutrition** transition," particularly during the last few decades of the twentieth century. In Mexico and Central America, as elsewhere, this transition has been fueled by **globalization** and urbanization. Major dietary changes include an increased use of animal products and processed foods that include large amounts of sugar, refined flour, and hydrogenated fats. At the same time, a decline in the intake of whole grains, fruit, and vegetables has been documented. While the increased variety has improved micronutrient status for many low-income groups, the inclusion of more animal fat and refined foods has contributed to a rapid increase in obesity and chronic disease throughout the region.

These changes are more evident among immigrants to the United States, where adoption of U.S. products has been shown to have both positive and negative impacts on nutritional status. Studies that compared diets of Mexican residents to newly arrived Mexican-American immigrants and to second-generation Mexican Americans have documented both nutritionally positive and negative changes with acculturation. On the positive side, acculturated Mexican Americans consume less lard and somewhat more fruit, vegetables, and milk than either newly arrived immigrants or Mexican residents. On the negative side, they also consume less tortilla, beans, soups, stews, gruels, and fruit-based drinks, with greater use of meat, sweetened ready-to-eat breakfast cereals, soft drinks, candy, cakes, ice cream, snack chips, and salad dressings.

Conclusion

The traditional diet of Mexico and Central America is based on corn and beans, but offers a wide **diversity** of preparations. Coupled with locally available fruits, vegetables, meat and dairy products, the diet can be highly nutritious. However, poverty frequently limits access to an adequate variety of quality foods, resulting in **malnutrition**. At the same time, the increasing use of processed foods is contributing to obesity, diabetes, and other chronic conditions in this region. The balance between improving access to variety and maintaining dietary quality poses a challenge for public health. SEE ALSO HISPANICS AND LATINOS, DIET OF; SOUTH AMERICANS, DIET OF.

Katherine L. Tucker

malnutrition: chronic lack of sufficient nutrients to maintain health

Bibliography

Guendelman, Sylvia, and Abrams, Barbara (1995). "Dietary Intake among Mexican-American Women: Generational Differences and a Comparison with White Non-Hispanic Women." *American Journal of Public Health* 85(1):20–25.

Romero-Gwynn, Eunice; Gwynn, Douglas; Grivetti, Louis; McDonald, Roger; Stanford, Gwendolyn; Turner, Barbara; West, Estella; and Williamson, Eunice (1993). "Dietary Acculturation among Latinos of Mexican Descent." *Nutrition Today* 28(4):6–12.

Romieu, Isabelle; Hernandez-Avila, Mauricio; Rivera, Juan A.; Ruel, Marie T.; and Parra, Socorro (1997). "Dietary Studies in Countries Experiencing a Health Transition: Mexico and Central America." *American Journal of Clinical Nutrition* 65(4, Suppl):1159S–1165S.

Sanjur, Diva (1995). *Hispanic Foodways, Nutrition, and Health*. Boston: Allyn and Bacon.

Tucker, Katherine L., and Buranapin, Supawan (2001). "Nutrition and Aging in Developing Countries." *Journal of Nutrition* 131:2417S–2423S.

Central Europeans and Russians, Diets of

A health gap separates Central and Eastern Europe from the United States, Canada, Japan, and the Western part of Europe. This East-West gap in health started during the 1960s. Almost half of this gap was due to **cardiovascular** disease (CVD) mortality differentials. There has been a marked increase of CVD in Central and Eastern Europe, which is only partially explainable by the high **prevalence** of the three traditional CVD risk factors (**hypercholesterolemia**, **hypertension**, and smoking) in these countries. There is an extreme nonhomogeneity of the former Soviet bloc, and the data from each country must be analyzed individually. The aim here is to present the latest available data, which show the health status of various regions of postcommunist Europe. All data used are taken from the World Health Organization (WHO) Health for All Database (as updated in June 2003). The last available data from most countries are from the year 2002.

As premature mortality was considered the most important information, the standardized death rate (SDR) for the age interval 0–64 years was used (SDR is the age-standardized death rate calculated using the direct method; it represents what the crude death rate would have been been if the population had the same age distribution as the standard European population).

cardiovascular: related to the heart and circulatory system

prevalence: describing the number of cases in a population at any one time

hypercholesterolemia: high levels of cholesterol in the blood

hypertension: high blood pressure

Central Europe (Poland, Hungary, Czech Republic, Slovakia)

Total, CVD and **cancer** mortality in Central Europe was relatively low at the beginning of the 1960s, but then an increase occurred. While the differences in 1970 between the nations of the European Union (EU) and the

cancer: uncontrolled cell growth

heart disease: any disorder of the heart or its blood supply, including heart attack, atherosclerosis, and coronary artery disease

Central European communist countries were not great, from the mid-1970s on, the relative trends in CVD mortality in EU countries and Central Europe showed a marked change: mortality in Central Europe increased, whereas in EU countries it decreased steadily. Between 1985 and 1990, the male CVD mortality in Central Europe was more than two times higher than in EU countries. A substantial proportion of this divergence was attributable to ischemic **heart disease**. After the collapse of Communism, however, a decrease in CVD mortality in Central Europe was observed.

The Former Soviet Union (Russian Federation)

The most significant changes in CVD mortality have been observed in the region of the former Soviet Union (USSR). Between the years 1980 and 1990, male premature mortality was relatively stable in all regions of the USSR, and two to three times higher than in EU nations, or average. After the collapse of the USSR, CVD mortality began to rise dramatically in all the new independent states within the territory of the former USSR. In 1994 the male CVD mortality in Russia and Latvia was more than five times higher than the EU average. Women in these countries have been affected to almost the same degree as men, and the CVD mortality trends were strongest among young adults and middle-aged individuals. Cancer mortality was stable during this period, however. In 1994 the life expectancy of Russian men was almost twenty years less than that of men in Japan and some European countries. After 1994, however, there was a sudden drop in mortality both in males and females, followed by a further increase.

Lifestyle and Nutrition

Communist period (1970–1989). The socioeconomic situation in the democratic part of Europe and in the United States after World War II was substantially different than that in the Soviet bloc. The United States and the European democratic states were prosperous countries with effective economies and a rich variety of all kinds of foods. The communist states, however, had ineffective centralized economies and lower standards of living. The amount of various foods, especially foods of animal origin, was almost always insufficient in the USSR and the majority of its satellite countries. Data on food consumption compiled by the Food and Agricultural Organization (FAO) confirm that meat consumption was, between 1961 and 1990, substantially lower in the USSR, Poland, Romania, and Bulgaria than in Western Europe or the United States. Similarly, the consumption of milk and butter in Bulgaria, Hungary, and Romania was significantly lower in comparison with Western and Northern Europe.

The increase of CVD mortality within the Soviet bloc seems to be only partially associated with a high prevalence of traditional risk factors. Efforts to apply the experience gained from successful preventive projects in Finland or the United States without analyzing the specificity of risk factors in this region, could lead to an incorrect formulation of priorities when determining preventive measures. The contribution of physical activity remains an open issue, but due to technical backwardness (lower number of cars, lower mechanization, etc.), the physical activity of people working in industry, agriculture, and services was generally higher in Eastern Europe than in the West.

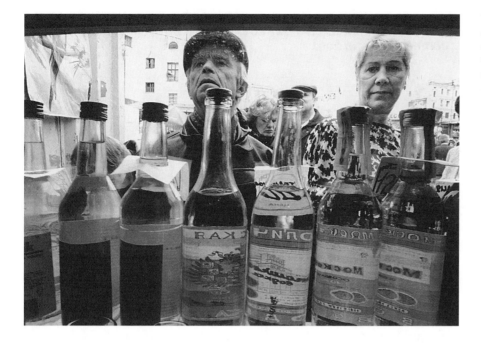

Some authors believe that economic conditions were the principal determinant of the gap in health status between the East and West. The close relationship between the gross national product per capita and life expectancy is well known, but the inhabitants of Central Europe were less healthy than their wealth predicted. The dramatic changes that occurred after the onset of communism created a toxic psychosocial environment. A loss of personal perspectives, **chronic stress**, tension, anger, hostility, social isolation, frustration, hopelessness, and apathy led to a lowered interest in health and to a very high **incidence** of alcoholism and suicide. People living for many decades in the informationally polluted environment rejected even useful health education.

It is widely believed that chronic stress can aggravate the development of chronic diseases. However, the reasons for the high cancer and CVD mortality in Eastern Europe are (with the significant exception of male smoking) not yet known. It is possible that in communist countries the effect of traditional risk factors has been intensified unidentified factors. Hypothetically, such factors can comprise psychosocial disorders, alcoholism, environmental pollution and specific **nutritional deficiencies** (e.g., very low intake of **antioxidant vitamins**, folic acid, and bioflavonoids). Very low blood levels of antioxidants, especially of vitamin C and selenium, were found in various regions of Central and Eastern Europe between 1970 and 1990.

Postcommunist period (after 1989). Thanks to its geographical location, Central Europe was best prepared for the democratic changes that occurred after 1989. After the collapse of communism, the decrease in CVD mortality in politically and economically more consolidated countries occured. The positive changes in Central European countries can be explained by higher consumption of healthful food, including a substantial increase in the consumption of fruit and vegetables, a decrease in butter and fatty milk consumption, and an increase in the consumption of vegetable oils and

chronic: over a long period

stress: heightened state of nervousness or unease

incidence: number of new cases reported each year

nutritional deficiency: lack of adequate nutrients in the diet

antioxidant: substance that prevents oxidation, a damaging reaction with oxygen

vitamin: necessary complex nutrient used to aid enzymes or other metabolic processes in the cell

MALE AND FEMALE LIFE EXPECTANCY AT BIRTH IN EUROPE DURING 2000 AND 2001		
Country	Males	Females
Russia	59.1	72.3
Ukraine	62.3	73.6
Hungary	68.3	76.8
Romania	67.7	75.0
Bulgaria	68.6	75.4
Poland	70.3	78.5
Slovakia	69.7	77.7
Czech Republic	72.1	78.7
Portugal	72.6	79.7
Spain	75.2	82.4
United Kingdom	75.7	80.5
Germany	75.2	81.3
Italy	76.2	82.6
Sweden	77.5	82.3
Switzerland	77.0	82.8
France	75.2	82.8

SOURCE: World Health Organization

plasma: the fluid portion of the blood, distinct from the cellular portion

free radical: highly reactive molecular fragment, which can damage cells

high-quality margarines. There was also a rapid improvement in the availability and quality of modern CVD health care.

Finnish and Russian epidemiologists compared the **plasma** ascorbic-acid concentrations among men in North Karelia (Finland) and in the neighboring Russian district. Almost all Russian men had levels suggesting a severe vitamin C deficiency, while more than 95 percent Finns had normal vitamin C levels. Comparison of fifty-year-old men in Sweden and Lithuania found significantly lower plasma concentrations of some antioxidant vitamins (beta-carotene, lycopene, gamma-tocopherol) in Lithuanian men. They also had substantially lowered resistance of low-density lipoprotein to oxidation than Swedish men. It is probable that in Russia an imbalance arose in which factors enhancing the production of **free radicals** (alcoholism, smoking, and pollution) dominated protective antioxidant factors.

High prevalence of smoking and alcoholism has also been an important factor in high CVD mortality rates in Russia. A substantial proportion of CVD deaths in Russia, particularly in the younger age groups, have been sudden deaths due to cardiomyopathies related to alcoholism. Alcoholism has evidently played a key role in the extremely high incidence of CVD mortality, as well as in the numbers of accidents, injuries, suicides, and murders. There is no way to determine a reliable estimation of the actual consumption of alcohol in Russia, since alcohol is being smuggled into the country on a large scale.

Normalization in the Russian Federation will likely be more difficult than in Central Europe. Trends in lifestyle, smoking, food selection, alcohol consumption, and other areas will be determined by both economic and political factors. The successfulness of the economic transformation, which provides hope for a sensible life, will be a key factor in improving health status in postcommunist countries. A significant decrease in cardiovascular and cancer mortality in Central Europe provides hope for the Russian Federation. Unfortunately, differences in life expectancy between these countries and Western Europe are still very great.

Emil Ginther

Internet Resource

World Health Organization."Health for All Database: Mortality Indicators by Cause, Age, and Sex." Available from <http://www.euro.who.int/hfadb>

Childhood Obesity

There have always been **overweight** children. Historically, chubby babies and toddlers were more likely to survive infections and contagious diseases, and overweight children and family members were often signs of affluence and financial security in a community. Thus, in some cultures, overweight was a valued body type.

Today, being overweight puts a child at risk of developing **chronic** diseases such as **type II diabetes**, **hypertension**, and high **cholesterol** levels. **Obesity** can promote degenerative joint disease, which will result in painful knees, hips, feet, and back, and it can severely limit physical activity. These are health concerns previously seen only in adults, usually in those over age forty. Obesity can be measured using a tool called **body mass index** (BMI). The BMI of an individual can be derived from tables or calculated using a formula (weight in kilograms divided by height in meters squared). In the year 2000, the U.S. Centers for Disease Control and Prevention (CDC) released updated growth charts incorporating BMI percentiles for children, beginning with children two years of age and extending the curves to age twenty. Using these gender-specific graphs, children, adolescents, and young adults are at risk for overweight at the 85th through 89.9th percentiles and are classified as overweight at the 95th percentile or greater. Using this criteria, children and teens are not labeled "**obese**"; technically, they are only "at risk of overweight" or "overweight." In much of the scientific literature, however, the terms are used interchangeably.

Nutritionists and researchers have been tracking data that clearly shows an increasing trend of overweight children in the United States. Monitoring the proportion of overweight children was identified as one of the ten leading health indicators in Healthy People 2010. All ethnic, racial, gender, and age groups have shown increases. For example, in the 1963–1970 National Health Examination Survey (NHES), the **prevalence** of overweight among white six to eleven years old was 5.1 percent and 5.3 percent for African-American girls of the same age. The prevalence of overweight in this same age group doubled for white girls (10.2%) and tripled for African-American girls (16.2%) in the 1988–1991 National Health and Nutrition Examination Survey (NHANES III). Preliminary data from 1999 NHANES suggests that the percentage of overweight children has continued to increase in recent years. It is estimated that 13 percent of children ages six to eleven years and 14 percent of adolescents ages twelve to nineteen years are overweight. This represents a 2-3 percentage point increase from NHANES III.

African-American and Hispanic teens are more likely to be at risk or overweight than white or Asian adolescents. Combined data from nine large studies (including NHANES II and NHANES III) of 66,772 children between five to seventeen years old indicates that the highest percentage of overweight exists among Hispanic boys and African-American and Hispanic girls.

overweight: weight above the accepted norm based on height, sex, and age

chronic: over a long period

type II diabetes: inability to regulate the level of sugar in the blood due to a reduction in the number of insulin receptors on the body's cells

hypertension: high blood pressure

cholesterol: multi-ringed molecule found in animal cell membranes; a type of lipid

obesity: the condition of being overweight, according to established norms based on sex, age, and height

body mass index: weight in kilograms divided by square of the height in meters; a measure of body fat

obese: above accepted standards of weight for sex, height, and age

prevalence: describing the number of cases in a population at any one time

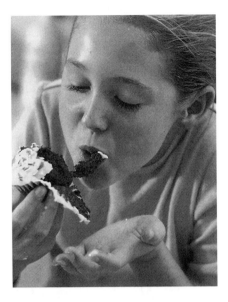

The National Institutes of Health have declared childhood obesity an epidemic in the United States. As with adults, the primary causes of children's obesity are too many calories and not enough exercise. Healthier meals and frequent physical activity are the proper method of prevention. [© Larry Williams/Corbis. Reproduced by permission.]

genetic: inherited or related to the genes

biological: related to living organisms

diabetes: inability to regulate level of sugar in the blood

fat: type of food molecule rich in carbon and hydrogen, with high energy content

fast food: food requiring minimal preparation before eating, or food delivered very quickly after ordering in a restaurant

fiber: indigestible plant material that aids digestion by providing bulk

calorie: unit of food energy

sedentary: not active

sleep apnea: difficulty breathing while sleeping

dyslipidemia: disorder of fat metabolism

Studies also show an increase in overweight rates among Native American children between 1970 and 2000. Second- and third-generation Asian-American children are more likely to be overweight, and certain Asian-American and Pacific Islander groups (Pacific Islanders, Koreans, Asian Indians) are noted to have higher overweight risks than other Asian Americans.

According to Dr. Mikael Fogelholm (at the May 2003 European Conference on Obesity), "the prevalence of obesity among adolescents worldwide has increased more rapidly than in middle-age adults." Outside the United States, obesity rates range from 2 percent in some developing countries to as high as 80 percent on remote Pacific Islands. In the United States, one child in four is now classified as overweight or at risk for becoming overweight. It is generally agreed that the longer and more overweight a child is, the more likely it is that the condition will continue into adulthood. Predisposing factors are complex and include a mix of **genetic**, social, cultural, environmental, and lifestyle factors.

Statistics show that a child with two obese parents has an 80 percent risk of becoming overweight, a child with only one obese parent has a 40 percent risk, and a child with normal weight parents has a 7 percent risk of becoming overweight. Twins who were adopted by different families were found to be more similar in weight to the **biological** parents than to their adoptive parents. Although the exact cause is still unknown, prenatal factors such as maternal obesity, excess pregnancy weight gain, and **diabetes** may also predispose a child to becoming overweight.

Other risk factors include meal patterns (e.g., skipping breakfast, meals and snacks eaten outside of the home, infrequent family dinners), unhealthful dietary intake (e.g., high **fat** intake, low intake of fruit and vegetables, **fast-food** meals, low **fiber** intake, high soft-drink intake), psychosocial factors such as acculturation and parenting style, and declining rates of physical activity. Based on data from NHANES II and III, among children twelve to seventeen years of age the prevalence of overweight increases 2 percent for each additional hour of TV viewed daily.

Prevention is the best treatment. Restricting **calories** can lead to stunted growth, adversely affect bone density, and even lead to eating disorders. Intervention strategies should involve the family and focus on permanent lifestyle changes under the supervision of a primary care physician or a registered dietitian. Parents can begin by limiting dining out to special occasions and by making time to enjoy regular meals at home together as a family. Time involved in **sedentary** activities such as playing video games or using the computer should be monitored and supervised, and the whole family should be encouraged to participate in thirty to sixty minutes of vigorous activity each day. To be successful, the entire family must be willing and ready to institute the many gradual, permanent changes needed.

Pharmacological and surgical treatments are associated with long-term risks and serious complications, and they constitute, at best, a last resort for severely overweight adolescents. Prolonged weight maintenance is recommended for many overweight children and allows a gradual decline in BMI as the child grows in height. However, if medical complications related to obesity already exist (**sleep apnea**, hypertension, **dyslipidemia** and orthopedic problems) weight loss of approximately one pound per month is recommended. SEE ALSO EATING DISORDERS; EATING DISTURBANCES; OBESITY; SCHOOL-AGED CHILDREN, DIET OF.

Nadine Pazder

Bibliography

Barlow, S., and Dietz, W. (1998). "Obesity Evaluation and Treatment: Expert Committee Recommendations." *Pediatrics* 102(3):1–11.

Ebbeling, Cara B.; Pawlak, Dororta B.; and Ludwig, David S. (2002). "Childhood Obesity: Public-Health Crisis, Common Sense Cure." *Lancet* 360:473–482.

Meerschaert, Carol (2002). "Managing Obesity in Children." *Soy Connection* 10(4):2. Also available from <http://www.talksoy.com>

Internet Resources

The Center for Weight and Health, University of California, Berkley (2001). "Pediatric Overweight: A Review of the Literature." Available from <http://www.cnr.berkeley.edu>

Centers for Disease Control and Prevention. "CDC Growth Charts." Available from <http://www.cdc.gov/growthcharts>

International Association for the Study of Obesity. Available from <http://www.iaso.org>

National Institutes of Health Weight Control Information Network (2002). "Youths' Weight and Eating Patterns Fall Short of Healthy People 2010 Objectives." *WIN NOTES* Winter 2002/2003. Available from <http://www.niddk.nih.gov/health>

College Students, Diets of

When students first enter college, their diets often deteriorate and they often gain weight. There are many factors responsible for these changes. However, there are also several actions that can be taken to avoid the weight gain and decline in **diet** quality that may occur during the college years.

The term "freshman 15" refers to the number of pounds many students gain during their first year in college. This weight gain is related to **stress**, a **sedentary** lifestyle, and changes in food intake and diet patterns, and it is not unique to American college students—international students attending American universities become heavier, too.

Meal and Snack Patterns and Serving Sizes

Meals are often skipped by college students, and management of weight and food intake is often nonexistent or disordered. Class and work schedules change daily, as well as every semester. However, structured eating patterns help students' academic performance. A study by Mickey Trockel, Michael Barnes, and Dennis Eggett, for example, found a positive relationship between eating breakfast and first-year college students' grade-point averages.

Lifestyle changes, peer pressure, limited finances, and access to food also contribute to erratic eating patterns. College students have little variety in their diet and often turn to high-fat snacks. A common error is underestimating serving sizes, meaning they often eat more than they think they are eating.

Food and Nutrient Intakes of College Students

Of the three nutrients that provide **calories** (**carbohydrates**, **proteins**, and fats), carbohydrate (particularly sugar) and fat intake often exceeds recommended levels. College students also tend to have a low intake of dietary **fiber**,

diet: the total daily food intake, or the types of foods eaten

stress: heightened state of nervousness or unease

sedentary: not active

calorie: unit of food energy

carbohydrate: food molecule made of carbon, hydrogen, and oxygen, including sugars and starches

protein: complex molecule composed of amino acids that performs vital functions in the cell; necessary part of the diet

fiber: indigestible plant material that aids digestion by providing bulk

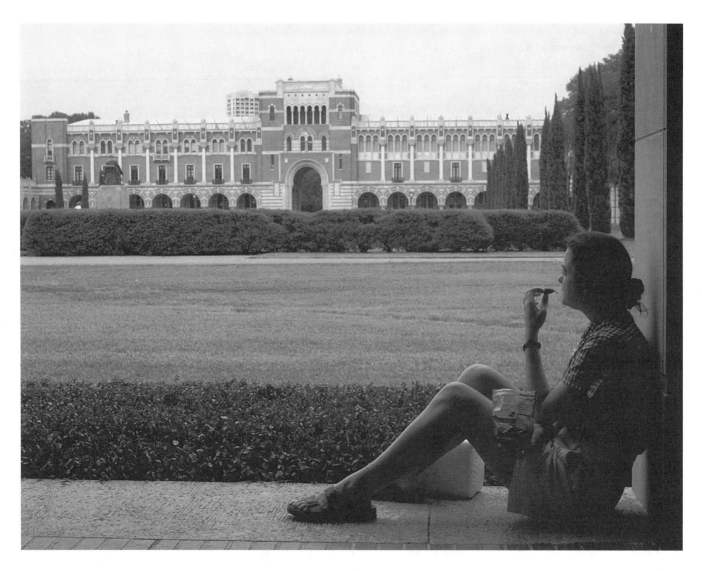

Irregular class schedules, part-time jobs, and variable homework loads can disrupt normal eating patterns among college students, leading to unhealthy habits that may be hard to break. Despite these difficulties, it is important for students to find time for nutritious and varied foods. [AP/Wide World Photos. Reproduced by permission.]

vitamin: necessary complex nutrient used to aid enzymes or other metabolic processes in the cell

mineral: an inorganic (non-carbon-containing) element, ion, or compound

calcium: mineral essential for bones and teeth

iron: nutrient needed for red blood cell formation

zinc: mineral necessary for many enzyme processes

energy: technically, the ability to perform work; the content of a substance that allows it to be useful as a fuel

anorexia nervosa: refusal to maintain body weight at or above what is considered normal for height and age

which is important for intestinal health. In terms of **vitamins**, a low vitamin C status has been associated with college students' low intake of fruits and vegetables (with levels of vitamin C being even lower among smokers). In terms of **minerals**, **calcium**, **iron**, and **zinc** intake are low, while sodium intake is generally higher than recommended.

Male college students are more likely to meet dietary intake recommendations for the meat, poultry, fish, dry beans, and nuts group; from the bread, cereal, rice, and pasta group; and from the vegetable food group than are females. Males seem to consume more food overall, and thus have a higher **energy** (calorie) intake. Female college students tend to eat too few breads, grains, and dairy products. In addition, it is estimated that about 10 percent of college students drink more than fifteen alcoholic beverages per week, further impairing the quality of their diet.

Eating disorders such as **anorexia** and **bulimia** are more prevalent among college females than among the general population. This is related to body image dissatisfaction—females that are underweight, as measured by their **body mass index** (BMI), sometimes consider themselves to be **overweight**. The **incidence** of anorexia and bulimia may increase when there is excessive preoccupation with weight, academic achievement, body image, and eating, as well as during stressful periods, such as final exams.

The **prevalence** of disordered eating is especially high among female athletes. College athletes may manipulate diet and fluid intake, putting their health at risk. They may also jeopardize their health by taking dangerous or excessive amounts of supplements as a result of misinformation, or of pressure from coaches or peers. Athletes may feel pressured to restrict their food intake if they are on an athletic scholarship or competing in weight-classification sports such as wrestling. Female athletes may be underweight or have an extremely low amount of body fat. The *female athlete triad* (disordered eating, **amenorrhea**, and **osteoporosis**) is estimated to occur in 15 to 62 percent of female college athletes.

Recommendations for Improvement

There are many actions that college students can take to eat in a healthful way and enjoy their college years without jeopardizing their health from excessive weight gain or weight loss. Among some recommendations are:

- Get at least eight hours of sleep a night. Lack of sleeps affects one's ability to concentrate and makes one feel tired. Sleep deprivation also seems to be connected with weight problems.

- Avoid skipping meals. When a meal is skipped, the subsequent hunger may cause one to overeat.

- Eat breakfast, which helps concentration and increases the likelihood of consuming calcium, folic acid, and vitamin C. These nutrients are often low in the diet of college students.

- Manage portion sizes. If portion sizes are underestimated, one may eat more calories than are needed. Also, the availability of a wide variety and mass quantities of "dorm" food (pizza, soda, etc.) may promote overeating and a significant increase of total energy intake.

- Drink water and eat fruit throughout the day. Water is calorie-free and fruits help manage urges to eat and contribute fiber, vitamins, and minerals.

- Exercise regularly. Physical activity helps burn off calories, helps manage stress, and promotes mental and physical stamina.

- Become familiar with the campus **environment** and the foods that are available. Most colleges and universities have a variety of eateries, each with a different format, theme, and food options.

- Try the low-calorie, low-fat, and vegetarian options available around campus. As part of a well-planned diet, these items can help manage total energy intake and introduce one to items that can become part of a regular diet.

- Keep low-fat and low-calorie snacks in the dorm room. This will help manage calorie intake when snacking, especially when eating late at night.

bulimia: uncontrolled episodes of eating (bingeing) usually followed by self-induced vomiting (purging)

body mass index: weight in kilograms divided by square of the height in meters; a measure of body fat

overweight: weight above the accepted norm based on height, sex, and age

incidence: number of new cases reported each year

prevalence: describing the number of cases in a population at any one time

amenorrhea: lack of menstruation

osteoporosis: weakening of the bone structure

environment: surroundings

Most universities offer a variety of meal plans. Students who take the time to acquaint themselves with the various foods available around campus, and who strive for nutritional balance, may find their academic performance improves along with their physical health. *[AP/Wide World Photos. Reproduced by permission.]*

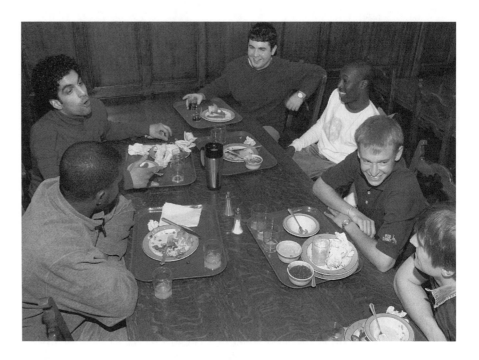

wellness: related to health promotion

Many universities have required or optional meal plans, which provide access to campus food for a flat rate paid either by semester or academic year. Per meal, these plans are a good value and provide access to a regular food resource. Among the things to consider are the hours the facilities are open, their proximity to student housing and classes, the quality and variety of items, and whether favorite foods are regularly available.

Universities can also take a variety of steps to promote healthful food behaviors. Campus and residence hall **wellness** programs can provide students with information and point-of-purchase information at dining halls can help students make on-the-spot decisions that support healthful choices. Education programs for university personnel can help them recognize and properly refer at-risk students.

College students will eat healthful foods if they are available. During the college years, students form a foundation and create eating habits that impact future health, so it is important to practice healthful eating during these years. SEE ALSO ADULT NUTRITION; EATING DISORDERS; EATING DISTURBANCES.

Judith C. Rodriguez

Bibliography

Anding, Jenna D.; Suminski, Richard R.; and Boss, Linda (2000). "Dietary Intake, Body Mass Index, Exercise, and Alcohol: Are College Women Following the Dietary Guidelines for Americans?" *Journal of American College Health* 49:167–171.

Johnston, Carol S.; Solomon, Elizabeth; and Conte, Corinne (1998). "Vitamin C Status of a Campus Population: College Students Get a C Minus." *Journal of American College Health* 46:209–213.

Schwitser, Alan M.; Bergholz, Kim; Dore, Terri; and Salimi, Lamieh (1998). "Eating Disorders among College Women: Prevention, Education, and Treatment Responses." *Journal of American College Health* 46(5):199–207.

Selkowitz, Ann (2000). *The College Student's Guide to Eating Well on Campus*. Bethesda, MD: Tulip Hill Press.

Tavelli, Suzanne; Beerman, Kathy; Shultz, Jill E.; and Heiss, Cindy (1998). "Sources of Error and Nutritional Adequacy of the Food Guide Pyramid." *Journal of American College Health* 47(2):77–87.

Trockel, Mickey T.; Barnes, Michael D.; and Egget, Dennis L. (2000). "Health Related Variables and Academic Performance among First-Year College Students: Implications for Sleep and Other Behaviors." *Journal of American College Health* 49(3):125–131.

Internet Resources

Grieger, Lynn. "15 Diet Tips to Beat the 'Freshman 15' (At Any Age!)." Available from <http://www.ivillage.com/diet>

Hobart, Julie A., and Smucker, Douglas R. "The Female Athlete Triad." Available from <http://www.aafp.org>

Commodity Foods

The United States Department of Agriculture (USDA) administers several programs that distribute commodity foods, which are foods that the federal government has the legal authority to purchase and distribute in order to support farm prices. The first commodity distribution program began during the Great Depression of the 1930s, when it was known as the Needy Family Program. This was the main form of food assistance for low-income people in the United States until the Food Stamp Program was expanded in the early 1970s. The Needy Family Program distributed surplus agricultural commodities such as cheese, butter, and other items directly to low-income people. Today, the Food and Nutrition Service (FNS), an agency of the U.S. Department of Agriculture, administers the nation's commodity food distribution programs. The programs continue to improve the nutrition status of low-income people, while providing a means for using surplus agricultural commodities from U.S. farm programs.

Commodity Supplemental Food Program

The Commodity Supplemental Food Program (CSFP) works to improve the health of low-income pregnant and breastfeeding women, other new mothers up to one year postpartum, infants, children up to age six, and low-income elderly persons sixty years of age and older by supplementing their diets with commodity foods. Eligible people cannot participate in USDA's Special Supplemental Program for Women, Infants, and Children (WIC) and CSFP at the same time.

The USDA purchases food and makes it available to state agencies and Indian tribal organizations, along with funds for administrative costs. The commodity foods provided to participants do not provide a complete **diet**, but are designed to supplement the nutritional needs of participants and may include canned fruit juice, canned fruits and vegetables, farina, oats, ready-to-eat cereal, nonfat dry milk, evaporated milk, egg mix, dry beans, peanut butter, canned meat, poultry or tuna, dehydrated potatoes, pasta, rice, cheese, butter, honey, and infant cereal and formula. Distribution sites make packages available on a monthly basis.

diet: the total daily food intake, or the types of foods eaten

As of 2003, the program operates in thirty-two states and the District of Columbia. An average of more than 410,000 people participated in the program each month in 2002, including more than 337,000 elderly people and more than 73,000 women, infants, and children.

Food Distribution Program on Indian Reservations (FDPIR)

The FDPIR provides monthly food packages of commodity foods to low-income American Indian households living on or near Indian reservations. Currently there are some 243 tribes receiving benefits under the FDPIR. Household eligibility for the program is based on income and resource standards set by the federal government. Many people participate in FDPIR as an alternative to the Food Stamp Program because they lack easy access to food stamp offices or authorized grocery stores. Households cannot participate in FDPIR and the Food Stamp Program in the same month.

Each month, participant households receive a food package to help them maintain a nutritionally balanced diet. Participants can select from over seventy products, including items such as frozen ground beef and chicken; canned meats, poultry, and fish; canned fruits and vegetables; canned soups and spaghetti sauce; macaroni and cheese; pasta; cereal; rice and other grains; cheese; egg mix and nonfat dry and evaporated milk; dried beans; dehydrated potatoes; canned juices and dried fruit; peanuts and peanut butter; flour, cornmeal, and crackers; corn syrup; and vegetable oil and shortening.

The Emergency Food Assistance Program (TEFAP)

The Emergency Food Assistance Program is the largest of the commodity food donation programs. TEFAP was designed to reduce the level of government-held surplus commodities by distributing them to low-income households to supplement the recipients' purchased food. Local agencies may also use the commodities to prepare and serve meals in congregate settings, such as soup kitchens.

Most states set eligibility criteria at between 130 and 150 percent of the poverty line. In many states, food stamp participants are automatically eligible for TEFAP. The types of foods USDA purchases for TEFAP distribution vary depending on the preferences of states and agricultural market conditions. Typical foods include canned and dried fruits, fruit juice, canned vegetables, dry beans, meat, poultry, fish, rice, oats, grits, cereal, peanut butter, nonfat dried milk, dried egg mix, pasta products, vegetable oil, and corn syrup.

Food Assistance for Disaster Relief

Food assistance for disaster relief is furnished to state relief agencies and organizations (e.g., Red Cross, Salvation Army) in times of emergency, such as hurricanes, earthquakes, floods, and winter storms. FNS may provide commodity foods for distribution to shelters and mass feeding sites, or distribute commodity food packages directly to persons in need.

Disaster relief organizations request food assistance through state agencies that run USDA's food and nutrition assistance programs. Emphasis is on food that requires little or no preparation, including such items as canned juice, canned meat, and canned fruits and vegetables. Baby food and infant formula are provided as needed.

Commodity Distribution to Other Programs

The USDA also donates food commodities to a variety of programs. The largest donations go to school food programs at more than 94,000 public

---

The Food and Nutrition Service

The goal of the Food and Nutrition Service (FNS) is to eliminate hunger amid the prosperity of the United States. The FNS administers 15 nutrition assistance programs at a cost of more than $40 billion per year. While these programs have been extremely successful in reducing widespread hunger in the United States, the U.S. Department of Agriculture estimates that approximately 3.5 percent of American households continue to experience hunger at some time during the year because they can't afford enough food.

—Paula Kepos

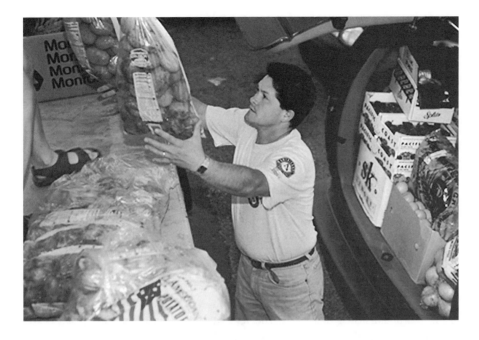

Workers prepare to redistribute surplus foods purchased by the U.S. Department of Agriculture. The USDA's commodity foods programs serve a dual purpose, maintaining the price of certain food products and ensuring that at-risk populations get the food they need. *[Photograph by Ken Hammond. USDA. Reproduced by permission.]*

and private nonprofit schools. During 2002, the USDA spent over $700 million on over a billion pounds of commodity foods for Schools/Child Nutrition Commodity Programs. Commodity food donations are also made to the Child and Adult Care Food Program and the nutrition programs for the elderly administered by the Department of Health and Human Services. Food commodities are also distributed to nonprofit, charitable institutions that serve meals to low-income people on a regular basis. These include homes for the elderly, hospitals, soup kitchens, food banks, Meals On Wheels programs, temporary shelters, and summer camps or orphanages not participating in any federal child nutrition program.

For these programs, states select a variety of foods from a list of one hundred different kinds of products. Typical foods include fruits and vegetables; meats; cheese; dry and canned beans; fruit juices; vegetable shortening and vegetable oils; peanut products; rice, pasta products, flour, and other grain products. Additional foods may be offered to states periodically, if they become available as agricultural surpluses. Additional products donated in previous years have included applesauce, beef roasts, dried fruit products, fresh pears, frozen apricots, nonfat dry milk, orange juice, pork products, salmon, and turkey. SEE ALSO NATIVE AMERICANS, DIET OF; NUTRITION PROGRAMS IN THE COMMUNITY; SCHOOL FOOD SERVICE; WIC PROGRAM.

Marie Boyle Struble

Bibliography

Boyle, Marie A. (2003). "Food Insecurity and the Food Assistance Programs." In *Community Nutrition in Action: An Entrepreneurial Approach*, 3rd edition. Belmont, CA: Wadsworth/Thomson Learning.

Food Research and Action Center (2002). *State of the States: A Profile of Food and Nutrition Programs Across the Nation*. Washington, DC: Author.

Internet Resources

U.S. Department of Agriculture, Food and Nutrition Service. "Nutrition Program Fact Sheets." Available from <http://www.fns.usda.gov>

U.S. Department of Agriculture, Food and Nutrition Service. "Food Distribution Programs." Available from <http://www.fns.usda.gov/fdd>

U.S. Department of Agriculture, Food and Nutrition Service. "Healthy Eating in Indian Country Fliers." Available from <http://www.fns.usda.gov/fdd>

Comprehensive School Health Program

The Comprehensive School Health Program (CSHP) is a national program in the United States that makes efforts in schools to improve the health of children. Since schools profoundly influence the health of young people, the CSHP is very important. The program is supported by a national health organization, the American School Health Association (ASHA), which is actively involved in improving the health of school-age children.

School-Age Children

cardiovascular: related to the heart and circulatory system

cancer: uncontrolled cell growth

diet: the total daily food intake, or the types of foods eaten

fat: type of food molecule rich in carbon and hydrogen, with high energy content

obesity: the condition of being overweight, according to established norms based on sex, age, and height

The major causes of death in America, such as **cardiovascular** disease and **cancer**, are greatly related to lifestyle, behavior, education, and prevention efforts are best focused on physical activity and **diet**. School-age children often have poor diets, making this a critical area for CSHPs to focus on. Few students are meeting the Dietary Guidelines for Americans. Their diets generally lack fruit and vegetables and contain an excess of foods that are high in **fat**. Childhood **obesity** has reached epidemic proportions, with greater numbers of people becoming affected earlier in their lives. This is an important issue for school health programs, since it has been well documented that the health of school-age children is directly related to their educational success.

American School Health Association

The American School Health Association (ASHA) recognizes that schools can do more than any single agency to help young people. This national organization unites the many professionals who are committed to improving the well being of school-age children. With more than 2,000 members, ASHA is comprised of counselors, health educators, physical educators, school nurses, school physicians, and administrators. Over half of members practice in K-12 schools or advise and oversee health-services programs or health education. The ASHA's mission is to protect and improve the well-being of children. To achieve this mission, ASHA members support the CSHP.

The Comprehensive School Health Program

environment: surroundings

nutrition: the maintenance of health through proper eating, or the study of same

The CSHP is an "organized set of policies, procedures, and activities designed to protect and promote the health and well-being of students and staff" (Cottrell, Girvan, and McKenzie, p. 67). This program traditionally includes three components: health education, a healthful school **environment**, and health services. It was expanded in 1987 (see Allensworth and Kolbe) to include physical education, **nutrition** services, counseling services, community and family involvement, and health promotion for faculty. These eight components promote the health of students, faculty, and the

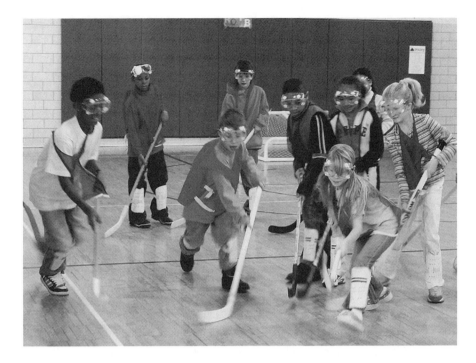

Physical education is one component of the Comprehensive School Health Program. The benefits of regular physical activity are numerous, and include enhanced bone, joint, and muscle fitness, weight control, and stress relief. *[Photo by Denay Wilding.]*

community. Since students spend a major part of their lives in school, schools are a good place to influence healthful living before harmful habits are established.

The first component, health education, suggests a planned health curriculum for students in grades K-12. The major content areas suggested for instruction are: community health, consumer health, environmental health, family life, mental and emotional health, injury prevention and safety, nutrition, personal health prevention, control of disease, and substance use and abuse. The individual states and local districts decide the actual content to be taught. Teachers are encouraged to teach healthful behaviors and provide students with skills to live healthier lives.

The second component, a healthful school environment, promotes a healthful physical and emotional environment. It is important that schools are safe and secure for all those who attend and work there. This component includes issues regarding safety, school security, a school's emotional and social atmosphere, the physical environment, and sexual harassment. Each year, many children are hurt on playgrounds, are exposed to environmental hazards, and witness violence among peers. The CSHP works towards making schools as safe as possible.

The third component, school health services, encourages promoting and protecting the health of every child. This may include on-site health clinics, school nurses, school physicians, and providing immunizations and screenings for vision, hearing, healthy weight, and head lice. With clinics and medical professionals located in schools, students have the opportunity for convenient medical care. Many clinics provide both treatment and educational services. For families who cannot afford medical care, this may be their only means to health care.

The fourth component, physical education, promotes regular exercise in schools as part of a healthful lifestyle. Approximately 75 percent of all junior high schools and high schools offer physical education classes lasting twenty minutes or more, three times per week. Physical education is important to develop strength and improve body image.

The fifth component, nutrition services, encourages balanced, appealing, and varied meals and snacks for students. The CSHP realizes the importance of good nutrition to prevent future illnesses.

The sixth component, counseling services, supports evaluations and counseling for students. By including services from guidance counselors and social workers, students' mental and emotional health is addressed.

The seventh component, community and family involvement, encourages the involvement of parents and the community in the schools. This program recognizes the need for schools to have good relationships with parents and community groups, which can be very beneficial in assisting schools and students with making decision and providing resources.

The final component, health promotion for faculty and staff, promotes a healthy staff. The many benefits of a healthy staff include less sick days, increased productivity, and positive role models for students.

wellness: related to health promotion

The CSHP encourages all schools to address their students' health on various levels. The program's mission is to promote **wellness**, motivate health improvement, and offer educational opportunities for students, families, and community members. By implementing the planned, ongoing services of the CSHP, schools have the ability to improve both education and the health of students and school personnel. SEE ALSO AMERICAN SCHOOL HEALTH ASSOCIATION; SCHOOL-AGE CHILDREN, DIET OF.

Elise M. Howard-Barr

Bibliography

Allensworth, Diane D., and Kolbe, Lloyd J. (1987). "The Comprehensive School Health Program: Exploring an Expanded Concept." *Journal of School Health* 57(10):409–412.

Butler, J. Thomas, ed. (2001). *Principles of Health Education and Health Promotion*, 3rd edition. Belmont, CA: Wadsworth.

Cottrell, Randal R.; Girvan, James T.; and McKenzie, James F., eds. (2002). *Principles and Foundations of Health Promotion and Education*, 2nd edition. San Francisco: Benjamin Cummings.

Internet Resource

American School Health Association. "About ASHA." Available from <http://www.ashaweb.org/>

Convenience Foods

Convenience foods are foods that have had preparation steps incorporated into their processing, or have been completely prepared during processing. This decreases preparation steps and time for the consumer. The "convenience" can mean the premixing of the ingredients for a cake or offering a fully prepared frozen meal. The term convenience food is generic and can apply to just about any food, but it is generally used in reference to canned items, instant foods or mixes, frozen foods or meals, and fast foods. Although they can be more costly than home-cooked meals, the trend is toward their increased use throughout the world. SEE ALSO DIETARY TRENDS, AMERICAN; DIETARY TRENDS, INTERNATIONAL; FAST FOODS.

Judith C. Rodriguez

Bibliography

Anderson, J., and Deskins, B. (1995). *The Nutrition Bible.* New York: William Morrow.

Labensky, S.; Ingram, G. G.; Labensky, S. R. (1997). *Webster's New World Dictionary of Culinary Arts.* Upper Saddle River, NJ: Prentice Hall.

Corn- or Maize-Based Diets

Maize, the American Indian word for corn, literally means "that which sustains life." After wheat and rice, it is the most important cereal grain in the world, providing **nutrients** for humans and animals. It also serves as a basic raw material for the production of starch, oil, **protein**, alcoholic beverages, food sweeteners, and fuel. Maize has the highest average yield per hectare.

Maize is an important food in Asia, Africa, Latin America, and parts of the former Soviet Union. Each country has one or more maize dishes that are unique to its culture. Examples are *ogi* (Nigeria), *kenkey* (Ghana), *koga* (Cameroon), *tô* (Mali), *injera* (Ethiopia), and *ugali* (Kenya). Most of these products are processed in traditional ways. In Africa, ground maize is cooked into a paste or mush and eaten while still warm, accompanied by a thick low-alcoholic beer. In some areas of Africa, maize mush is fried or baked. In Central and Latin American, maize is consumed in the form of maize bread or tortillas.

Maize is also used as animal feed and raw material for industrial use. In industrialized countries, a larger proportion of the grain is used as livestock feed and as industrial raw material for food and nonfood uses. On the other hand, the bulk of maize produced in developing countries is used as human food, although its use as animal feed is increasing. Maize is the largest food crop of the United States, which is responsible for 40 percent of the world's production.

Maize constitutes an important source of **carbohydrates**, protein, vitamin B, and **minerals**. As an **energy** source, it compares favorably with root and **tuber** crops, and it is similar in energy value to dried **legumes**. Furthermore, it is an excellent source of carbohydrate and is complete in nutrients compared to other cereals.

Varieties of Maize

Six general varieties of maize or corn are differentiated by the characteristics of the kernel. Dent corn is the leading type of corn grown on U.S. farms. The sides of the kernel consist of hard, so-called horny starch, and the crown contains soft starch. As the grain matures, this soft starch shrinks, forming the characteristic dent. In flint corn, the horny starch extends over the top of the kernel, so there is no denting. Popcorn, a light, highly popular snack throughout the United States, is a variant of flint corn with small kernels of great hardness. When heated, the moisture in the kernels expands, causing the kernels to pop open. Flour corn contains a preponderance of soft or less densely packed starch, and it is readily ground into meal. Sweet corn is

nutrient: dietary substance necessary for health

protein: complex molecule composed of amino acids that performs vital functions in the cell; necessary part of the diet

carbohydrate: food molecule made of carbon, hydrogen, and oxygen, including sugars and starches

mineral: an inorganic (non-carbon-containing) element, ion or compound

energy: technically, the ability to perform work; the content of a substance that allows it to be useful as a fuel

tuber: swollen plant stem below the ground

legumes: beans, peas, and related plants

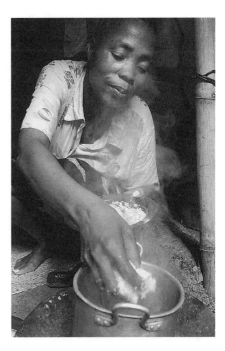

Many Africans depend on some variation of this mush, which is made with water and ground maize. It can be eaten as a porridge or a dumpling, depending on the thickness of the batter and the cooking method. *[AP/Wide World Photos. Reproduced by permission.]*

133

the type commonly grown in the United States for human consumption. The sugar produced by the sweet-corn plant is not converted to starch during growth, as it is in other types. Pod corn is seldom used as food but is often grown as a decorative plant—each kernel is enclosed in its own set of diminutive husks. Another decorative corn, commonly called Indian corn, consists of multicolored varieties of flour and flint types.

Protein Quality

amino acid: building block of proteins, necessary dietary nutrient

The nutritional quality of maize is determined by the **amino acid** makeup of its protein. Maize is deficient in two essential amino acids: lysine and tryptophan, making it a poor protein food. The kernel is made up of the endosperm, the germ, the pericap, and the tip cap. The protein concentration is highest in the germ, but the quality is better in the endosperm. The germ proteins contribute significantly to essential amino acids, so maize food products without the germ, including quality protein maize (QPM) endosperm, are lower in protein quality compared to the whole kernel.

vitamin: necessary complex nutrient used to aid enzymes or other metabolic processes in the cell

nitrogen: essential element for plant growth

metabolic: related to processing of nutrients and building of necessary molecules within the cell

The germ contributes most of the oil, sugar, **vitamins**, and minerals of the kernel. The germ also has a lower leucine to isoleucine ratio, giving it a higher biological value. Biological value is defined as the amount of absorbed **nitrogen** needed to provide the necessary amino acids for the different **metabolic** functions in the body.

The high consumption of maize by the human population and the well-established lysine and tryptophan deficiencies in maize protein motivated researchers to develop the QPM to increase concentrations of these essential amino acids in its protein. Newer varieties provide higher protein content (18%) by increasing the prolamine (zein) fraction in maize endosperm. An example of QPM is one opaque-2 maize.

QPM varieties have almost double the percentages of lysine and tryptophan compared to normal maize, but are similar in overall protein content. However, the QPM varieties have a greatly reduced amount of the major storage protein, zein. The biological value of common maize is 45 percent whereas the QPM is about 80 percent. Hence the production and consumption of QPM maize in countries that use maize as their chief grain crop would have a beneficial effect on the nutritional state of the people and significant economic implications from the better use of what is produced and consumed.

Compared to normal maize, production of QPM varieties may have some disadvantages. QPM varieties have softer, floury endosperms, providing a slightly lower yield and making the plant more susceptible to storage insects. Furthermore, QPM varieties have lower zein content, which is associated with lysine deficiency and a higher imbalance of essential amino acids. Hence they are considered to be of a lower quality. They are also susceptible to weevils in storage.

Minerals and Vitamins

niacin: one of the B vitamins, required for energy production in the cell

The nutritional disease pellagra, which is caused by a deficiency in **niacin**, is associated with maize-based diets in the Americas and Africa. While niacin is readily available in corn, it exists in a bound form (niacytin) that is not biologically available to monogastric (single-stomach) animals. Furthermore,

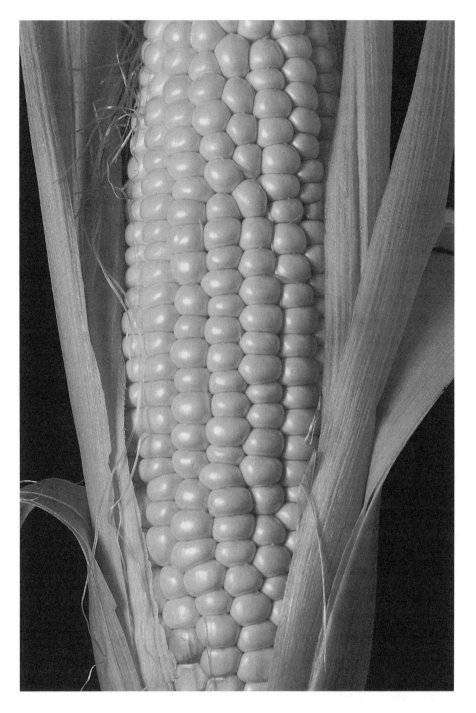

most of the niacin in the kernel (63%) occurs in the outermost layer of the endosperm. This layer is often removed with the pericarp during dehulling. In Mexico, Guatemala, and other countries, maize is treated with an alkaline solution of lime, which releases the niacin and helps prevent pellagra. Furthermore, pellagra seldom occurs among people in Latin America, since they eat tortillas—tortilla preparation greatly increases the **bioavailability** of the niacin in maize.

bioavailability: availability to living organisms, based on chemical form

Persons suffering from pellagra usually appear to be poorly nourished, and they are often weak and underweight. They also exhibit dermatitis, diarrhea, and **dementia**. If untreated, pellagra can result in death. Niacin supplements

dementia: loss of cognitive abilities, including memory and decision-making

are available to aid in the treatment of the disease. There are also several methods of increasing niacin content in maize-based diets, including:

- Complementing maize-based diets with nuts and fish, which are rich in niacin.

- Preparing maize in a way that retains the outer layer of the endosperm, contributing more niacin to the **diet**.

- Cooking maize in alkaline solution to increase niacin availability, a procedure commonly used in Latin America in the preparation of tortillas.

Maize is a good source of vitamin B and B_{12}. Yellow maize can provide substantial amounts of vitamin A, and the maize germ is rich in vitamin E. Furthermore, maize oil contains a high level of **polyunsaturated fatty acids** and natural **antioxidants** (Okoruwa, 1996). However, of the three major cereal grains (wheat, maize, and rice), maize has the lowest concentration of protein, **calcium**, and niacin.

Dietary preferences, processing, and mode of preparation affect the contributions of maize in human **nutrition**. For example, the nutritive value of the grain may increase or decrease depending upon the method in which it is processed (the milling of maize reduces the concentration of protein, **lipids**, and **fiber**). Diets that rely heavily on corn may require the consumption of complementary foods to supplement its deficiency in certain amino acids and vitamins. SEE ALSO NATIVE AMERICANS, DIET OF; RICE-BASED DIETS.

Ranjita Misra

diet: the total daily food intake, or the types of foods eaten

polyunsaturated: having multiple double bonds within the chemical structure, thus increasing the body's ability to metabolize it

fatty acids: molecules rich in carbon and hydrogen; a component of fats

antioxidant: substance that prevents oxidation, a damaging reaction with oxygen

calcium: mineral essential for bones and teeth

nutrition: the maintenance of health through proper eating, or the study of same

lipid: fats, waxes and steroids; important components of cell membranes

fiber: indigestible plant material which aids digestion by providing bulk

Bibliography

Latham, Michael C. (1997). *Human Nutrition in the Developing World.* Rome: FAO Publishing.

Internet Resources

Eastern and Central Africa Maize and Wheat Research Network. "About ECAMAW." Available from <http://www.asareca.org/ecamaw>

Okoruwa, Augustine (1996). "Nutrition and Quality of Maize." International Institute of Tropical Agriculture. Available from <http://www.iita.org/info>

Food and Agriculture Organization of the United Nations. *Maize in Human Nutrition.* Available from <http://www.fao.org/docrep>

Cravings

Most people, at some time, have a strong desire for some particular food, such as ice cream or pizza. Such a desire for a particular food, even when one is not hungry, is called a craving. There are a number of theories as to why people crave certain foods, including:

- Self-imposed food restriction.

- A **psychological** desire for a "comfort" food.

- Hormonal changes.

- Gender differences.

- Response to **stress**.

psychological: related to thoughts, feelings, and personal experiences

stress: heightened state of nervousness or unease

Food Restriction. The theory of food restriction holds that people desire those foods that they feel should be avoided. According to the dietitian Debra Waterhouse, food cravings do not cause weight gain, but denying the cravings does. This creates a vicious cycle. For example, a person may feel guilty for wanting a giant cinnamon roll that he or she smells upon entering a shopping mall. The urge is avoided, but a couple of hours later, the person may want the cinnamon roll more than ever, give in to the craving, and quickly eat the entire cinnamon roll. This leads to even stronger feelings of guilt, along with the resolve not to eat anything remotely similar for some period of time. Soon, however, the craving strikes again. The cycle becomes one of denial leading to deprivation, then to overindulgence, and then back to denial. This denial-deprivation-overindulgence pattern confirms the negative view of all food as either good or bad. It would be better, however, to imagine a world where foods are not designated as bad and not allowed, but where reasonable portions of any food can be part of a healthful **diet**. Portion control is the key.

Comfort Foods. Certain foods are usually served during holidays or special occasions. These foods become associated with comfort and happy times, eliciting feelings of relaxation and reduced stress, and are thus called "comfort foods." Some common comfort foods are ice cream, macaroni and cheese, meatloaf, pudding, cookies, and chicken. One's cultural background plays a large part in comfort-food choices. Mood also plays a roll in cravings for comfort food. Women are more likely to eat when they are sad, mad, or anxious, while men look to food when bored or lonely.

Those who find themselves reaching for comfort foods frequently should ask themselves if they are truly hungry, or whether they are using food to soothe their mood. For those who are feeding emotions with food, it is helpful to begin to replace the food with healthier activities, such as taking a walk, participating in a favorite form of exercise, or reading a good book.

Hormones and Cravings. How do **hormone** changes affect food cravings? For women, these cravings can be more intense than for men. Hormonal changes tied to the menstrual cycle are often a cause of cravings. Immediately prior to the menstrual period, the body's **estrogen** level drops, as does the **serotonin** level in the brain.

Serotonin is a **neurotransmitter**, or brain chemical, that plays a role in maintaining a relaxed feeling. When the level decreases, irritability and mood swings increase as does the craving for carbohydrate- and fat-rich foods such as chocolate, cookies, cake, potato chips, and roasted nuts. There is nothing wrong with eating a piece of chocolate, of course, but when chocolate and other craved foods become the mainstay of the diet and healthier choices get overlooked, then the cravings have gotten out of control and health may be compromised.

Gender Differences. Is there a difference between the sexes when it comes to food cravings? According to Waterhouse, the foods most frequently craved or preferred by men include hot dogs, eggs, and meat, which are all **protein** foods, while women reach for chocolate, ice cream, and bread. She attributes these differences to sex hormones and body composition. Men have larger amounts of the hormone **testosterone** and about forty pounds

---

Pregnancy Cravings

Is there any truth to the belief that pregnant women suffer intense cravings for particular foods, sometimes in odd combinations? Absolutely. According to medical researchers, pregnant women experiencing changes in hormones and an increased need for calories frequently exhibit changes in the types of foods they prefer. Common cravings include fruit, milk products, salty foods, chocolate, and other sweets. In the early stages of pregnancy, women often have a strong aversion to bitter tastes, which scientists think may serve as a warning against ingesting toxic plants or fruits during the period when a fetus is most vulnerable. In later stages of pregnancy, women often exhibit preferences for salty foods (which satisfy their increased need for sodium) and sour foods (which contribute to a varied diet). Thus the lure of pickles and potato chips.

—Paula Kepos

---

diet: the total daily food intake, or the types of foods eaten

hormone: molecules produced by one set of cells that influence the function of another set of cells

estrogen: hormone that helps control female development and menstruation

serotonin: chemical used by nerve cells to communicate with one another

neurotransmitter: molecule released by one nerve cell to stimulate or inhibit another

protein: complex molecule composed of amino acids that performs vital functions in the cell; necessary part of the diet

testosterone: male sex hormone

Women may crave ice cream when they're feeling anxious, and men may hunger for hot dogs when they get bored. These food cravings can be quieted by eating regular, healthy meals. *[Photograph by Mark Peterson. Corbis. Reproduced by permission.]*

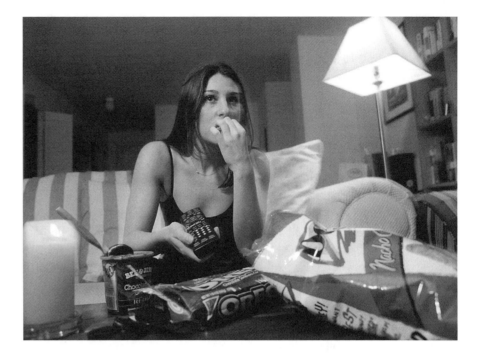

more muscle mass than women. They eat increased amounts of protein to build, repair, and synthesize muscle.

Stress Response. Many people today lead stressful lives, which can lead to stress eating. Increased stress results in a need for carbohydrates to provide **energy** for the stress response, also known as the *fight-or-flight* response (a defense reaction of the body that prepares it to fight or flee by triggering certain **cardiovascular**, hormonal, and other changes). When coping with stress, a person needs increased energy to deal with the demands placed on the body. Carbohydrates provide a fairly rapid source of fuel to the body by raising blood-glucose levels. However, when life becomes hectic and feels out of control, it is common to reach for any available food regardless of **calories** or nutritional content.

energy: technically, the ability to perform work; the content of a substance that allows it to be useful as a fuel

cardiovascular: related to the heart and circulatory system

calorie: unit of food energy

Conquering Cravings

Life will always have its stresses, but dealing with stress in a healthful, nutritional way can have a positive impact on self-esteem, energy level, emotional outlook, and weight. There are a number of positive ways to deal with cravings, including:

- Start the day off with breakfast, which helps prevent overwhelming hunger later in the day.

- Eliminate feelings of guilt related to labeling food as either good or bad. Some choices are healthier than others, but snacks and treats can be consumed in reasonable amounts.

- Plan ahead for each new week. Think about one's school, work, and activity schedule and how healthful snacks can be incorporated into it.

- Keep healthful snacks close at hand, both at home and at work.

- Try not to go for long periods of time without eating.

- Combine lean protein foods with high-fiber carbohydrate sources to provide energy that lasts for several hours, such as a slice of vegetable pizza or a bean burrito.

Cravings can be the exception instead of the rule when it comes to one's diet. Developing a lifestyle that includes healthful food selections and regular meals and snacks can help control cravings. The extra time it takes in planning meals or snacks, whether eating at home or eating on the run, is easily made up for in increased energy and improved mood. SEE ALSO EATING DISORDERS; PICA; WEIGHT MANAGEMENT.

Susan Mitchell

Bibliography

Waterhouse, Debra (1995). *Why Women Need Chocolate*. New York: Hyperion.

Mitchell, Susan, and Christie, Catherine (1997). *I'd Kill for a Cookie*. New York: Dutton.

Internet Resources

American Dietetic Association. "Eating in Stressful Times." Available from <http://www.eatright.org/pr.html>

Hellmich, Nanci. "Stress Can Put on Pounds." *USA Today*. Available from <http://usatoday.com/news>

Cultural Competence

Despite notable progress in the overall health of Americans, there are continuing disparities in health status among African Americans, Hispanics, Native Americans, and Pacific Islanders, compared to the U.S. population as a whole. In addition, the health care system is becoming more challenged as the population becomes more ethnically diverse. Therefore, the future health of the U.S. population as a whole will be influenced substantially by improvements in the health of racial and ethnic minorities.

Cultural, ethnic, linguistic, and economic differences impact how individuals and groups access and use health, education, and social services. They can also present barriers to effective education and health care interventions. This is especially true when health educators or health care practitioners stereotype, misinterpret, make faulty assumptions, or otherwise mishandle their encounters with individuals and groups viewed as different in terms of their backgrounds and experiences. The demand for culturally competent health care in the United States is a direct result of the failure of the health care system to provide adequate care to all segments of the population.

Cultural Competence, Cultural Sensitivity, and Culturally Effective Health Care

The term *cultural competence* refers to the ability to work effectively with individuals from different cultural and ethnic backgrounds, or in settings where several cultures coexist. It includes the ability to understand the language, culture, and behaviors of other individuals and groups, and to make appropriate recommendations. Cultural competence exists on a continuum from incompetence to proficiency.

Cultural sensitivity, which is a necessary component of cultural competence, means that health care professionals make an effort to be aware of

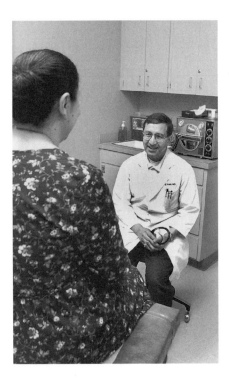

Cultural competence cannot be achieved through short workshops or classes. A long-term commitment is required to learn a second language and become familiar with other cultures to deliver effective health care for the ethnically diverse U.S. population. *[AP/Wide World Photos. Reproduced by permission.]*

diversity: the variety of cultural traditions within a larger culture

pluralistic: of many different sources

monocultural: from a single culture

the potential and actual cultural factors that affect their interactions with a client. It also means that they are willing to design programs and materials, to implement programs, and to make recommendations that are culturally relevant and culturally specific.

The terms *cultural competence* and *culturally effective health care* are sometimes used synonymously. Culturally effective health care is, indeed, related to cultural competence and cultural sensitivity. However, it goes beyond these concepts in describing the dynamic relationship between provider and client. Effective communication between providers and clients may be even more challenging when linguistic barriers exist.

Becoming Culturally Competent

Cultural competence is a developmental process that requires a long-term commitment. It is not a specific end product that occurs after a two-hour workshop, but it is an active process of learning and practicing over time. Becoming culturally competent is easier to talk about than to accomplish. Individuals working with different ethnic and cultural groups can become more culturally competent by advancing through three main stages: developing awareness, acquiring knowledge, and developing and maintaining cross-cultural skills.

Developing Awareness. Developing cultural awareness includes recognizing the value of population **diversity**. It also means an honest assessment of one's biases and stereotypes.

Acquiring Knowledge. One can never learn everything about another culture. However, acquiring knowledge about other groups is the foundation of cultural competence. In addition to understanding other cultures, it is essential to understand how different cultural groups view one's own culture. Knowledge of another culture includes assessments of facts not only about relevant norms, values, worldviews, and the practicality of everyday life, but also about how one's culture and the services one provides are viewed.

Developing and Maintaining Cross-Cultural Skills. Even though the United States is a **pluralistic** society, most health professionals have been trained in a **monocultural** tradition. In addition, many continue to practice as if ethnic and cultural differences are insignificant. Cross-cultural skills are developed through formal coursework, informal interaction and networking, and experience.

Organizational Responsibilities

It is important for health care organizations and professional preparation programs to articulate a commitment to cultural competence and to initiate cultural-competence initiatives. Many organizations are getting social and legal pressures to do this from different segments of the population. In addition to the social impact of diversity, these organizations are beginning to realize that a commitment to diversity makes good business sense.

Professional preparation programs can play a significant role in providing the knowledge and skills for culturally competent health professionals. These programs can provide courses and other formats developed with the sole purpose of addressing cultural competence and/or cultural sensitivity.

Steps to Becoming Culturally Competent

Developing Awareness

- Admitting personal biases, stereotypes, and prejudices

- Becoming aware of cultural norms, attitudes, and beliefs

- Valuing diversity

- Willingness to extend oneself psychologically and physically to the client population

- Recognizing comfort level in different situations

Acquiring Knowledge

- Knowing how your culture is viewed by others

- Attending classes, workshops, and seminars about other cultures

- Reading about other cultures

- Watching movies and documentaries about other cultures

- Attending cultural events and festivals

- Sharing knowledge and experiences with others

- Visiting other countries

Developing and Maintaining Cross-Cultural Skills

- Making friends with people of different cultures

- Establishing professional and working relationships with people of different cultures

- Learning another language

- Learning verbal and nonverbal cues of other cultures

- Becoming more comfortable in cross-cultural situations

- Assessing what works and what does not

- Assessing how the beliefs and behaviors of the cultural group affect the client or family

- Learning to negotiate between the person's beliefs and practices and the culture of your profession

- Being more flexible

- Attending continuing education seminars and workshops

- Learning to develop culturally relevant and appropriate programs, materials, and interventions

- Learning to evaluate culturally relevant and appropriate programs, materials, and interventions

- Ongoing evaluation of personal feelings and reactions

- Overcoming fears, personal biases, stereotypes, and prejudices

They also can provide specific educational components on cultural competence and/or cultural sensitivity within the curricula, **internship** and residency programs, continuing education programs, and in-service programs. Organizations need to go beyond educating their employees and providing workshops on cultural sensitivity, however. They must also change institutional policies and procedures.

internship: training program

The Office of Minority Health and the Department of Health and Human Services made specific recommendations for culturally effective health care in the document, "Assuring Cultural Competence in Health Care: Recommendations for National Standards and an Outcomes-Focused Research Agenda." Some of these recommendations include:

- Developing and implementing a strategy to recruit, retain, and promote qualified, diverse, and culturally competent administrative, **clinical**, and support staff

- Promoting and supporting the necessary attitudes, behaviors, knowledge, and skills for staff to work respectfully and effectively with patients and each other in a culturally diverse work environment

clinical: related to hospitals, clinics, and patient care

- Developing a comprehensive strategy to address culturally and linguistically appropriate services, including strategic goals, plans, policies, and procedures

- Hiring and training interpreters and bilingual staff

- Providing a bilingual staff or free interpretation services to clients with limited English skills

- Translating and making available signage and commonly used educational materials in different languages

- Developing structures and procedures to address cross-cultural ethical and legal conflicts, complaints, or grievances by patients and staff

- Preparing and distributing an annual progress report documenting the organizations' progress in implementing these standards, including information on programs, staffing, and resources

While cultural competence has increased significantly, there is still much to be done on the personal, organizational, and societal levels. Education and training to enhance the provision of culturally effective health care must be integrated into lifelong learning. Through these activities, current and future health professionals will be prepared to meet the needs of clients from all segments of the population.

Delores C. S. James

Bibliography

American Academy of Pediatrics (1999). "Culturally Effective Pediatric Care: Education and Training Issues." *Pediatrics* 103:167–170.

Chin, Jean Lauu (2000). "Culturally Competent Health Care." *Public Health Report* 115:25–33

Kumanyika, Shiriki, and Morssink, Christian (1999). "Working Effectively in Cross-Cultural and Multicultural Settings." In *Nutrition and the Community*, 4th edition, ed. Anita Owen, Patricia Splett, and George Owen. Boston: WCB McGraw-Hill.

Internet Resource

Office of Minority Health. "Assuring Cultural Competence in Health Care: Recommendations for National Standards and an Outcomes-Focused Research Agenda." Available from <http://www.omhrc.gov/clas>

Dehydration

Dehydration is the excessive loss of water from the body. Water can be lost through urine, sweat, feces, respiration, and through the skin. Symptoms of dehydration in order of severity are: thirst, **nausea**, chills, clammy skin, increased heart rate, muscle pain, reduced sweating, dizziness, headache, shortness of breath, dry mouth, **fatigue**, lack of sweating, hallucinations, fainting, and loss of consciousness. Dehydration can affect mental alertness, renal function, circulation, and total physical capacity.

The following can help to avoid dehydration:

1. Drink before feeling thirsty

2. Drink enough fluid to have pale yellow urine

3. Avoid caffeine and alcohol, which act as **diuretics**

dehydration: loss of water

nausea: unpleasant sensation in the gut that precedes vomiting

fatigue: tiredness

diuretic: substance that depletes the body of water

142

4. Drink two to three cups of fluid two hours before exercise or heavy outside work in hot temperatures

5. Drink one to two cups of fluid every fifteen minutes during exercise or heavy outside work in hot temperatures

6. Avoid exercising during midday heat, and wear appropriate clothing that allows airflow around the body

Athletes, elderly persons, young children, and those with specific illnesses that affect fluid balance, such as severe diarrhea, are at higher risk for dehydration than the average person. SEE ALSO MALNUTRITION; ORAL REHYDRATION THERAPY; SPORTS NUTRITION.

Mindy Benedict

Bibliography

Dorland's Pocket Medical Dictionary, 23d edition (1982). Philadelphia: W. B. Saunders.

Berning, Jacqueline R., and Steen, Suzanne Nelson (1998). *Nutrition for Sport and Exercise*, 2nd edition. Gaithersburg, MD: Aspen.

Diabetes Mellitus

Diabetes mellitus is a common **metabolic** disorder resulting from defects in **insulin** action, insulin production, or both. Insulin, a **hormone** secreted by the pancreas, helps the body use and store **glucose** produced during the digestion of food. Characterized by **hyperglycemia**, symptoms of diabetes include frequent urination, increased thirst, **dehydration**, weight loss, blurred vision, **fatigue**, and, occasionally, coma. Uncontrolled hyperglycemia over time damages the eyes, nerves, blood vessels, kidneys, and heart, causing organ dysfunction and failure. A number of risk factors are attributed to the **incidence** of diabetes, including family history, age, ethnicity, and **social group** characteristics, as well as **behavioral**, lifestyle, **psychological**, and clinical factors.

The World Health Organization estimates that 150 million people had diabetes worldwide in 2002. This number is projected to double by the year 2025. Much of this increase will occur in developing countries and will be due to population growth, aging, unhealthful diets, **obesity**, and **sedentary** lifestyles. In the United States, diabetes is the sixth leading cause of death. While 6.2 percent of the population has diabetes, an estimated 5.9 million people are unaware they have the disease. In addition, about 19 percent of all deaths in the United States for those age twenty-five and older are due to diabetes-related complications.

The **prevalence** of diabetes varies by age, gender, race, and ethnicity. In the United States, about 0.19 percent of the population less than twenty years of age (151,000 people) have diabetes, versus 8.6 percent of the population twenty years of age and older. In addition, adults sixty-five and older account for 40 percent of those with diabetes, despite composing only 12 percent of the population. Considerable variations also exist in the prevalence of diabetes among various racial and ethnic groups. For example, 7.8 percent of non-Hispanic whites, 13 percent of non-Hispanic blacks, 10.2 percent of Hispanic/Latino Americans, and 15.1 percent of American Indians and Alaskan Natives have diabetes. Among Asian Americans and Pacific

diabetes: inability to regulate level of sugar in the blood

metabolic: related to processing of nutrients and building of necessary molecules within the cell

insulin: hormone released by the pancreas to regulate level of sugar in the blood

hormone: molecules produced by one set of cells that influence the function of another set of cells

glucose: a simple sugar; the most commonly used fuel in cells

hyperglycemia: high level of sugar in the blood

dehydration: loss of water

fatigue: tiredness

incidence: number of new cases reported each year

social group: tribe, clique, family, or other group of individuals

behavioral: related to behavior, in contrast to medical or other types of interventions

psychological: related to thoughts, feelings, and personal experiences

obesity: the condition of being overweight, according to established norms based on sex, age, and height

sedentary: not active

prevalence: describing the number of cases in a population at any one time

The standard method of measuring blood glucose level is called a *fingerstick,* which is a small blood sample taken from the fingertip. Diabetics must monitor their blood glucose levels daily in order to avoid dire complications such as kidney disease, blindness, stroke, and poor blood circulation. *[Photograph by Tom Stewart. Corbis. Reproduced by permission.]*

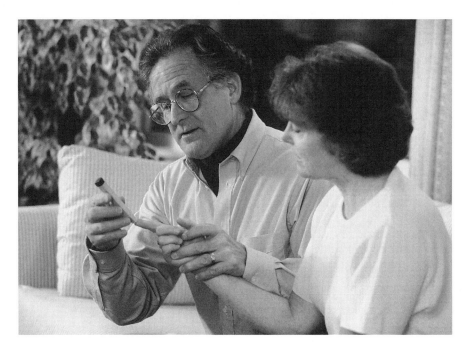

Islanders, the rate of diabetes varies substantially and is estimated at 15 to 20 percent. The prevalence of diabetes is comparable for males and females—8.3 and 8.9 percent respectively. Nevertheless, the disease is more devastating and more difficult to control among women, especially African-American and non-Hispanic white women. In fact, the risk for death is greater among young people (3.6 times greater for people from 25 to 44 years of age) and women (2.7 times greater for women ages 45 to 64 than men of the same age).

Types of Diabetes

Diabetes mellitus is classified into four categories: type 1, type 2, gestational diabetes, and other. In type 1 diabetes, specialized cells in the pancreas are destroyed, leading to a deficiency in insulin production. Type 1 diabetes frequently develops over the course of a few days or weeks. Over 95 percent of people with type 1 diabetes are diagnosed before the age of twenty-five. Estimates show 5.3 million people worldwide live with type 1 diabetes. Although the diagnosis of type 1 diabetes occurs equally among men and women, an increased prevalence exists in the white population. Type 1 diabetes in Asian children is relatively rare.

diet: the total daily food intake, or the types of foods eaten

toxins: poison

Family history, **diet**, and environmental factors are risk factors for type 1 diabetes. Studies have found an increased risk in children whose parents have type 1 diabetes, and this risk increases with maternal age. Environmental factors such as viral infections, **toxins**, and exposure to cow's milk are being contested as causing or modifying the development of type 1 diabetes.

Type 2 diabetes is characterized by insulin resistance and/or decreased insulin secretion. It is the most common form of diabetes mellitus, accounting for 90 to 95 percent of all diabetes cases worldwide. Risk factors for type 2 diabetes include family history, increasing age, obesity, physical inactivity, ethnicity, and a history of gestational diabetes. Although type 2 diabetes is frequently diagnosed in adult populations, an increasing number of children and adolescents are currently being diagnosed. Type 2 diabetes is also more common in blacks, Hispanics, Native Americans, and women, especially women with a history of gestational diabetes.

Genetics and environmental factors are the main contributors to type 2 diabetes. Physical inactivity and adoption of a Western lifestyle (particularly choosing foods with more animal **protein**, animal fats, and processed **carbohydrates**), especially in indigenous people in North American and within ethnic groups and migrants, have contributed to weight gain and obesity. In fact, obesity levels increased by 74 percent between 1991 and 2003. Increased body **fat** and abdominal obesity are associated with insulin resistance, a precursor to diabetes. Impaired glucose tolerance (IGT) and impaired fasting glucose (IFG) are two prediabetic conditions associated with insulin resistance. In these conditions, the blood glucose concentration is above the normal range, but below levels required to diagnose diabetes. Subjects with IGT and/or IFG are at substantially higher risk of developing diabetes and **cardiovascular** disease than those with normal glucose tolerance. The conversion of individuals with IGT to type 2 diabetes varies with ethnicity, **anthropometric** measures related to obesity, fasting blood glucose (a measurement of blood glucose values after not eating for 12 to 14 hours), and the two-hour post-glucose load level (a measurement of blood glucose taken exactly two hours after eating). In addition to IGT and IFG, higher than normal levels of fasting insulin, called *hyperinsulinemia*, are associated with an increased risk of developing type 2 diabetes. Insulin levels are higher in African Americans than in whites, particularly African-American women, indicating their greater predisposition for developing type 2 diabetes.

The complexity of inheritance and interaction with the environment makes identification of **genes** involved with type 2 diabetes difficult. Only a small percentage (2–5%) of diabetes cases can be explained by single gene defects and are usually atypical cases. However, a "thrifty gene," although not yet identified, is considered predictive of weight gain and the development of type 2 diabetes. Thrifty-gene theory suggests that indigenous people who experienced alternating periods of feast and **famine** gradually developed a way to store fat more efficiently during periods of plenty to better survive famines. Regardless of the thrifty gene, the contribution of **genetic** mutations in the development of type 2 diabetes has not been established, due to the number of genes that may be involved.

Gestational diabetes mellitus (GDM) is defined as any degree of glucose intolerance with onset or first recognition during pregnancy. This definition applies regardless of whether insulin or diet modification is used for treatment, and whether or not the condition persists after pregnancy. GDM affects up to 14 percent of the pregnant population—approximately 135,000 women per year in United States. GDM complicates about 4 percent of all pregnancies in the U.S. Women at greatest risk for developing GDM are **obese**, older than twenty-five years of age, have a previous history of abnormal glucose control, have first-degree relatives with diabetes, or are members of ethnic groups with a high prevalence of diabetes. Infants of a woman with GDM are at a higher risk of developing obesity, impaired glucose tolerance, or diabetes at an early age. After a pregnancy with GDM, the mother has an increased risk of developing type 2 diabetes.

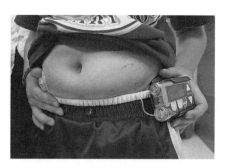

Type 1 diabetics are more likely than other diabetics to require insulin injections to regulate blood glucose levels. Insulin pumps like the one shown here can provide an extra measure of control by administering a very accurate dose of insulin on a set schedule. *[Photograph by Paul Sakuma. AP/Wide World Photos. Reproduced by permission.]*

genetics: inheritance through genes

protein: complex molecule composed of amino acids that performs vital functions in the cell; necessary part of the diet

carbohydrate: food molecule made of carbon, hydrogen, and oxygen, including sugars and starches

fat: type of food molecule rich in carbon and hydrogen, with high energy content

cardiovascular: related to the heart and circulatory system

anthropometric: related to measurement of characteristics of the human body

gene: DNA sequence that codes for proteins, and thus controls inheritance

famine: extended period of food shortage

genetic: inherited or related to the genes

obese: above accepted standards of weight for sex, height, and age

drugs: substances whose administration causes a significant change in the body's function

plasma: the fluid portion of the blood, distinct from the cellular portion

hemoglobin: the iron-containing molecule in red blood cells that carries oxygen

ketoacidosis: accumulation of ketone bodies along with high acid levels in the body fluids

energy: technically, the ability to perform work; the content of a substance that allows it to be useful as a fuel

triglyceride: a type of fat

ketones: chemicals produced by fat breakdown; molecule containing a double-bonded oxygen linked to two carbons

pneumonia: lung infection

electrolyte: salt dissolved in fluid

Other forms of diabetes are associated with genetic defects in the specialized cells of the pancreas, drug or chemical use, infections, or other diseases. The most notable of the genetically linked diabetes is *maturity onset diabetes of the young* (MODY). Characterized by the onset of hyperglycemia before the age of twenty-five, insulin secretion is impaired while minimal or no defects exist in insulin action. **Drugs**, infections, and diseases cause diabetes by damaging the pancreas and/or impairing insulin action or secretion.

Diabetes Complications

People with diabetes are at increased risk for serious long-term complications. Hyperglycemia, as measured by fasting **plasma** glucose concentration or glycosylated **hemoglobin** (HbA1c), causes structural and functional changes in the retina, nerves, kidneys, and blood vessels. This damage can lead to blindness, numbness, reduced circulation, amputations, kidney disease, and cardiovascular disease. Type 1 diabetes is more likely to lead to kidney failure. About 40 percent of people with type 1 diabetes develop severe kidney disease and kidney failure by the age of fifty. Nevertheless, between 1993 and 1997, more than 100,000 people in the United States were treated for kidney failure caused by type 2 diabetes.

African Americans experience higher rates of diabetes-related complications such as eye disease, kidney failure, and amputations. They also experience greater disability from these complications. The frequency of diabetic retinopathy (disease of the small blood vessels in the retina causing deterioration of eyesight) is 40 to 50 percent higher in African Americans than in white Americans. In addition, the rate of diabetic retinopathy among Mexican Americans is more than twice that of non-Hispanic white Americans. Furthermore, African Americans with diabetes are much more likely to undergo a lower-extremity amputation than white or Hispanic Americans with diabetes. Little is known about these complications in Asian and Pacific Islander-Americans.

Diabetic **ketoacidosis** (DKA) and hyperosmolar hyperglycemia state (HHS) are serious diabetic emergencies and the most frequent cause of mortality. Both DKA and HHS result from an insulin deficiency and an increase in counter-regulatory hormones (a.k.a. hyperglycemia). Hyperglycemia leads to glycosuria (glucose in the urine), increased urine output, and dehydration. Because the glucose is excreted in the urine, the body becomes starved for **energy**. At this point, the body either continues to excrete glucose in the urine making the hyperglycemia worse (HHS), or the body begins to break down **triglycerides** causing the release of **ketones** (by-products of fat breakdown) into the urine and bloodstream (DKA). The mortality rate of patients with DKA is less than 5 percent while the mortality rate of HHS patients is about 15 percent. Infection (urinary tract infections and **pneumonia** account for 30 to 50 percent of cases), omission of insulin, and increased amounts of counter-regulatory hormones contribute to DKA and HHS. Type 1 and type 2 diabetic patients may experience DKA and HHS. However, DKA is more common in type 1 diabetic patients, while HHS is more common in type 2 diabetic patients. Treatment of DKA and HHS involves correction of dehydration, hyperglycemia, ketoacidosis, and **electrolyte** deficits and imbalances.

Diabetes, Heart Disease, and Stroke

Many people with diabetes are not aware that they are at particularly high risk for heart disease and stroke, which can result from the poor blood flow that is a symptom of diabetes. In addition, people with type 2 diabetes have higher rates of hypertension and obesity, which are additional risk factors. Diabetics are two to four times more likely to have a heart attack than nondiabetics, and at least 65 percent of people with diabetes die from heart attack or stroke. While deaths from heart disease have been declining overall, deaths from heart disease among women with diabetes have increased, and deaths from heart disease among men with diabetes have not declined nearly as rapidly as they have among the general male population. The National Diabetes Education Program has launched a campaign to bring the problem to public attention. Patients are advised to work with medical personnel to control their glucose level, blood pressure, and cholesterol level and, of course, to avoid smoking.

Treatment for Diabetes

Treatment for diabetes involves following a regimen of diet, exercise, self-monitoring of blood glucose, and taking medication or insulin injections. Although type 1 diabetes is primarily managed with daily insulin injections, type 2 diabetes can be controlled with diet and exercise. However, when diet and exercise fail, medication is added to stimulate the production of insulin, reduce insulin resistance, decrease the liver's output of glucose, or slow **absorption** of carbohydrate from the **gastrointestinal** tract. When medication fails, insulin is required.

Following the diagnosis of diabetes, a diabetic patient undergoes medical **nutrition** therapy. In other words, a registered dietician performs a nutritional assessment to evaluate the diabetic patient's food intake, metabolic status, lifestyle, and readiness to make changes, along with providing dietary instruction and goal setting. The assessment is individualized and takes into account cultural, lifestyle, and financial considerations. The goals of medical nutrition therapy are to attain appropriate blood glucose, lipid, **cholesterol**, and triglyceride levels, which are critical to preventing the **chronic** complications associated with diabetes. For meal planning, the diabetic exchange system provides a quick method for estimating and maintaining the proper balance of carbohydrates, fats, proteins, and **calories**. In the exchange system, foods are categorized into groups, with each group having food with similar amounts of carbohydrate, protein, fat, and calories. Based on the individual's diabetes treatment plan and goals, any food on the list can be exchanged with another food within the same group.

Exercise and blood glucose monitoring are also critical components of a diabetic patient's self-management. Exercise improves blood glucose control, increases sensitivity to insulin, reduces cardiovascular risk factors, contributes to weight loss, and improves well-being. Exercise further contributes to a reduction in the risk factors for diabetes-related complications. Daily self-monitoring of blood glucose levels allows diabetic patients to evaluate and make adjustments in diet, exercise, and medications. Self-monitoring also assists in preventing **hypoglycemic** episodes.

Diabetes mellitus is a chronic and debilitating disease. Attributed to genetics, physical inactivity, obesity, ethnicity, and a number of environmental

absorption: uptake by the digestive tract

gastrointestinal: related to the stomach and intestines

nutrition: the maintenance of health through proper eating, or the study of same

cholesterol: multi-ringed molecule found in animal cell membranes; a type of lipid

chronic: over a long period

calorie: unit of food energy

hypoglycemic: related to low level of blood sugar

factors, diabetes requires lifestyle changes and medication adherence in order to control blood glucose levels. Due to the damage caused by hyperglycemia, diabetic patients also experience a number of complications related to the disease. With good self-management practices, however, individuals with diabetes can live a long and productive life. SEE ALSO CARBOHYDRATES; EXCHANGE SYSTEM; GLYCEMIC INDEX; HYPERGLYCEMIA; HYPOGLYCEMIA; INSULIN.

Julie Lager

Bibliography

American Diabetes Association (2003) "Gestational Diabetes Mellitus." *Diabetes Care* 26(1):S103–S105.

American Diabetes Association (2003) "Hyperglycemic Crises in Patients with Diabetes Mellitus." *Diabetes Care* 26(1):S109–S117.

American Diabetes Association (2003) "Physical Activity/Exercise and Diabetes Mellitus." *Diabetes Care* 26(1):S73–77.

American Diabetes Association (2003) "Standards of Medical Care for Patients with Diabetes Mellitus." *Diabetes Care* 26(1):S33–S50.

Atkinson, Mark A., and Eisenbarth, George S. (2001). "Type 1 Diabetes: New Perspectives on Disease Pathogenesis and Treatment." *Lancet* 358:221–229.

Black, Sandra A. (2002). "Diabetes, Diversity, and Disparity: What Do We Do with the Evidence?" *American Journal of Public Health* 92(4):543–548.

Chiasson, Jean-Louis; Aris-Jilwan, Nahla; Belanger, Raphael; Bertrand, Sylvie; Beauregard, Hugues; Ekoe, Jean-Marie; Fournier, Helene; and Havrankova, Jana (2003). "Diagnosis and Treatment of Diabetic Ketoacidosis and the Hyperglycemic Hyperosmolar State." *Canadian Medical Association Journal* 168(7):859–866.

Green, Anders (1996). "Prevention of IDDM: The Genetic Epidemiologic Perspective." *Diabetes Research and Clinical Practice* 34:S101–S1006.

Mandrup-Paulson, Thomas (1998). "Recent Advances: Diabetes." *British Medical Journal* 316(18):1221–1225.

Mokdad, Ali H.; Ford, Earl S.; Bowman, Barbara A.; Dietz, William, H.; Vinicor, Frank; Bales, Virginia, S.; and Marks, James S. (2003). "Prevalence of Obesity, Diabetes, and Obesity-Related Health Risk Factors, 2001." *Journal of the American Medical Association* 289(1):76–79.

Jovanovic, Lois, and Pettitt, David J. (2001). "Gestational Diabetes Mellitus." *Journal of the American Medical Association* 283(20):2516–2518.

Kitabchi, Abbas E.; Umpierrez, Guillermo E.; Murphy, Mary Beth; Barrett, Eugene J.; Kreisberg, Robert A.; Malone, John I.; and Wall, Barry M. (2001). "Management of Hyperglycemic Crises in Patients with Diabetes." *Diabetes Care* 24(1):131–153.

Simpson, R. W.; Shaw, J. E.; and Zimmet, P. Z. (2003). "The Prevention of Type 2 Diabetes—Lifestyle Change or Pharmacotherapy? A Challenge for the 21st Century." *Diabetes Research and Clinical Practice* 59:165–180.

Yki-Jarvinen, Hannele (1998). "Toxicity of Hyperglycemia in Type 2 Diabetes." *Diabetes/Metabolism Reviews* 14:S45–S50.

Internet Resources

American Diabetes Association. "Basic Diabetes Information." Available from <http://www.diabetes.org>

Centers for Disease Control and Prevention. "Diabetes Public Health Resource." Available from <http://www.cdc.gov/diabetes>

National Diabetes Information Clearinghouse (NDIC). "Diabetes." Available from <http://diabetes.niddk.nih.gov>

World Health Organization. "Fact Sheets: Diabetes Mellitus." Available from <http://www.who.int>

Diarrhea

Diarrhea, a condition that has a major impact on global health, is highly correlated with nutritional status. It is an important area of focus due not only to its high worldwide **prevalence** and health costs, but also because it can be significantly reduced by appropriate interventions and treatment.

Diarrhea has various causes and symptoms, resulting in a wide range of definitions for this illness. The U.S. National Institutes of Health (NIH) defines diarrhea as loose, watery stools occurring more than three times a day, which is the most common definition. The term **acute** *diarrhea* is used to describe an episode lasting less than three weeks. *Persistent diarrhea* is an episode that lasts more than fourteen days, and **chronic** *diarrhea* is the term for recurring episodes of diarrhea. *Dysentery* is diarrhea that contains blood. The severity of diarrhea ranges from **asymptomatic** to severe **dehydration** resulting in death.

Causes of Diarrhea

Diarrhea can present in many ways because it has many potential causes. Most cases of diarrhea are caused by some type of infection. For example, surveillance studies in rural Bangladesh have cited infection as the cause of 86 percent of the cases of diarrhea in that population. This is the case in much of the developing world. Regardless of the cause, diarrhea results from an alteration of the lining of the wall of the **intestines**. Normal digestion occurs when there is a balance of fluid and **nutrients** across the **bowel** wall. Disruption of this process can be caused directly by organisms, **toxins**, or immune reactions. Any imbalance alters the composition of the stool and the motility (motion) of the bowel wall, resulting in an increased loss of fluid and nutrients. Dehydration is the result of loss of body fluids and **electrolytes**. A loss of 5 percent of body weight can result in a rapid heart rate, dizziness, decreased urination, disorientation, and even coma. A 10 percent loss of body weight caused by severe diarrhea can lead to **acidosis**, **shock**, and death.

People in developing countries suffer most from infectious forms of diarrhea. Most infections pass through a fecal-oral route. This results from environmental causes such as poor sanitation, decreased access to clean water, and a poor understanding of transmission and treatment of disease. These are conditions that arise most frequently in the developing world, though they affect both rural and urban populations. Improvements in these areas result in a dramatic reduction of cases of infectious diarrhea, as shown in studies in numerous developing nations, such as India, Gambia, and elsewhere, where poor **socioeconomic status** affects a large percentage of the population. *Traveler's diarrhea* is the result of exposure to such infectious agents when visiting countries where sanitation is inadequate.

Diarrhea in Developing Nations

Diarrhea is a major cause of death in much of the world, particularly in developing nations, where the effect is greatest among the young. The World Health Organization (WHO) attributes 3.5 million deaths a year to diarrhea, with 80 percent of these deaths occurring in children under the age of five, and most occurring in children between six months and three years of age. Children are the most susceptible because a smaller amount of fluid

prevalence: describing the number of cases in a population at any one time

acute: rapid-onset and short-lived

chronic: over a long period

asymptomatic: without symptoms

dehydration: loss of water

intestines: the two long tubes that carry out the bulk of the processes of digestion

nutrient: dietary substance necessary for health

bowel: intestines and rectum

toxins: poison

electrolyte: salt dissolved in fluid

acidosis: elevated acid level in the blood

shock: state of dangerously low blood pressure and loss of blood delivered to the tissues

socioeconomic status: level of income and social class

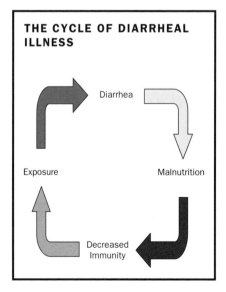

THE CYCLE OF DIARRHEAL ILLNESS

Diarrhea

Malnutrition

Decreased Immunity

Exposure

CAUSES OF DIARRHEA

Causes	Examples
Viral infections	Rotavirus, Norwalk virus
Bacterial infections	E. coli, Vibrio cholerae, Campylobacter, Shigella
Parasites	Giardia, Entamoeba
Helminths (intestinal worms)	Strongyloides
Allergic	Lactose intolerance, celiac sprue, medication side effects
Autoimmune	Ulcerative colitis, Crohn's disease
Malabsorptive	Pancreatic deficiency, biliary disease
Nutritional	Zinc deficiency, vitamin A deficiency, enteral feedings consisting of liquid nutritional formulas delivered straight to the bowels
Functional	Irritable bowel syndrome, short bowel syndrome, cancer

energy: technically, the ability to perform work; the content of a substance that allows it to be useful as a fuel

malnutrition: chronic lack of sufficient nutrients to maintain health

absorption: uptake by the digestive tract

immune system: the set of organs and cells, including white blood cells, that protect the body from infection

malnourished: lack of adequate nutrients in the diet

zinc: mineral necessary for many enzyme processes

catabolism: breakdown of complex molecules

protein: complex molecule composed of amino acids that performs vital functions in the cell; necessary part of the diet

undernutrition: food intake too low to maintain adequate energy expenditure without weight loss

calorie: unit of food energy

wean: cease breastfeeding

loss is necessary to result in significant dehydration, because they have fewer internal resources, and because their **energy** requirements are higher.

Children in developing nations suffer from an average of four cases of diarrhea a year. Most of these cases are infectious diarrhea. Infectious diarrhea also contributes to **malnutrition** due to a decreased nutritional intake and diminished **absorption** of vital nutrients during the acute episode and recovery period. Malnutrition, in turn, decreases the ability of the **immune system** to fight further infections, making diarrheal episodes more frequent.

Studies have shown that poor nutritional status can double the risk of contracting diarrhea when exposed to an infectious agent. In addition, the duration of the acute episode can be up to three times as long in **malnourished** children. In addition, reduced immunity and deficiencies of nutrients such as vitamin A and **zinc**, which are common in malnourished individuals, can increase the health risks from diarrhea. Diarrhea also causes decreased appetite and food intake, decreased absorption of nutrients from the food that is ingested, and increased **catabolism** of body **proteins**. The resulting **undernutrition** stunts future mental and physical development.

Eating patterns before and after diarrheal episodes play an important role in this cycle. In developing countries, environmental factors, such as pervasive bacterial contamination of water used for drinking, cooking, and cleaning, contribute to continued exposure to agents that cause diarrhea. Maternal practices related to feeding are also a factor. Reduced breastfeeding rates in developing nations mean that fewer children receive the protective and nutritional benefits of breast milk. Nursing allows for the delivery of milk high in fats, proteins, and **calories** in a sterile fashion. When illness causes mothers to **wean** their children too early, nutritious breast milk is replaced with cereals and gruels that are often low in calories and proteins and are made with contaminated water. Commercial formulas are also often diluted with contaminated water and put in bottles that are not sterile.

A lack of maternal education often leads to the common practice of withholding food during acute episodes of diarrhea out of fear that eating will exacerbate the symptoms. Because of the nutritional losses from diarrhea, children actually need up to a 30 percent increase in calories and a 100 percent increase in protein intake during the acute and recovery stages of diarrhea. Studies have shown that children who receive increased nourishment during this time suffer less from the acute and long-term effects of diarrhea. The WHO recommends the continuation of breastfeeding throughout an acute episode, as well as the use of mixed food cereals high in calories and protein. There is also evidence to support zinc supplementation, which can reduce the **morbidity** rates from diarrhea.

morbidity: illness or accident

Treatment

The mainstay of treatment for diarrhea is rehydration to replace the fluid and electrolyte losses. This is the cornerstone of oral rehydration therapy (ORT), which has greatly reduced the morbidity and mortality from diarrheal illnesses throughout the world. Rehydration must be combined with the fulfillment of increased nutritional demands. **Antibiotics** have a very limited role in effectively reducing morbidity and mortality from diarrhea, and antimotility and absorbent agents have virtually no role.

antibiotic: substance that kills or prevents the growth of microorganisms

It is evident that the morbidity and mortality from diarrhea results from a complex interplay of environmental hazards, risk factors, and treatment response. Interventions to reduce the global impact of diarrhea must therefore be multifactorial in their approach. This is an illness that imposes a large health burden on society, but has avenues for effective intervention. SEE ALSO MALNUTRITION; ORAL REHYDRATION THERAPY.

Seema Pania Kumar

Bibliography

Basch, Paul (1999). *Textbook of International Health.* New York: Oxford University Press.

Chen, Lincoln, and Scrimshaw, Nevin (1983). *Diarrhea and Malnutrition: Interactions, Mechanisms, and Interventions.* New York: Plenum Press.

Semba, Richard, and Bloem, Martin (2000). *Nutrition and Health in Developing Countries.* Totowa, NJ: Humana Press.

Internet Resources

National Institutes of Health. <http://www.nih.gov>

World Health Organization. <http://www.who.int>

Diet

The term *diet* refers to a person's pattern of eating and drinking. Diet is influenced by many factors, including income, culture, religion, geographic location, and lifestyle. A balanced diet contains food from several food groups and supplies the body with the **energy** and essential **nutrients** it needs (as defined by the Food Guide Pyramid and **Dietary Reference Intakes**).

energy: technically, the ability to perform work; the content of a substance that allows it to be useful as a fuel

nutrient: dietary substance necessary for health

Dietary Reference Intakes: set of guidelines for nutrient intake

The Food Guide Pyramid lists food categories and serving recommendations. Dietary Reference Intake values provide a range of dietary recommendations, including the **Recommended Dietary Allowances** (RDAs), which provide the daily intake needed to meet the needs of "nearly all healthy persons." Dietary recommendations, and how they are represented, vary around the world. Most, however, convey a common message: balance,

Recommended Dietary Allowances: nutrient intake recommended to promote health

variety, and moderation in food choices. SEE ALSO EATING HABITS; DIETARY REFERENCE INTAKES; FOOD GUIDE PYRAMID; RECOMMENDED DIETARY ALLOWANCES.

Delores Truesdell

Bibliography

Brown, Judith (2002). *Nutrition through the Life Cycle.* Belmont, CA: Wadsworth.

Internet Resource

United States Department of Agriculture, Food and Nutrition Center. "Food Guide Pyramid." Available from <http://nal.usda.gov/fnic>

Dietary Assessment

A dietary assessment is a comprehensive evaluation of a person's food intake. It is one of four parts of a **nutrition** assessment done in a **clinical** setting. These four parameters of assessment include: (1) an assessment of **anthropometrics** (weight, height, weight-to-height ratio, head circumference, **body mass index**, etc.); (2) dietary assessment, which includes a **diet** history or food frequency analysis; (3) a physical examination with a medical history; and (4) **biochemical** exams or blood/urine tests.

Reviewing a person's dietary data may suggest risk factors for **chronic** diseases and help to prevent them. Laboratory tests may uncover **malnutrition** and detect problems before any side effects appear, such as the tiredness and apathy associated with iron-deficiency **anemia**. The strengths of a simple blood test and food intake record are that these are easy to do and are affordable and appropriate for most people.

Problems with using diet histories can occur because a person's memory about what he or she ate earlier may not be accurate. It can also be time-consuming to collect food intake records. There are also problems with interpreting food intakes, laboratory values, and appropriate weights and heights.

A final area of concern related to dietary assessment is what to do with the information once it has been gathered. Providing nutrition education and counseling to people of different ages and from different backgrounds requires a great deal of skill and a good understanding of diet quality, normal eating, and normal physical and psychosocial development. It is important to treat people as individuals with unique needs and concerns. Dietitians are trained to do this, but many health care workers are not trained to measure diet quality, define dietary moderation, or provide counseling. SEE ALSO NUTRITIONAL ASSESSMENT.

Delores Truesdell

nutrition: the maintenance of health through proper eating, or the study of same

clinical: related to hospitals, clinics, and patient care

anthropometric: related to measurement of characteristics of the human body

body mass index: weight in kilograms divided by square of the height in meters times 100; a measure of body fat

diet: the total daily food intake, or the types of foods eaten

biochemical: related to chemical processes within cells

chronic: over a long period

malnutrition: chronic lack of sufficient nutrients to maintain health

anemia: low level of red blood cells in the blood

Internet Resources

American Heart Association. "Healthy Lifestyle: Diet and Nutrition." Available from <http://www.americanheart.org>

U.S. Department of Agriculture (2000). "Dietary Guidelines for Americans," 5th edition. Available from <http://www.usda.gov/cnpp>

U.S. Department of Agriculture, Food and Nutrition Information Center. "Dietary Assessment." Available from <http://www.nal.usda/fnic>

Dietary Guidelines

The Dietary Guidelines for Americans are the foundation of national **nutrition** policy for the United States. They are designed to help Americans make food choices that promote health and reduce the risk of disease. The guidelines are published jointly by the U.S. Department of Agriculture (USDA) and U.S. Department of Health and Human Services (HHS). The first set of guidelines was published as *Nutrition and Your Health: Dietary Guidelines for Americans* in 1980. Since then, an advisory committee has been appointed every five years to review and revise the guidelines based on the latest research in nutrition and health.

Early Dietary Advice in the United States

The first half of the twentieth century was a period of enormous growth in nutrition knowledge. The primary goal of nutrition advice at this time was to help people select foods to meet their **energy** (**calorie**) needs and prevent **nutritional deficiencies**. During the Great Depression of the 1930s, food was rationed and people had little money to buy food. They needed to know how to select an adequate **diet** with few resources, and the USDA produced a set of meal plans that were affordable for families of various incomes. To this day, a food guide for low-income families—the Thrifty Food Plan—is issued regularly by the USDA and used to determine food stamp allotments. In addition to meal plans, the USDA developed food guides—tools to help people select healthful diets. Over the years the food guides changed, based on the current information available.

Food Guides versus Dietary Guidelines

Food guides are practical tools that people can use to select a healthful diet. Food guide recommendations, such as how many servings of grains to eat, are based on dietary guidelines that are overall recommendations for healthful diets. For example, the Dietary Guidelines for Americans include the recommendation that Americans "choose a variety of grains daily, especially whole grains." To help people reach this goal, the USDA's Food Guide Pyramid is built on a base of grain foods and recommends six to eleven servings daily with several servings from whole grains. Thus, the Food Guide Pyramid supports the recommendations of the Dietary Guidelines.

Evolution of the Dietary Guidelines

During the 1970s, scientists began identifying links between people's usual eating habits and their risk for **chronic** diseases such as **heart disease** and **cancer**. They realized that a healthful diet was important not only to prevent **nutrient** deficiencies, but because it might play a role in decreasing the risk for chronic diseases. Since heart disease and cancer were, and still are, major causes of death and disability in the United States, there was a need to help Americans select health-promoting diets.

The first major step in federal dietary guidance was the 1977 publication of *Dietary Goals for the United States* by the Senate Select Committee on Nutrition and Human Needs, which recommended an increased intake of **carbohydrates** and a reduced intake of **fat, saturated fat, cholesterol,**

nutrition: the maintenance of health through proper eating, or the study of same

energy: technically, the ability to perform work; the content of a substance that allows it to be useful as a fuel

calorie: unit of food energy

nutritional deficiency: lack of adequate nutrients in the diet

diet: the total daily food intake, or the types of foods eaten

chronic: over a long period

heart disease: any disorder of the heart or its blood supply, including heart attack, atherosclerosis, and coronary artery disease

cancer: uncontrolled cell growth

nutrient: dietary substance necessary for health

carbohydrate: food molecule made of carbon, hydrogen, and oxygen, including sugars and starches

fat: type of food molecule rich in carbon and hydrogen, with high energy content

saturated fat: a fat with the maximum possible number of hydrogens; more difficult to break down that unsaturated fats

cholesterol: multi-ringed molecule found in animal cell membranes; a type of lipid

fiber: indigestible plant material that aids digestion by providing bulk

salt, and sugar. There was heated debate among nutrition scientists when the Dietary Goals were published. Some nutritionists believed that not enough was known about effects of diet and health to make suggestions as specific as those given.

In 1980, the first edition of Dietary Guidelines for Americans was released by the USDA and HHS. The seven guidelines were: (1) Eat a variety of foods; (2) Maintain ideal weight; (3) Avoid too much fat, saturated fat, and cholesterol; (4) Eat foods with adequate starch and **fiber**; (5) Avoid too much sugar; (6) Avoid too much sodium; and (7) If you drink alcohol, do so in moderation. The second edition, released in 1985, made a few changes, but kept most of the guidelines intact. Two exceptions were the weight guideline, which was changed to "Maintain desirable weight" and the last guideline, in which "alcohol" was changed to "alcoholic beverages."

Following publication of the second edition of the Dietary Guidelines, two influential reports concerning diet and health were issued. The *Surgeon General's Report on Nutrition and Health* was published in 1988, and the National Research Council's report *Diet and Health—Implications for Reducing Chronic Disease Risk* was published in 1989. These two reports supported the goal of the Dietary Guidelines to promote eating habits that can help people stay healthy. In 1990, the third edition of the guidelines took a more positive tone than previous editions, using phrases such as "Choose a diet..." or "Use ... only in moderation," rather than "Avoid too much..." This was seen as a positive step by many nutrition educators.

The fourth edition was the first to include the Food Guide Pyramid, which had been introduced in 1992. It also was the first edition to address vegetarian diets and the recently introduced "Nutrition Facts" panel for food labels. The fifth edition, issued in 2000, expanded the number of guidelines to ten and organized them into three messages: "Aim for Fitness, Build a Healthy Base, and Choose Sensibly" (ABC).

The Dietary Guidelines for Americans have evolved since they were first published in 1980. Their recommendations represent the latest research in diet and health promotion, and, as new research emerges, the guidelines will continue to change to reflect new insights into diet and health. People can take steps toward healthier lifestyles by following the recommendations of the Dietary Guidelines and using tools like the Food Guide Pyramid to guide their food choices. SEE ALSO DIETARY TRENDS, AMERICAN; FOOD GUIDE PYRAMID.

Linda Benjamin Bobroff

The 2000 Dietary Guidelines for Americans

Aim for Fitness

- Aim for a healthy weight
- Be physically active each day

Build a Healthy Base

- Let the Pyramid guide your food choices
- Choose a variety of grains daily, especially whole grains
- Choose a variety of fruits and vegetables daily
- Keep food safe to eat

Choose Sensibly

- Choose a diet that is low in fat and cholesterol and moderate in fat
- Choose beverages and foods to moderate your intake of sugar
- Choose and prepare foods with less salt
- If you drink alcoholic beverages, do so in moderation

Bibliography

Cronin, Frances J., and Shaw, Anne M. (1988). "Summary of Dietary Recommendations for Healthy Americans." *Nutrition Today* 23:26–34.

National Research Council (1989). *Diet and Health: Implications for Reducing Chronic Disease Risk.* Washington, DC: National Academy Press.

U.S. Department of Agriculture, and U.S. Department of Health and Human Services (1980). *Nutrition and Your Health: Dietary Guidelines for Americans.* (Home and Garden Bulletin 232.) Washington, DC: U.S. Government Printing Office.

U.S. Department of Agriculture, and U.S. Department of Health and Human Services (2000). *Nutrition and Your Health: Dietary Guidelines for Americans,* 5th ed. Washington, DC: Government Printing Office.

U.S. Department of Health and Human Services, Public Health Service (1988). *The Surgeon General's Report on Nutrition and Health.* (DHHS [PHS] Publication No. 88-50210.) Washington, DC: U.S. Government Printing Office.

Dietary Reference Intakes

Dietary Reference Intakes (DRIs) are a set of **nutrient** reference values. They are used to help people select healthful diets, set national **nutrition** policy, and establish safe upper limits of intake. DRIs include four sets of nutrient standards: Estimated Average Requirement (EAR), Recommended Dietary Allowance (RDA), Adequate Intake (AI), and Tolerable Upper Intake Level (UL). Starting in the mid-1990s, DRIs began to replace RDAs and Recommended Nutrient Intakes for Canadians, which had been the standards for the United States and for Canada, respectively.

Each component of the DRIs has a unique purpose. The EARs are average nutrient requirements for a population group (e.g., females ages 19–30). They are used in nutrition research and to set nutrition policy. RDA values are based on the EARs. RDA values represent a level of nutrient intake that would meet the needs of about 97 percent of people in a particular group.

If there is not enough information to set RDA values, then an AI may be established for that nutrient. The AI is based on information about average intake of the nutrient by a healthy group of people. RDA and AI are both used to plan healthful diets for individuals.

Not only is it important to know how much of a nutrient is needed for good health, it is also critical to know how much of a nutrient is too much. The UL is the highest intake of a nutrient that does not pose a threat to health for most people. Intake higher than the UL can cause adverse health effects, especially over time. SEE ALSO DIETARY ASSESSMENT; RECOMMENDED DIETARY ALLOWANCES; NUTRIENTS.

Linda Benjamin Bobroff

nutrient: dietary substance necessary for health

nutrition: the maintenance of health through proper eating, or the study of same

Bibliography

Insel, Paul; Turner, R. Elaine; and Ross, Don (2001). *Nutrition.* Sudbury, MA: Jones and Bartlett.

Sizer, Frances, and Whitney, Eleanor (2000). *Nutrition Concepts and Controversies,* 8th edition. Belmont, CA: Wadsworth/Thomson Learning.

Internet Resource

Food and Nutrition Information Center, U.S. Department of Agriculture. "Dietary Reference Intakes (DRI) and Recommended Dietary Allowances (RDA)." Available from <http://www.nal.usda.gov/fnic>

Dietary Supplements

The demand for dietary supplements in the United States catapulted what was once a cottage industry into a $14 billion per year business in the year 2000. In 1994, the U.S. Congress formally defined the term *dietary supplement* as a product taken by mouth that contains a "dietary ingredient" intended to supplement the **diet**. The dietary ingredients in these products may include **vitamins**, **minerals**, herbs, **amino acids**, **enzymes**, organ tissues, glandulars, and **metabolites**. Dietary supplements can also be extracts or concentrates, and may be found in many forms, such as tablets, capsules, liquids, or powders.

The use of dietary supplements is widespread—they are taken by half of American adults. But the use of supplements is not limited to adults. A study

diet: the total daily food intake, or the types of foods eaten

vitamin: necessary complex nutrient used to aid enzymes or other metabolic processes in the cell

mineral: an inorganic (non-carbon-containing) element, ion, or compound

amino acid: building block of proteins, necessary dietary nutrient

enzyme: protein responsible for carrying out reactions in a cell

metabolite: the product of metabolism, or nutrient processing within the cell

Baby Boomers and Nutritional Supplements

Informed, prosperous, and health-conscious, the baby boomers are known as a generation that plans to fight vigorously against the encroachments of age. During the 1990s, as the boomers began reaching their fifties, they increasingly turned to supplements to ward off osteoporosis, memory loss, and a host of other ailments. With increased demand, the vitamins, minerals, and herbs they sought migrated from health food stores to mass merchandisers. Between 1997 and 2002 the supplement industry experienced a 34 percent jump in sales, to more than $19 billion annually.

—*Paula Kepos*

food additive: substance added to foods to improve nutrition, taste, appearance or shelf-life

drugs: substances whose administration causes a significant change in the body's function

efficacy: effectiveness

calcium: mineral essential for bones and teeth

osteoporosis: weakening of the bone structure

scurvy: a syndrome characterized by weakness, anemia, and spongy gums, due to vitamin C deficiency

antioxidant: substance that prevents oxidation, a damaging reaction with oxygen

published in the November 2001 *Journal of the American Dietetic Association* showed that dietary supplement use is prevalent among students as well, with 17.6 percent of 1,532 eighth-graders reporting the use of a vitamin-mineral supplement. Herbs, one type of dietary supplement, are widely used throughout the world. In China, traditional medicine encompasses a holistic approach to healing, and herbal remedies are routinely included in self-care. The World Health Organization (WHO) estimates that in developing countries up to 80 percent of indigenous populations rely on herbs for primary health care needs. In France and Germany, 30 to 40 percent of all medical doctors rely on herbal preparations as their primary medicines.

Regulation of Dietary Supplements

In 1994 the U.S. Congress passed the Dietary Supplement Health and Education Act (DSHEA), which President Bill Clinton signed into law the same year. One provision of DSHEA clarified the definition for dietary supplements outlined above. DSHEA also mandated the establishment of the Office of Dietary Supplements (ODS) within the National Institutes of Health. The ODS coordinates research on dietary supplements and acts as a clearinghouse for regulatory issues. It also maintains an excellent resource for consumers, the International Bibliographic Information on Dietary Supplements (IBIDS), which is a database that contains citations published in scientific journals on the topic of dietary supplements. The public can access IBIDS on the ODS website.

DSHEA established a new regulatory framework for supplement safety and for the labeling of dietary supplements by the U.S. Food and Drug Administration (FDA). Dietary supplements are regulated under food law, but with certain provisions that apply only to dietary supplements. For example, dietary supplements escape the stringent approval process that **food additives** and **drugs** must go through before being marketed to the public, unless the manufacturer of a dietary supplement makes a claim for therapeutic **efficacy**.

DSHEA also gave manufacturers the freedom to provide information about product benefits on labels through three types of claims. *Health claims* describe a relationship between a food substance and a disease or health-related condition. For example, the health claim "diets high in **calcium** may reduce the risk of **osteoporosis**" has been authorized by the FDA and may appear on the labels of dietary supplements. *Structure function claims* may state a benefit related to a nutrient-deficiency disease (such as **scurvy**, which is caused by a deficiency of vitamin C), as long as the statement tells how widespread the disease is. These claims may also describe the role of a nutrient intended to affect a structure or function—for example, "**antioxidants** maintain cell integrity," or "calcium builds strong bones." *Nutrient content claims* describe the level of a nutrient or dietary substance in a product, using FDA-regulated terms such as "good source," "high," or "free." For example, if a label claims a dietary supplement is fat-free, the supplement must contain less than 0.5 grams of fat per serving.

However, information on supplement labels cannot be false or misleading. For example, statements that a product will treat, cure, or diagnose a disease are reserved for drugs. That is why the label of the popular herbal extract echinacea may boast that the herb "supports good immune function" but will not claim to "cure your cold."

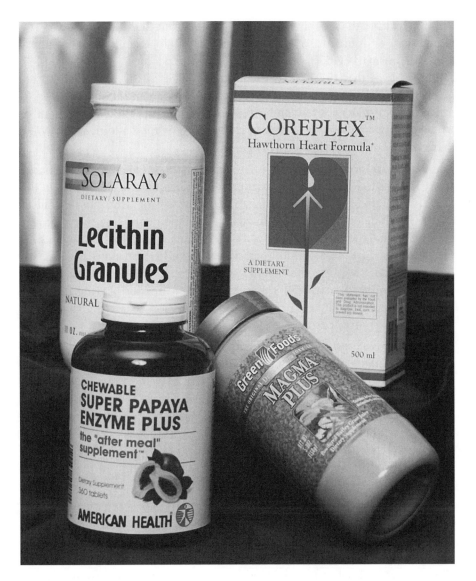

Because they are not regulated as strictly as drugs, dietary supplements can cause unpredictable side effects. For example, studies have shown an increased risk of prostate cancer among men who take beta-carotene supplements and drink alcohol, and an increased risk of lung cancer among people who take beta-carotene supplements and smoke. *[Photograph by Robert J. Huffman. Field Mark Publications. Reproduced by permission.]*

In Germany, herbs and herbal products are regulated in a different way than in the United States. In 1978, the German Federal Health Agency established the German Commission E to investigate the safety and efficacy of herbal remedies commonly used in Germany. The commission weighed evidence from the literature, from anecdotal reports, and from clinical studies. They subsequently developed monographs on over 400 herbs. These monographs are now used worldwide as essential references on herbal therapy. The commission also established indications (how an herb is used medicinally) and dosage recommendations, resulting in the successful mainstreaming of herbs into medical practice. German physicians frequently prescribe the herbs ginkgo biloba, hawthorn, St. John's wort, horse chestnut, and saw palmetto. Unlike U.S. law, German law allows herb manufacturers to market herbs with drug claims if the herb is proven safe and effective.

Controversies Surrounding the Use of Dietary Supplements

Opponents of DSHEA claim that the issue of public safety is their primary concern. Steven H. Zeisel, of the University of North Carolina School of

Public Health and School of Medicine, writes that "DSHEA modifies the regulatory environment so that it becomes possible, even likely, that products will be marketed that inadvertently harm people" (Zeisel, p. 1855). Zeisel believes that the DSHEA legislation makes it easy for small enterprises to market products without investing the time and money needed to prove their product's safety and efficacy. He contrasts the development of a new dietary supplement to that of a new drug or food additive, for which there is a formal process to evaluate safety.

A manufacturer developing a new drug or food additive must conduct safety studies following FDA procedures. Results must be submitted to the FDA for review and approval before the ingredient or drug can be sold to the public. This is not the case for dietary supplements, however, because under DSHEA they are legally in a class by themselves. The FDA must simply be notified of the new product, and the notification must provide information that supports the manufacturer's claim that its product is safe. Once the product is marketed, the FDA is responsible for proving that a dietary supplement is unsafe before it can take action to restrict that product's use or remove it from the marketplace.

Another issue critics of DSHEA cite is the scant quality control of dietary supplements. Quality control is important to assure consumers that a product contains the ingredients stated on the label in the stated amounts. Neither the FDA nor any other federal or state agency routinely tests dietary supplements for quality prior to sale. But some manufacturers of dietary supplements do adhere to Good Manufacturing Practices (GMPs) and make every effort to produce a quality product. Also, the FDA has assisted the industry by proposing GMPs that focus on ensuring the identity, purity, quality, strength, and composition of dietary supplements.

DSHEA supporters fear that increased regulation of dietary supplements will decrease access to beneficial products. National opinion surveys show that many supplement users feel so strongly about the potential health benefits of supplements that they would continue to use them even if the supplements were shown to be ineffective in clinical studies. Consumers value freedom of choice, and many view regulation as an attempt by the government and medical establishment to monopolize treatment options. Clearly, a balance needs to be reached between preserving freedom of choice and ensuring that dietary supplements are safe and effective. SEE ALSO ALTERNATIVE MEDICINES AND THERAPIES; FOOD LABELS; HEALTH CLAIMS; QUACKERY; VITAMINS, FAT-SOLUBLE; VITAMINS, WATER-SOLUBLE.

Jackie Shank

Bibliography

Blendon, R. J.; DesRoches, C. M.; Benson, J. M.; Brodie, M.; and Altman, D. E. (2001). "American's Views on the Use and Regulation of Dietary Supplements." *Archives of Internal Medicine* 161(6):805–10.

Dwyer, Johanna T.; Garceau, Anne O.; Evans, Marguerite; Li, Donglin; Lytle, Leslie; Hoelscher, Deanna; Nicklas, Theresa A.; and Zive, Michelle (2001). "Do Adolescent Vitamin-Mineral Supplement Users Have Better Nutrient Intakes than Nonusers? Observations from the CATCH Tracking Study." *Journal of the American Dietetic Association* 101(11):1340–1346.

Fleming, Thomas, ed. (1998). *PDR for Herbal Medicines.* Montvale, NJ: Medical Economics.

Sarubin, Allison (2000). *The Health Professional's Guide to Popular Dietary Supplements.* Chicago: American Dietetic Association.

Skidmore-Roth, Linda (2001). *Mosby's Handbook of Herbs & Natural Supplements*. St. Louis, MO: Mosby.

Somer, Elizabeth (1996). *The Essential Guide to Vitamins and Minerals*, 2nd edition. New York: HarperPerennial.

Zeisel, Steven H. (1999). "Regulation of Nutraceuticals." *Science* 285:1853–55.

Internet Resources

National Institutes of Health, Office of Dietary Supplements. <http://ods.od.nih.gov>

U.S. Food and Drug Administration Center for Food Safety and Applied Nutrition (2001). "Overview of Dietary Supplements." Available from <http://www.cfsan.fda.gov/~dms>

Dietary Trends, American

Americans have become more aware of what they eat, and how it might affect their health. Concerns about the safety of the food supply are on the rise, and increasing nutritional awareness has led to an increase in vegetarian, organic, and health-food options in supermarkets. "Lite" food is in, and indulgence is out. But are Americans practicing what they preach? A closer look at American dietary trends reveals that parts of the American **diet** are still lacking in nutritional quality, despite consumer demand for healthier options.

diet: the total daily food intake, or the types of foods eaten

Dietary Patterns

Fruit and vegetable intake, although rising, is still below the five servings per day recommended in the USDA's Dietary Guidelines for Americans. The average American eats one and one-half servings of vegetables and one serving of fruit per day. Since the beginning of the twentieth century, consumption of milk and eggs has been declining, while cheese consumption has gone up. Meat, poultry, and fish intake has climbed dramatically. Grain and cereal consumption has also risen. Vegetable fats are increasingly being used instead of animal fats, but total **fat** consumption is still high.

fat: type of food molecule rich in carbon and hydrogen, with high energy content

Sixty percent of Americans eat snack food regularly, consuming about 20 percent of their **calories** from snacks. Because half of young adults skip breakfast, and one-fourth skip lunch, between-meal eating contributes significantly to the daily **nutrient** intakes of Americans. Children, in particular, require several small meals per day, as their stomachs cannot hold large amounts of food at one time. Carefully chosen snacks can add to good dietary habits. Most Americans, however, do not snack wisely.

calorie: unit of food energy

nutrient: dietary substance necessary for health

More than 30 percent of men and more than 40 percent of women take a daily multivitamin/mineral supplement. Doses of about 100 percent of the Daily Value (DV) of most nutrients are common in these supplements. Although **nutrition** experts agree that the average American does not need supplements, there is little harm in taking them. Problems can arise, however, when individual nutrients are taken. Megadoses of certain **minerals** and relatively low supplemental doses of certain fat-soluble **vitamins** can lead to toxicity. For example, a surplus of vitamin A can lead to cheilitis (cracking and inflammation of the lips), dryness of the nasal **mucosa** and eyes, hair loss, and, eventually, liver damage. Megadoses of **vitamin D** can lead to the calcification of soft tissues, such as the lungs, heart, and kidneys.

nutrition: the maintenance of health through proper eating, or the study of same

mineral: an inorganic (non-carbon-containing) element, ion or compound

vitamin: necessary complex nutrient used to aid enzymes or other metabolic processes in the cell

mucosa: moist exchange surface within the body

vitamin D: nutrient needed for calcium uptake and therefore proper bone formation

159

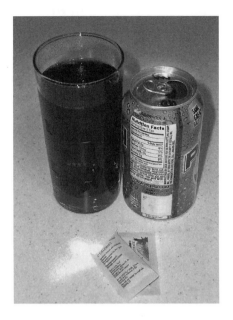

An average American consumes more than fifty pounds of artificial sweeteners per year, which is a 300 percent increase since 1965. Much of the increase is due to the popularity of diet soft drinks.
[Photograph by Kelly A. Quin. Reproduced by permission.]

overweight: weight above the accepted norm based on height, sex, and age

calcium: mineral essential for bones and teeth

convenience food: food that requires very little preparation for eating

fast-food: food requiring minimal preparation before eating, or food delivered very quickly after ordering in a restaurant

Sweet, Quick, and Easy

Since 1965, artificial sweetener use has increased threefold. At the same time, there has been a 14 percent increase in sugar use. It seems Americans are using sugar substitutes in addition to, rather than in place of, sugar. The current consumption of all types of sweeteners is 150 pounds per capita, 99 pounds of which is sugar. According to the USDA Food Guide Pyramid, sugar and sweets should be consumed sparingly. America's preference for sweets only adds to the growing problem of an **overweight** population.

Most sweeteners are consumed in soft drinks. According to the United States Department of Agriculture (USDA) 1998 Continued Survey of Food Intakes by Individuals (CSFII), soft-drink intake has surpassed both men's and women's milk intake (since the 1989–1991 survey). Given that milk is the primary dietary **calcium** source, this trend has contributed to low calcium levels. Total soft-drink use has increased by 300 percent since the 1950s. In 1974 alone, nearly 4.5 billion cases of soft drinks were sold. It has since become nearly impossible to estimate the annual soft-drink consumption of the United States.

The introduction of the Swanson TV dinner in 1953 started the trend for **convenience foods**. In addition, fewer meals are prepared at home as more women have joined the workforce. About 25 percent of calories eaten by adult men and women are eaten away from home (according to the 1998 CSFII, which covered the years 1994–1996). "Home-cooked" meals now often come prewashed, precooked, prebaked, preprocessed, and presliced. Toaster ovens, microwaves, and other home appliances have further reduced preparation times.

The completion of the national highway system in the 1950s triggered the rise of McDonald's and other road-side hamburger chains across the nation. Many meals eaten away from home now come from **fast-food** eateries. In 1978, fast-food sales totaled $9 billion—a figure that rose to $106 billion in 1998. Fast-food restaurants have beaten sit-in restaurants in sales since 1994. In addition, serving sizes have continued to increase dramatically, and fast-food diets are low in calcium, riboflavin, vitamin A, folic acid, and vitamin C, as well as being high in fat and **saturated fat**.

Portion Sizes, Caloric Intake, and Obesity

Scientists have begun to trace the link between portion sizes and increased obesity in the United States. According to the Centers for Disease Control and Prevention, between 1971 and 2000 American women increased the number of calories they consumed by 22 percent (from 1,542 to 1,877 per day), while men increased their intake by 7 percent (from 2,450 to 2,618 calories). Government recommendations, by contrast, are a mere 1,600 calories a day for women and 2,200 a day for men. Many of the additional calories consumed have come from carbohydrates, which has led some scientists to theorize that an increased emphasis on reducing saturated fat in diets led people to believe they could consume all the carbohydrates they wanted. Moreover, many more meals are now consumed outside the home, and serving sizes at national restaurant chains have become two to five times larger than they were in the 1970s. Cookbook publishers have followed suit by increasing portion sizes in recipes. During the thirty-year period covered by the study, obesity rates doubled, and two-thirds of Americans are now considered overweight.

—*Paula Kepos*

AMERICAN DIETARY TRENDS, BY DECADE

	Historical Events	Food Trends of the Time
1950–1959	- Mothers returning to the home after the war effort - Postwar baby boom - Construction of the national highway system	- Packaged meals available - First TV dinner (Swanson), 1953 - Rise of hamburger chains along highways; Oscar Mayer "Wiener-Mobile"
1960–1969	- Growing middle class with money to spend - Growing social unrest over the Vietnam War in late 1960s	- Introduction of Julia Child's French cooking - "Hippies" bring back demand for unprocessed, made-from-scratch foods - Vegetarian trend starts
1970–1979	- End of Vietnam War - Watergate scandal - Growing inflation - Major influx of Asians due to Immigration Act of 1965	- Continued demand for organic and fresh: "California Cuisine" - Elaborate dinner parties with ethnic dishes - Growing appetite for Asian cuisine
1980–1989	- Stock market plummet of 1987	- "Nouvelle Cuisine" is the thing du jour–diners willing to pay more to eat less - Return to simplicity in late 1980s - Exploration of different tastes (e.g., TexMex, Ethiopian, Southwestern)
1990–1999	- Introduction of the Internet puts foods at consumers fingertips	- Everything reduced-fat, low-fat, fat-free - Naturally healthy cuisines (Mediterranean) - New movement toward simplicity

Nutritional Adequacy

Many adult women fail to meet the **Recommended Dietary Allowances** (RDAs) for calcium, vitamin E, vitamin B$_6$, magnesium, and **zinc**. Adult men fall short on vitamin E, magnesium, and zinc. Men consume about 4,000 milligrams of sodium each day, while women consume about 3,000. Both exceed the recommended level of no more than 2,400 milligrams of sodium per day.

All age groups above age two exceed the recommended intake of fat (no more than 30 percent of calories) and saturated fat (no more than 10 percent of calories). **Cholesterol** consumption is within the recommendation of no more than 300 milligrams per day. **Iron** intake is often low, especially in adolescents and adult women, and iron-deficiency **anemia** is higher in these groups than in any other. Low calcium intake is of particular concern in adolescent girls and pregnant women.

The main shortcoming of the American diet is the surplus of **energy** (calories). Over one third of adult Americans are **obese** (and many more are overweight), and a growing number of children are overweight. The reason for this increasing trend is two-fold: energy consumption is up, and activity levels are down.

The Third National Health and Nutrition Examination Survey (NHANES III), carried out between 1988 and 1994, showed an increase of between 100 and 300 calories in daily energy intake since NHANES II (1976 to 1980). In addition, a 1993 survey of 87,000 adults undertaken by the Center for Disease Control and Prevention (CDC) showed that 58.1 percent of Americans engaged in little or no physical activity. This lack of exercise, coupled with increased food intake, contributes to many **chronic** diseases, such as **cardiovascular** disease, certain types of **cancer**, and **diabetes**.

Although awareness about proper diet has increased, most Americans do not follow the recommended guidelines for healthful eating. Fast-food

saturated fat: a fat with the maximum possible number of hydrogens; more difficult to break down that unsaturated fats

Recommended Dietary Allowances: nutrient intake recommended to promote health

zinc: mineral necessary for many enzyme processes

cholesterol: multi-ringed molecule found in animal cell membranes; a type of lipid

iron: nutrient needed for red blood cell formation

anemia: low level of red blood cells in the blood

energy: technically, the ability to perform work; the content of a substance that allows it to be useful as a fuel

obese: above accepted standards of weight for sex, height, and age

chronic: over a long period

cardiovascular: related to the heart and circulatory system

cancer: uncontrolled cell growth

diabetes: inability to regulate level of sugar in the blood

and convenience-food consumption, snacking, supplementation, and soft-drink use have all increased. Many Americans do not meet the RDAs for key nutrients, yet they exceed their caloric requirements, leading to an increasingly overweight population. Future trends will likely include a higher demand for safer, quicker, and more convenient fast foods that also provide the health benefits Americans need. SEE ALSO CONVENIENCE FOODS; FAST FOODS; OBESITY; RECOMMENDED DIETARY ALLOWANCE.

Kirsten Herbes

Bibliography

Duyff, Roberta L. (1998). *The American Dietetic Association's Complete Food & Nutrition Guide.* Minneapolis, MN: Chronimed.

Mahan, L. Kathleen, and Escott-Stump, Sylvia, eds. (2000). *Krause's Food, Nutrition, & Diet Therapy,* 10th edition. Philadelphia: W. B. Saunders.

McIntosh, Elaine N. (1995). *American Food Habits in Historical Perspective.* Westport, CT: Praeger.

Root, Waverley, and de Rochemont, Richard (1995). *Eating in America: A History.* Hopewell, NJ: Ecco Press.

Internet Resources

Clagett Farm. "From Farm to Table: Dietary Trends." Available from <http://www.clagettfarm.org>

Food Surveys Research Group. "What We Eat in America." Available from <http://www.barc.usda.gov/bhnrc/foodsurvey>

National Center for Health Statistics. "Survey and Data Collection Systems." Available from <http://www.cdc.gov/nchs>

Tufts Center on Nutrition Communication. "Nutrition Navigator." Available from <http://www.navigator.tufts.edu>

Wilkinson Enns, Cicilia; Goldman, Joseph D.; and Cook, Annetta (1997). "Trends in Food and Nutrition Intakes by Adults: NCFS 1977-78, CSFII 1989-91, and CSFII 1994-95." Family Economics and Nutrition Review 10(4):2–15. Available from <http://www.barc.usda.gov/bhnrc/foodsurvey>

Dietary Trends, International

What foods an individual eats is affected by the ability to access foods. Economic status, geography, and politics have influenced the diets of people throughout history. Poverty is linked to **malnutrition**, while economic growth and a rise in population pose new nutritional problems. Ironically, diets high in complex **carbohydrates** and **fiber** in poor economic times give way to consumption of foods high in sugars and **fat** when economic conditions improve.

Between 1995 and 1997, among countries that showed an increase in per capita incomes, average caloric consumption also showed a significant increase. Between 1970 and 1972, and between 1996 and 1997, world consumption of **calories** from complex carbohydrates fell by 30 percent while the consumption of calories from meat increased by a third (33%) and those from vegetable oil by almost half (46.2%). As nations become wealthier, people move from eating "a poor man's **diet**" of high levels of grains, fruits, and vegetables to consuming diets with more fats and sugar. Fat still remains the food for the rich—with more income, people start to eat more meat and poultry, and vegetable oils become more available. Combined with cane and corn sugars, vegetable oils are used to produce baked goods and snack foods high in calories.

malnutrition: chronic lack of sufficient nutrients to maintain health

carbohydrate: food molecule made of carbon, hydrogen, and oxygen, including sugars and starches

fiber: indigestible plant material that aids digestion by providing bulk

fat: type of food molecule rich in carbon and hydrogen, with high energy content

calorie: unit of food energy

diet: the total daily food intake, or the types of foods eaten

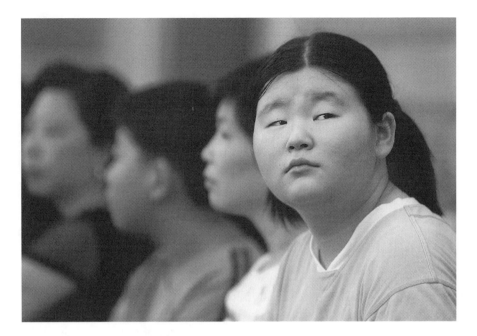

Young Chinese attend a weight-loss lecture in Shanghai. A trend toward obesity in many nations is accompanied by obsession over body image. During 2002, several citizens of Asian nations died and hundreds were sickened when they took a popular diet pill that was known to cause health problems. *[AP/Wide World Photos. Reproduced by permission.]*

The Westernization of Dietary Patterns

Toward the end of the twentieth century, economic growth among developing countries caused the phenomenon of the Westernization of traditional eating patterns. Industrialization and modern transportation brought baking technology and Western food styles to developing countries. New and tasty foods high in fat, sugar, and salt became the choice of the new rich. Trendy fast foods, soft drinks, and meat products replaced traditional ethnic foods.

Fortunately, in many emerging societies the poor are still unable to afford Western fast foods, and are thus spared the ills of high consumption of fats, meat, and sugars. For example, many people in India still spend more than half their income on food consumed at home, compared to the average American, who spends less than 8 percent of his or her disposable income on home-cooked food.

The American diet, much like that of many industrialized nations, derives its calories from fats, sugars, and animal products in foods prepared or processed away from home. One out of every three meals in America is consumed away from home. From 1990 to 2000 there was a 14 percent decrease in the number of meals eaten at home. In 1977 only 16 percent of all meals and snacks were eaten way from home. By 1995, this rose to 27 percent. In 1995, away-from-home foods provided 34 percent of total caloric intake, an increase from 18 percent in 1977. In addition, eating at home does not always mean cooking. Supermarkets and grocery stores provide thousands of ready-made meals, frozen foods, and processed meals that require little preparation at home.

Total fat consumption in the United States increased from 18 percent in 1977 to 38 percent in 1995. According to Lin and Frazao, away-from-home foods deliver more calories in fat and **saturated fat** and are lower in fiber and **calcium** than home-cooked foods. The average total calories consumed by Americans rose from 1,807 calories in 1987 to 2,043 calories in

saturated fat: a fat with the maximum possible number of hydrogens; more difficult to break down that unsaturated fats

calcium: mineral essential for bones and teeth

163

fast food: food requiring minimal preparation before eating, or food delivered very quickly after ordering in a restaurant

obesity: the condition of being overweight, according to established norms based on sex, age, and height

overweight: weight above the accepted norm based on height, sex, and age

obese: above accepted standards of weight for sex, height, and age

chronic: over a long period

heart disease: any disorder of the heart or its blood supply, including heart attack, atherosclerosis, and coronary artery disease

hypertension: high blood pressure

hyperlipidemia: high levels of lipids (fats or cholesterol) in the blood

cancer: uncontrolled cell growth

stroke: loss of blood supply to part of the brain, due to a blocked or burst artery in the brain

type II diabetes: Inability to regulate the level of sugar in the blood due to a reduction in the number of insulin receptors on the body's cells

incidence: number of new cases reported each year

food additive: substance added to foods to improve nutrition, taste, appearance or shelf-life

food poisoning: illness caused by consumption of spoiled food, usually containing bacteria

bacteria: single-celled organisms without nuclei, some of which are infectious

virus: noncellular infectious agent that requires a host cell to reproduce

toxins: poison

parasite: organism that feeds off of other organisms

1995. Since away-from-home foods deliver more fat and more calories, the trend of eating out can become a health hazard. People tend to eat more from restaurants and **fast-food** places because many eating establishments "supersize" their portions. Customers feel that they get their money's worth when they receive more food than they need.

Influence of Diet on Health

Childhood and adulthood **obesity** are on the rise. Between 1988 and 1994, 11 percent of U.S. children and adolescents aged six to nine years of age were **overweight** or **obese**. During this same period, 35 percent of the American adult population aged twenty and over were obese, compared to 25 percent during the years 1976 through 1980. The rising trend in obesity pervades the Middle East, the Caribbean, Europe, Latin America, Brazil, Japan, South East Asia, Australia, and China.

Since being overweight is associated directly with many **chronic** illnesses, such as **heart disease**, **hypertension**, **hyperlipidemia**, **cancer**, **stroke**, and **type II diabetes**, an increase in the **incidence** of overweight and obesity is a serious concern. The top three leading causes of death in the United States during the 1990s were heart disease, cancer, and stroke. Diabetes ranked seventh in 1997—it was not even in the top ten in 1987. The U.S. Surgeon General reported in 1998 that type II diabetes, an adult health problem related to obesity, was being seen in children as young as four years old. Diabetes among adults increased by 70 percent between 1990 and 1998 among individuals 30 to 39 years of age; by 41 percent among individuals 40 to 49; and by 31 percent among those 50 to 59. By 1998, 16 million American adults suffered from diabetes. In addition to the health threat, obesity can cause emotional pain due to social stigmatization, discrimination, and lowered self-esteem. In 2000, the World Health Organization estimated that there are 1.2 billion obese individuals around the world.

Food Safety

The increase in the number of fast-food restaurants, supermarkets, and restaurants in developing countries, and the rising trend of eating meals away from home, present a global challenge to ensure that food is appealing and safe. Many countries have agencies that set and regulate standards for food safety. In the United States, the U.S. Department of Agriculture (USDA) has the task of regulating and inspecting meats and poultry during slaughter and processing, while the Food and Drug Administration (FDA) is responsible for conducting tests, setting standards, and enforcing laws regulating food quality and processing. FDA inspectors check restaurants to make sure that they practice food safety regulations. FDA officials also review the safety of chemicals that manufacturers use as **food additives**. Importing foods from countries where food safety is not strictly monitored presents a global health threat.

The biggest problem with food safety is **food poisoning**. Some **bacteria** and **viruses** that cause food poisoning are: *Escherichia coli*, *Salmonella*, *Listeria monocytogenes*, *Shigella*, *Campylobacter*, and *yersinia*. Bacteria, viruses, **toxins, parasites**, and chemical contaminants can all cause food-borne illnesses, and it takes only a small amount of contaminated food to cause severe food illnesses.

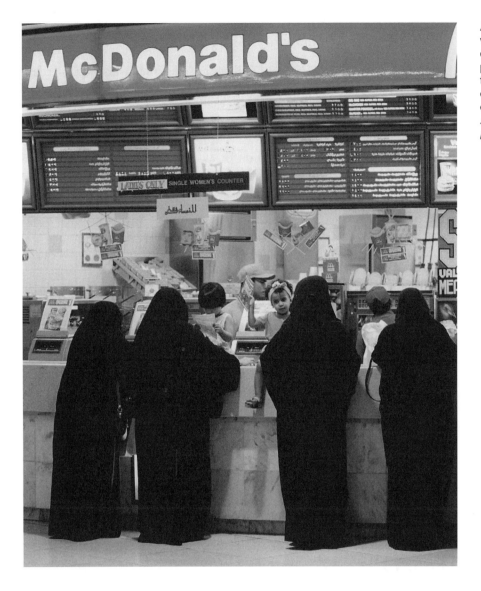

Abaya-wearing women in Saudi Arabia wait in the ladies-only line to order a quick meal. In developing nations, the popularity of fast-food alternatives to traditional cuisines has prompted debate over the nutritional and cultural impacts of Westernization. *[Photograph by Saleh Rifai. AP/Wide World Photos. Reproduced by permission.]*

Signs and symptoms of food-borne illness may present within thirty minutes of eating contaminated food, or they may not show up for up to three weeks. While some food-borne illnesses may last for a couple of days, some may last for weeks. Severe cases can be life threatening. SEE ALSO CONVENIENCE FOODS; FAST FOODS; OBESITY.

Kweethai C. Neill

Bibliography

Centers for Disease Control and Prevention (1997). "Update: Prevalence of Overweight Among Children, Adolescents, and Adults—United States, 1988–1994." *Mortality and Morbidity Weekly Report* 46:199–202.

Lin, B. H., and Frazao, E. (1977). "The Nutritional Quality of Foods at and Away from Home." *Food Review* 20:33–40.

Internet Resources

Centers for Disease Control and Prevention (2000). "Major Increase in Diabetes among Adults Occurred Nationwide between 1990 and 1998." Available from <http://www.cdc.gov>

International Obesity Task Force. "The Global Epidemic of Obesity." Available from <http://www.iotf.org/publications/Newsletter/spring97.htm>

Dietetic Technician, Registered (DTR)

nutrition: the maintenance of health through proper eating, or the study of same

diet: the total daily food intake, or the types of foods eaten

A dietetic technician, registered (DTR) is a professional who is knowledgeable about food, **nutrition**, and **diet** therapy, which is the use of diet and nutrition in the treatment of diseases. A person seeking DTR credentials must complete a two-year associate's degree in an accredited dietetic technician (DT) program, a minimum of 450 hours of supervised practice experience (gained under the direction of an accredited DT program), and successfully complete the national registration examination for DTR.

The goal of a DTR is to provide safe and effective food and nutrition services to the public. DTRs work independently or with registered dietitians in a variety of settings, such as hospitals, food service operations, and public health. Thus, they may provide nutrition services to individuals, manage food service operations, or provide nutrition education. SEE ALSO AMERICAN DIETETIC ASSOCIATION; CAREERS IN DIETETICS.

Susan Himburg

Bibliography

Payne-Palacio, June, and Canter, Deborah D. (2000). *The Profession of Dietetics: A Team Approach*, 2nd edition. Upper Saddle River, NJ: Prentice Hall.

Winterfeldt, Esther A.; Bogle, Margaret L.; and Ebro, Lea L. (1998). *Dietetics: Practice and Future Trends*. Gaithersburg, MD: Aspen.

Internet Resources

American Dietetic Association. "Careers in Dietetics." Available from <http://www.eatright.org/>

Florida Area Health Education Center. "Careers in Health." Available from <http://www.flahec.org/hlthcareers>

Dietetics

nutrient: dietary substance necessary for health

Dietetics is the study of food, food science, and nutrition, and of the interactions of food and **nutrients** in people and populations. It can also refer to the management of food service and the provision of health guidance in a variety of settings, including hospitals, nursing homes, health departments, clinics, and in private practice.

The study of dietetics prepares students to apply the principles of food, nutrition, and food service management to caring for the health of individuals and groups of people. Individuals who graduate from an approved dietetics program are eligible to take the RD (registered dietitian) examination. The goal of dietetics programs, which are offered at both undergraduate and graduate levels, is to promote health and decrease disease by training health care professionals in nutrition science, thus enabling them to foster good nutritional health for individuals and diverse populations across the lifespan. These programs also provide information on health care policy and administration, delivery systems, reimbursement issues, and regulations. SEE ALSO AMERICAN DIETETIC ASSOCIATION; CAREERS IN DIETETICS; DIETETIC TECHNICIAN, REGISTERED; DIETITIAN; NUTRITIONIST.

Delores Truesdell

Bibliography

Payne-Palacio, June, and Canter, Deborah D. (2000). *The Profession of Dietetics: A Team Approach*, 2nd edition. Upper Saddle River, NJ: Prentice Hall.

Internet Resource

American Dietetic Association. "Careers in Dietetics." Available from <http://www.eatright.org>

Dieting

The term *dieting* refers to restrictive eating or nutritional remedies for conditions such as iron-deficiency **anemia**, **gastrointestinal** diseases, pernicious anemia, **diabetes**, **obesity**, or **failure to thrive**. Someone can be on a heart-healthy **diet** that encourages the consumption of reasonable amounts of whole grains and fresh fruits, vegetables, beans, and fish, but limits foods high in **saturated fat** and sodium, or one can be on a weight loss diet. Examples of weight loss diets include: the Atkins New Diet Revolution, the Calories Don't Count Diet, the Protein Power Diet, the Carbohydrate Addict's Diet, and Weight Watchers. There is a lack of research, however, on whether these diets (except for Weight Watchers) are helpful, especially over the long term (defined as two to five years from the date of weight loss).

The recommended approach to dieting for weight loss is to eat in moderation so as to control calories (do not go below 1,200 per day) and to increase activity to lead to a gradual, safe weight loss. A recommended method is to decrease calories each day by 125 (the amount in a small soft drink or full cup of juice) and to increase **energy** expenditure by 125 (walking for about 30 minutes). That is, a 250-calorie deficit a day should result in about a one- to two-pound weight loss over the course of a month. The goal is to slowly change eating and exercise routines and maintain a lifelong healthy weight. Quicker weight losses are hard to maintain. Most people can lose weight on any diet, even on fad diets, but the trick is to keep the weight off.

So-called fad diets are diets that come and go in the marketplace and are typically deficient in various ways. For example, they may lack variety (e.g., the Grapefruit Diet, the Cabbage Soup Diet), be too low in calories and protein (the Rice Diet), and/or simply too bizarre (the Rotation Diet for food **allergies**). People should be especially wary of any "breakthrough" quick-fix diets. If a diet sounds too good to be true, it probably is.

Delores Truesdell

anemia: low level of red blood cells in the blood

gastrointestinal: related to the stomach and intestines

diabetes: inability to regulate level of sugar in the blood

obesity: the condition of being overweight, according to established norms based on sex, age, and height

failure to thrive: lack of normal developmental progress or maintenance of health

diet: the total daily food intake, or the types of foods eaten

saturated fat: a fat with the maximum possible number of hydrogens; more difficult to break down that unsaturated fats

energy: technically, the ability to perform work; the content of a substance that allows it to be useful as a fuel

allergy: immune system reaction against substances that are otherwise harmless

Bibliography

Alford, B. B.; Blankenship, A. C.; and Haen, R. D. (1990). "The Effects of Variations in Carbohydrate, Protein, and Fat Content of the Diet upon Weight Loss, Blood Values, and Nutrient Intake of Adult Obese Women." *Journal of the American Dietetic Association* 90:534–540.

Golay, A., et al. (1996). "Similar Weight Loss with Low- or High-Carbohydrate Diets." *American Journal of Clinical Nutrition* 63:174–176

Leeds, M. J. *Nutrition for Healthy Living.* WCB McGraw-Hill.

Ornish, D.; Scherwitz, L. W.; Billings, J. H.; et al. (1998). "Intensive Lifestyle Changes for Reversal of Coronary Heart Disease." *Journal of the American Medical Association* 280:2001–2007.

Internet Resource

Larsen, Joanne. "Fad Diets." Available from <www.dietitian.com>

Dietitian

nutrition: the maintenance of health through proper eating, or the study of same

physiology: the group of biochemical and physical processes that combine to make a functioning organism, or the study of same

internship: training program

entrepreneur: founders of new businesses

clinical: related to hospitals, clinics, and patient care

diabetes: inability to regulate level of sugar in the blood

cancer: uncontrolled cell growth

A dietitian is a professional nutritionist—an educated food and **nutrition** specialist who is qualified by training and examination to evaluate people's nutritional health and needs. Most dietitians are registered and are referred to as RDs. To become an RD, a person must earn an undergraduate degree in nutrition, food science, or food management, including courses in several other related subjects (chemistry, anatomy and **physiology**, management, psychology, etc.); complete a 900-hour **internship**; pass a national exam administered by the Commission on Dietetic Registration (the credentialing arm of the American Dietetic Association), and maintain up-to-date knowledge and registration by participating in required continuing education activities, such as attending workshops, doing research, taking courses, or writing professional papers.

Administrative dietitians are sometimes called dietary directors. They are **entrepreneurs**, disturbance handlers, resource allocators, and negotiators who work in local health departments or manage the **clinical** and food service systems in hospitals, correctional facilities, or long-term care institutions. Clinical dietitians or nutrition managers provide patient care in hospitals and in outpatient clinics especially related to **diabetes** and **cancer**. Nutrition-support-team dietitians coordinate nutrition care with other health care professionals; they may work in teaching hospitals, outpatient clinics, or in pediatric and diabetes clinics. In school food service, dietitians manage the overall operation, including the purchasing of food. In the food and pharmaceutical industry, dietitians conduct research, develop and market products, and represent companies at various food and health shows.

A clinical dietitian helps her patient design a nutritious weight-loss program. Such work is increasingly valuable in the United States, where three out of five adults are overweight or obese. *[© 1992 SIU Biomed Comm. Custom Medical Stock Photo. Reproduced by permission.]*

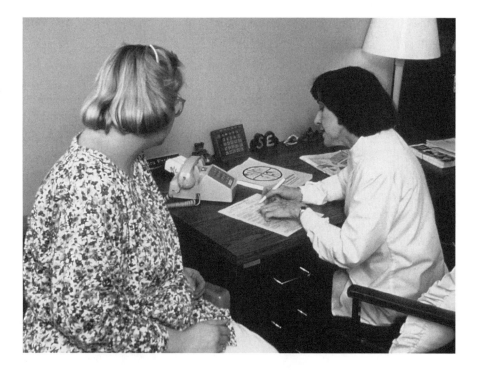

Some states require people who provide nutrition advice to be licensed, but not necessarily registered. Others allow anyone to use the title *nutritionist*. However, the title *registered dietitian* is usually used only by those who have completed the appropriate course work. The purpose of registration is to protect the health and welfare of the public by encouraging high standards of performance. SEE ALSO AMERICAN DIETETIC ASSOCIATION; CAREERS IN DIETETICS; DIETETICS.

Delores Truesdell

Bibliography

Hudson, Nancy R. (2000). *Management Practice in Dietetics*. Belmont, CA: Wadsworth.

Whitney, Eleanor N., and Rolfes, Sharon R. (2002). *Understanding Nutrition*, 9th edition. Belmont, CA: Wadsworth.

Digestion and Absorption

Digestion is the breakdown of food into smaller particles or individual **nutrients**. It is accomplished through six basic processes, with the help of several body fluids—particularly digestive juices that are made up of compounds such as saliva, mucus, **enzymes**, hydrochloric acid, bicarbonate, and **bile**.

The six processes of digestion involve: (1) the movement of food and liquids; (2) the lubrication of food with bodily secretions; (3) the mechanical breakdown of **carbohydrates**, fats, and **proteins**; (4) the reabsorption of nutrients—especially water; (5) the production of nutrients such as vitamin K and **biotin** by friendly **bacteria**; and (6) the excretion of waste products. Comprehension of the tasks or processes needed to break down food are essential to an understanding of how and when food really begins to function within the body. For example, not understanding that carbohydrates break down into **glucose** could lead one to believe that the best source of glucose is in liquid form such as a soft drink. This could cause one to miss out on the nutrients (and great taste) in fruits, vegetables, and grains. Likewise, not understanding the digestion process could lead a person to believe in the myth of "food combining," or perhaps to think it is normal to be hungry all the time. But, in fact, the digestive processes normal to human **physiology** can simultaneously handle carbohydrates, fats, and proteins—and allow people to go several hours between meals, especially if meals are balanced in **fiber** and the individual nutrients needed.

GI Tract Physiology

Digestion begins in the mouth with the action of salivary amylase. The food material then progresses past the esophagus and into the stomach. A bolus (soft mass) of chewed food moves by muscular wave actions, called *peristalsis*, from the mouth to the pharynx, and then past the epiglottis that covers the larynx. The epiglottis closes off the air passage so that one doesn't choke. The cardiac sphincter prevents reflux of stomach contents into the esophagus.

From the Stomach to the Small Intestine

Food mixtures leaving the stomach are called *chyme*, and this empties into the small intestine after about two to four hours in the stomach. The small

nutrient: dietary substance necessary for health

enzyme: protein responsible for carrying out reactions in a cell

bile: substance produced in the liver which suspends fats for absorption

carbohydrate: food molecule made of carbon, hydrogen, and oxygen, including sugars and starches

protein: complex molecule composed of amino acids that performs vital functions in the cell; necessary part of the diet

biotin: a portion of certain enzymes used in fat metabolism; essential for cell function

bacteria: single-celled organisms without nuclei, some of which are infectious

glucose: a simple sugar; the most commonly used fuel in cells

physiology: the group of biochemical and physical processes that combine to make a functioning organism, or the study of same

fiber: indigestible plant material that aids digestion by providing bulk

intestine is where most digestion takes place. A pyloric sphincter controls the rate of flow of chyme from the stomach into the small intestine.

Most digestion occurs in the upper portion of the small intestine, called the *duodenum*. Below the duodenum is the *jejunum*, and then there is the last segment, called the *ileum*. About 5 percent of undigested food products are broken down in the ileum. This is why some people can have a small part of their intestine removed and still seem to digest most foods with little problem.

Digestion of food that enters the small intestine is usually complete after three to ten hours. Once digestion is essentially finished, waste products leave the ileum with the help of fiber, and these solids then enter the large intestine (the colon). In the colon, water is reabsorbed; some nutrients are produced by friendly bacteria (vitamin K, biotin, vitamin B_{12}); fibers are digested to various acids and gases; and **minerals**, such as potassium and sodium, are reabsorbed (when needed). Any fiber that is not broken down—and small amounts of other undigested products—are excreted in the feces.

Protective Factors

During digestion in the stomach, large proteins break down into smaller protein forms, and harmful bacteria can become inactive. Hydrochloric acid is especially important for this because it lowers the **pH** of the stomach contents below 2. Along with the uncoiling of protein in the stomach, a little carbohydrate and lipid are broken down with the help of enzymes (called *amylase* and *lipase*, respectively).

In the stomach, carbohydrates in foods turn to starch, but it is not until the chyme reaches the small intestine and becomes more neutralized that starch turns to simple sugars that are then absorbed into the portal vein, which transports them to the liver. Also in the small intestine, lipids (mostly in the form of **triglycerides**) are emulsified and form **monoglycerides** and free **fatty acids** that can then go through the **lymph system** to the heart and bloodstream.

As previously mentioned, the mouth, stomach, small intestine, and colon are the major organs of digestion. However, the liver, gallbladder, and pancreas are also important to the process. The liver detoxifies foreign compounds, such as natural **toxicants** in foods and **drugs**. The liver also makes bile, an emulsifier, which enters the small intestine and prepares fats and oils for digestion. This bile is stored in the gallbladder prior to delivery to the small intestine. A **hormone** called *cholecystokinin* helps control the release of bile.

The pancreas makes pancreatic juice consisting of enzymes (amylases, lipases, and proteases) and bicarbonate, which helps neutralize acidic secretions produced during digestion. The pancreas delivers the pancreatic juice to the small intestine, in response to a signal of food in the intestine and the release of the hormone *secretin*. The pancreas also has another function, the secretion of the hormones *insulin* and *glucagon*, which helps maintain a steady state of blood sugar in the body (insulin decreases blood glucose concentration, while glucagon increases it).

Food moves from the mouth to the epiglottis, bypassing the trachea, into the esophagus, past the cardiac sphincter into the stomach, past the pyloric valve into the small intestine (duodenum, jejunum, ileum), and then

mineral: an inorganic (non-carbon-containing) element, ion, or compound

pH: level of acidity, with low numbers indicating high acidity

triglyceride: a type of fat

monoglyceride: breakdown product of fats

fatty acids: molecules rich in carbon and hydrogen; a component of fats

lymph system: system of vessels and glands in the body that circulates and cleans extracellular fluid

toxicant: harmful substance

drugs: substances whose administration causes a significant change in the body's function

hormone: molecules produced by one set of cells that influence the function of another set of cells

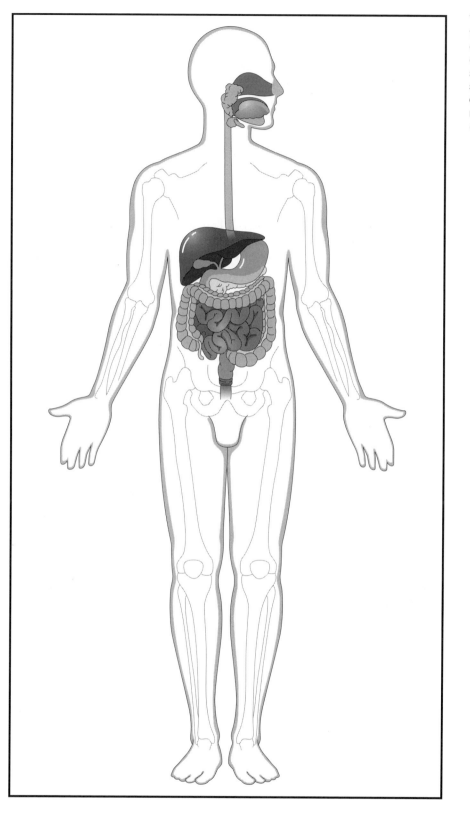

The tract running from the esophagus to the large intestine is called the alimentary canal, and it is where most digestion occurs. As food is pushed through the system, it encounters numerous specialized processes that act on it in different ways, extracting nutrients and rejecting waste. *[Illustration by Argosy. The Gale Group.]*

past the ileocecal valve into the colon. Waste then leaves the colon through the rectum and anus. When chyme reaches the small intestine, the pancreas and liver contribute to the digestion by providing products such as bicarbonate, enzymes, and bile.

molecule: combination of atoms that form stable particles

gastrointestinal: related to the stomach and intestines

vitamin: necessary complex nutrient used to aid enzymes or other metabolic processes in the cell

energy: technically, the ability to perform work; the content of a substance that allows it to be useful as a fuel

lactose intolerance: inability to digest lactose, or milk sugar

allergy: immune system reaction against substances that are otherwise harmless

amino acid: building block of proteins, necessary dietary nutrient

lipid: fats, waxes, and steroids; important components of cell membranes

gastric: related to the stomach

ulcer: erosion in the lining of the stomach or intestine due to bacterial infection

nervous system: the brain, spinal cord, and nerves that extend throughout the body

stress: heightened state of nervousness or unease

water-soluble: able to be dissolved in water

lymphatic system: group of ducts and nodes through which fluid and white blood cells circulate to fight infection

Absorption

Absorption is the movement of **molecules** across the **gastrointestinal** (GI) tract into the circulatory system. Most of the end-products of digestion, along with **vitamins**, minerals, and water, are absorbed in the small intestinal lumen by four mechanisms for absorption: (1) active transport, (2) passive diffusion, (3) endocytosis, and (4) facilitative diffusion. Active transport requires **energy**.

Nutrient absorption is efficient because the GI tract is folded with several surfaces for absorption and these surfaces are lined with villi (hairlike projections) and microvilli cells. As one nutrition textbook puts it, each person has a surface area "equivalent to the surface of a tennis court" packed into his or her gut (Insel et al., p. 81). Efficient absorption can be compromised due to **lactose intolerance**. Lactose intolerance is not uncommon in the world, affecting about 25 percent of the U.S. population and 75 percent of the worldwide population. It is usually due to the lack or absence of the enzyme *lactase*, which breaks down milk sugar.

Lactose intolerance is not a food **allergy**. Food allergies are serious, even life threatening, but most people with lactose intolerance can digest small amounts of milk, especially in yogurt and cheese.

Protein, carbohydrate, lipid, and most vitamin absorption occur in the small intestine. Once proteins are broken down by proteases they are absorbed as dipeptides, tripeptides, and individual **amino acids**. Carbohydrates, including both sugar and starch molecules, are broken down by enzymes in the intestine to disaccharides called *sucrose*, *lactose*, and *maltose*, and then finally into the end-products known as *glucose*, *fructose*, and *galactose*, which are absorbed mostly by active transport. Lipase, an enzyme in the pancreas and the small intestine, and bile from the liver, break down **lipids** into fatty acids and monglycerides; these end-products then are absorbed through villi cells as triglycerides.

Alcohol is not a nutrient, but 80 percent of consumed alcohol is absorbed in the small intestine. The other 20 percent is absorbed into the stomach. Alcohol is absorbed by simple diffusion, which explains why **gastric ulcers** are not uncommon in people who drink excessively.

Coordination and Transport of Nutrients into the Blood or to the Heart

Hormones and the **nervous system** coordinate digestion and absorption. The presence of food, or the thought or smell of food, can cause a positive response from these systems. Factors that can inhibit digestion include **stress**, cold foods, and bacteria.

After foods are digested and nutrients are absorbed, they are transported to specific places throughout the body. **Water-soluble** nutrients leave the GI tract in the blood and travel via the portal vein, first to the liver and then to the heart. Unlike the vascular system for water-soluble nutrients, the **lymphatic system** has no pump for fat-soluble nutrients; instead, these nutrients eventually enter the vascular system, though they bypass the activity of the liver at first. SEE ALSO BIOAVAILABILITY; EATING HABITS; INSULIN; NUTRITION.

Delores Truesdell

Bibliography

Insel, Paul; Turner, Elaine; and Ross, Don (2004). *Nutrition*, 2nd edition. Sudbury, MA: Jones and Bartlett.

Wardlaw, Kessel (2002). *Perspectives in Nutrition*, 5th edition. Boston: McGraw-Hill.

Whitney, E. N., and Rolfes, S. R. *Understanding Nutrition*, 9th edition. Belmont, CA: Wadsworth.

Disaster Relief Organizations

Natural disasters, as well as some human-caused disasters, lead to human suffering and create needs that the victims cannot alleviate without assistance. Examples of disasters include hurricanes, tornadoes, floods, earthquakes, drought, blizzards, **famine**, war, fire, volcanic eruption, a building collapse, or a transportation wreck. When any such disaster strikes, a variety of international organizations offer relief to the affected country. Each organization has different objectives, expertise, and resources to offer, and several hundred may become involved in a single major disaster. International disaster relief on such a large scale must be properly coordinated to avoid further chaos and confusion both during and after the disaster.

famine: extended period of food shortage

Assessment

In the event of a disaster, the government of the affected country must conduct a **needs assessment** to determine what emergency supplies and personnel are required. These needs should be communicated to those relief organizations that will potentially provide assistance. The process of requesting and receiving supplies is lengthy and includes many events that could delay the arrival of assistance. Requests for assistance must first be reviewed and approved by relief organizations, and then supplies and personnel must be collected and transported to the disaster site. Effective management of relief assistance depends on anticipating and identifying problems, and on delivering specific supplies and personnel at the times and places they are needed.

needs assessment: formal procedure for determining needs

Health Risks

Disasters often pose significant health threats. One of the most serious concerns after a disaster, especially a natural disaster, is sanitation. Disruptions in water supplies and sewage systems can pose serious health risks to victims because they decrease the amount and quality of available drinking water and create difficulties in waste disposal. Drinking water can be contaminated by breaks in sewage lines or the presence of animal cadavers in water sources. These factors can facilitate the spread of disease after a disaster. Providing **potable** drinking water to victims and adopting alternative methods of sanitation must be a priority after a disaster.

potable: safe to drink

Food shortages are often an immediate health consequence of disasters. Existing food stocks may be destroyed or disruptions to distribution systems may prevent the delivery of food. In these situations, food relief programs should include the following elements: (1) assessment of food supplies available after the disaster, (2) determination of the nutritional needs of victims, (3) calculation of daily food needs, and (4) surveillance of victims' nutritional

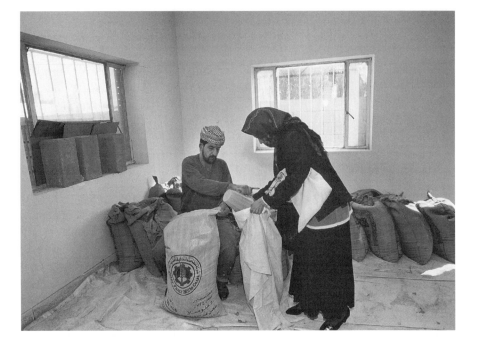

A woman gets her monthly distribution of food at a disaster-relief center in Baghdad. Following the 2003 war in Iraq, hundreds of relief agencies provided support to affected citizens. *[Photograph by Caroline Penn. Corbis. Reproduced by permission.]*

malnutrition: chronic lack of sufficient nutrients to maintain health

drugs: substances whose administration causes a significant change in the body's function

dehydration: loss of water

antibiotic: substance that kills or prevents the growth of microorganisms

bacteria: single-celled organisms without nuclei, some of which are infectious

anemia: low level of red blood cells in the blood

incidence: number of new cases reported each year

status. Some populations are particularly susceptible to **malnutrition**, such as children under five years of age and pregnant women. In addition to food, these populations should be given nutritional supplements whenever possible.

After a disaster, victims must be protected from hazardous climatic conditions, such as severe temperatures or precipitation. People should be kept dry, reasonably well clothed, and able to access emergency shelter.

Disasters can also cause disruptions to the health care infrastructure. Hospitals and health centers may suffer structural damage, or health personnel may be among the casualties, limiting the ability to provide health services to disaster victims. Emergency Health Kits that contain essential medical supplies and **drugs** are often provided to victims as part of the immediate response to disasters. Developed through the collaboration of various relief organizations, these kits are designed to meet the primary health care needs of people without access to medical facilities. Each kit covers the needs of about 10,000 persons for three months, at a cost of about fifty cents per person. The twelve essential drugs in the basic kit include anti-inflammatories, an antacid, a disinfectant, oral **dehydration** salts, an antimalarial, a basic **antibiotic** (effective against the most common **bacteria**), and an ointment for eye infections. These medicines can treat the most common illnesses of disaster victims, such as **anemia**, pain, diarrhea, fever, respiratory tract infections, eye and ear infections, measles, and skin conditions. The basic kit also includes simple medical supplies such as cotton, soap, bandages, thermometers, some medical instruments, health cards and record books, and items to help create a clean water supply.

Risk of Disease

Natural disasters do not usually result in infectious disease outbreaks. However, certain circumstances can increase the chance for disease transmission. Immediately after a disaster, most increases in disease **incidence** are caused

INTERNATIONAL DISASTER RELIEF ORGANIZATIONS AND AGENCIES

Organization or Agency Name	Services
Adventist Development and Relief Agency International (ADRA)	Provides immediate disaster relief; supports development programs in community development, construction, and agriculture
Church World Service (CWS)	Provides material aid to refugees and disaster victims; supports development programs in agriculture, energy, soil conservation, reforestation, preventive medicine, sanitation, and potable water supply
Cooperative for Assistance and Relief Everywhere (CARE)	Provides refugee and disaster relief; supports development programs in reforestation, conservation, and agriculture
Direct Relief International (DRI)	Specializes in emergency health care, providing pharmaceuticals, medical supplies, and equipment in famine, refugee, and disaster-affected areas
Disaster Preparedness and Emergency Response Association (DERA)	Assists international communities in disaster preparedness, response, and recovery; serves as a professional association linking disaster relief personnel
Food for the Hungry (FH)	Provides food aid and disaster relief supplies; provides technological support to eliminate hunger
League of Red Cross and Red Crescent Societies (LICROSS)	Coordinates relief activities for disaster victims; provides assistance to refugees; helps countries increase their capacity to respond to humanitarian needs of victims
Lutheran World Federation (LWF)	Provides emergency relief for disaster victims; supports refugee settlement programs and a variety of development assistance activities
OXFAM International (formerly Oxford Committee for Famine Relief)	Provides assistance to people affected by emergencies, disease, famine, earthquakes, war, and civil conflict; supports long-term development programs in impoverished nations
Salvation Army World Service Office (SAWSO)	Supports a variety of programs in disaster relief, community development, food production, public health, and social welfare
United Nations Children's Fund (UNICEF)	Provides disaster and refugee assistance, particularly to children; supports programs in sanitation and water supply; promotes training and education to improve child health care
United Nations Office for the Coordination of Humanitarian Affairs (OCHA)	Responsible for the coordination of UN assistance in humanitarian crises; provides support for international policy development; advocates humanitarian issues
United States Agency for International Development (USAID)	Provides humanitarian, economic, and development assistance to the international community; houses the Office of U.S. Foreign Disaster Assistance

by fecal contamination of water and food supplies. This contamination usually results in intestinal disease. Outbreaks of communicable diseases are directly associated with population density and displacement. If disaster victims live in overcrowded conditions or are forced to leave their homes, the risk of a disease outbreak increases. An increased demand on water and food supplies, elevated risk of contamination, and disruption of sanitation services all contribute to the risk of a disease outbreak.

In the longer term after a disaster, the risk for vector-borne diseases increases. Vector-borne diseases are spread to humans by insects and other arthropods, such as ticks or mosquitoes. Vector-borne diseases are of particular concern following heavy rains and floods. Insecticides may be washed away from buildings and the number of mosquito breeding sites may increase. In addition, wild or domestic animals that have been displaced can introduce infection to humans.

International disaster relief organizations play an important role in the response to disasters. They provide valuable supplies and personnel to victims and help to minimize the social, economic, and health consequences of a disaster. Health concerns, such as potential disease outbreak, malnutrition, and poor sanitation, should be addressed immediately after a disaster to avoid serious health consequences. International relief organizations help victims fulfill unmet needs and play a vital role in effective disaster management. SEE ALSO EMERGENCY NUTRITION NETWORK; FAMINE.

Karen Bryla

Bibliography

Gorman, R. F. (1994). *Historical Dictionary of Refugee and Disaster Relief Organizations.* Metuchen, NJ: Scarecrow Press.

Internet Resources

Pan American Health Organization. "Natural Disasters: Protecting the Public's Health." Available from <http://www.paho.org>

Grantmakers Without Borders. "International Emergency Relief Links." Available from <http://www.internationaldonors.org>

Disaster Center. "Disaster Relief Agencies." Available from <http://www.disaster center.com/agency.htm>

Pan American Health Organization. "Disasters and Humanitarian Assistance." Available from <http://www.paho.org/disasters>

UNICEF. "Emergency Health Kits." Available from <http://www.supply.unicef.dk/emergencies/healthkit.htm>

Eating Disorders

Eating disorders affect both the mind and the body. Although deviant eating patterns have been reported throughout history, eating disorders were first identified as medical conditions by the British physician William Gull in 1873. The **incidence** of eating disorders increased substantially throughout the twentieth century, and in 1980 the American Psychiatric Association formally classified these conditions as mental illnesses.

incidence: number of new cases reported each year

Diagnosis

Individuals with eating disorders are obsessed with food, body image, and weight loss. They may have severely limited food choices, employ bizarre eating **rituals**, excessively drink fluids and chew gum, and avoid eating with others. Depending on the severity and duration of their illness, they may display physical symptoms such as weight loss; **amenorrhea**; loss of interest in sex; low **blood pressure**; depressed body temperature; **chronic**, unexplained vomiting; and the growth of soft, fine hair on the body and face.

ritual: ceremony or frequently repeated behavior

amenorrhea: lack of menstruation

blood pressure: measure of the pressure exerted by the blood against the walls of the blood vessels

chronic: over a long period

176

There are various types of eating disorders, each with its own physical, **psychological**, and **behavioral** manifestations. They are classified into four distinct diagnostic categories by the American Psychiatric Association: **anorexia nervosa**, **bulimia** nervosa, **binge eating disorder**, and eating disorder not otherwise specified.

Anorexia nervosa. Clinically, anorexia nervosa is diagnosed as intentional weight loss of 15 percent or more of normal body weight. The anorexic displays an inordinate fear of weight gain or becoming fat, even though he or she may be extremely thin. Food intake is strictly limited, often to the point of life-threatening starvation. Sufferers may be unaware of or in denial of their weight loss, and may therefore resist treatment.

Peak ages of onset are between 12 and 13 and at age 17. Among women of menstruating age, menstruation ceases due to weight-related declines in female **hormones**.

This illness has two subtypes: the *restricting type*, in which weight loss is achieved solely via reduction in food intake, and the *binge eating/purging type*, in which anorexic behavior is accompanied by recurrent episodes of binge eating or purging.

Bulimia nervosa. Bulimia nervosa is characterized by repeated episodes of bingeing followed by compensatory behaviors to prevent weight gain. Compensatory behaviors include vomiting, diuretic and laxative abuse, fasting, or excessive exercise. Like the anorexic, the typical bulimic has an unusual concern about body weight and weight loss. Unlike the anorexic, he or she is acutely aware of this condition and has a greater sense of guilt and loss of self control.

Bulimia typically develops during the late teens and early twenties. In contrast to the typically emaciated anorexic, most bulimics are of normal body weight, although weight may fluctuate frequently. Physically, the bulimic may have symptoms such as erosion of tooth enamel, swollen salivary glands, potassium depletion, bruised knuckles, and irritation of the esophagus.

To qualify for a clinical diagnosis of bulimia nervosa, binge eating and related compensatory behaviors must take place at least two times a week for a minimum of three months. Sufferers are classified into one of two subtypes: the *purging type*, which employs laxatives, **diuretics**, or self-induced vomiting to compensate for bingeing, or the *nonpurging type*, which relies on behaviors such as excessive exercising or fasting to offset binges.

Binge eating disorder. Binge eating disorder is characterized by eating binges that are not followed by compensatory methods. This condition, which frequently appears in late adolescence or the early twenties, affects between 15 and 50 percent of individuals participating in diet programs and often develops after substantial diet-related weight loss. Of those affected, 50 percent are male.

Binge eating disorder is diagnosed when an individual recurrently (at least twice a week for a six month period) indulges in bingeing behavior. A clinical diagnosis also requires three or more of the following behaviors: (1) eating at an unusually rapid pace, (2) eating until uncomfortably full, (3) eating large quantities of food in the absence of physical hunger, (4) eating alone out

psychological: related to thoughts, feelings, and personal experiences

behavioral: related to behavior, in contrast to medical or other types of interventions

anorexia nervosa: refusal to maintain body weight at or above what is considered normal for height and age

bulimia: uncontrolled episodes of eating (bingeing) usually followed by self-induced vomiting (purging)

binge: uncontrolled indulgence

eating disorder: behavioral disorder involving excess consumption, avoidance of consumption, self-induced vomiting, or other food-related aberrant behavior

hormone: molecules produced by one set of cells that influence the function of another set of cells

diuretic: substance that depletes the body of water

depression: mood disorder characterized by apathy, restlessness, and negative thoughts

of shame, and (5) feelings of self-disgust, guilt, or **depression** subsequent to bingeing episodes.

Eating disorder not otherwise specified. The category *eating disorder not otherwise specified* (EDNOS) is used to diagnose individuals whose eating disorders are equally as serious as anorexia nervosa, bulimia nervosa, or binge eating disorder, but do not meet all of the diagnostic criteria for these illnesses. An example of EDNOS might be a female who fulfills all of the criteria for anorexia but is still having regular menstrual periods, or an individual with all of the signs of bulimia who binges and purges less than twice a week.

Prevalence

Originally considered to be a disease targeting affluent white women and adolescents, eating disorders are now prevalent among both males and females, affecting people of all ages and from many ethnic and cultural groups. As many as 70 million people worldwide are estimated to suffer from these conditions, with one in five women displaying pathological eating patterns.

Most eating-disorder research focuses on females, who represent 90 percent of all cases. The additional 10 percent are males, a group that is often underdiagnosed due a widespread misperception that this disease only affects females. This belief also makes males less likely to seek treatment, frequently resulting in poor recovery. Among males, body image is a driving factor in the development of eating problems. Gender identity may also play a role in the evolution of eating disorders, with homosexual males more prone to this disorder than the overall male population.

Risk Factors

biological: related to living organisms

stress: heightened state of nervousness or unease

Environmental, social, **biological**, and psychological factors all contribute to eating-disorder risk. Early childhood environment and parenting may have a substantial impact. Many sufferers report dysfunctional family histories, with parents who were either emotionally absent or overly involved in their upbringing. As a result, these children may not tolerate **stress** well, they may have low self-esteem, and they may have difficulty in interpersonal relationships. Children who have been abused either physically, sexually, or psychologically are also highly vulnerable to eating disorders, particularly bulimia. Those raised by eating-disordered parents may be at heightened risk due to repeated exposure to maladaptive food-related behaviors.

nutrition: the maintenance of health through proper eating, or the study of same

serotonin: chemical used by nerve cells to communicate with one another

neurotransmitter: molecule released by one nerve cell to stimulate or inhibit another

Professions, activities, and dietary regimens that emphasize food or thinness may also encourage eating disorders. For example, athletes, ballet dancers, models, actors, diabetics, vegetarians, and food industry and **nutrition** professionals may have higher rates of disordered eating than the general population. In addition to environmental and social influences, biological and psychological factors may also increase risk for eating disorders in some people. Low levels of **serotonin**, a **neurotransmitter** involved in appetite regulation and satiety, may be indicative of a predisposition to pathological eating behaviors. Similarly, as many as 50 to 75 percent of those who are diagnosed with eating disorders suffer from depression, a mental illness also associated with abnormalities in serotonin balance. Other psychiatric disturbances, such as bipolar depression, obsessive-compulsive disorder, seasonal affective disorder, post-traumatic stress disorder, attention-deficit–hyperactivity disorder, and addictive behaviors, are also common in people with eating disorders.

Causes

Societal influences also contribute to this illness. Increasingly, Westernized culture portrays thinness as a coveted physical ideal associated with happiness, vitality, and well-being, while **obesity** is perceived as unhealthy and unattractive. This has encouraged a growing sentiment of body dissatisfaction, particularly among young women. Endless images of unrealistically thin models and actors in all forms of media further promote body dissatisfaction—one of the strongest risk factors for the development of disordered eating.

Abnormal eating patterns are most likely to develop during the mid- to late teens, a period of considerable physical, psychological, and social change. While the exact events that lead to the evolution of these disorders are unknown, there are two common milestones that can trigger disordered eating, especially in those with a biological predisposition. The first is the occurrence of a traumatic event, such as the death of a loved one or a divorce. The other is the adoption of a strict diet, which may be even more pivotal than a personal trauma. In fact, rigorous dieting has been identified again and again as the most common initiating factor in the establishment of an uncontrollable pattern of disordered eating.

Treatment Modalities

Treatment is based on a combination of psychotherapy, medication, and nutritional counseling. Goals include restoration of healthy body weight, correction of medical complications, adoption of healthful eating habits and treatment of maladaptive food-related thought processes, treatment of co-existing psychiatric conditions, and prevention of relapse. Depending on the severity of the illness, therapy may be conducted on an outpatient, day treatment, or inpatient basis.

Outpatient therapy. Outpatient therapy provided by practitioners specializing in eating disorders is appropriate for highly motivated patients within 20 percent of their normal body weight and whose illness is mild or just developing. Treatment consists of cognitive-behavioral therapy, intensive nutritional counseling, support-group referrals, and medical monitoring. At the outset of treatment, a contract is established, outlining an anticipated rate of weight gain (usually between 0.5 and 2 pounds per week), target goal weight, and consequences if weight gain is not achieved. Vitamin and mineral supplementation and the use of liquid supplements to facilitate weight gain may also be indicated.

Day treatment programs. Day treatment programs are being used with increasing frequency in place of inpatient hospitalization. This form of therapy provides an intermediate level of care for patients who require frequent monitoring but do not require treatment twenty-four hours a day. It may be used for patients who are not responding to outpatient therapy or who are stepping down from inpatient hospitalization. Treatment, which may take place four or five days per week from morning until evening, is similar in structure to outpatient therapy, but is provided on a more intensive level.

obesity: the condition of being overweight, according to established norms based on sex, age, and height

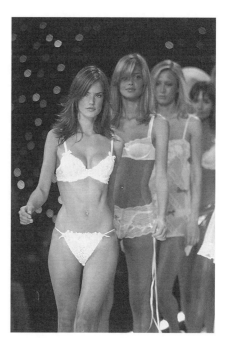

Idealized images of thinness can cause body dissatisfaction, which may lead to eating disorders. Such disorders may also be encouraged by professions that require a certain body type, such as modeling or gymnastics. *[Photograph by George De Sota. AP/Wide World Photos. Reproduced by permission.]*

Christy Henrich, a member of the U.S. gymnastics team, narrowly missed making the Olympics in 1988. Some say Henrich's anguish over that failure caused the eating disorder that killed her six years later, when she weighed less than fifty pounds. *[AP/Wide World Photos. Reproduced by permission.]*

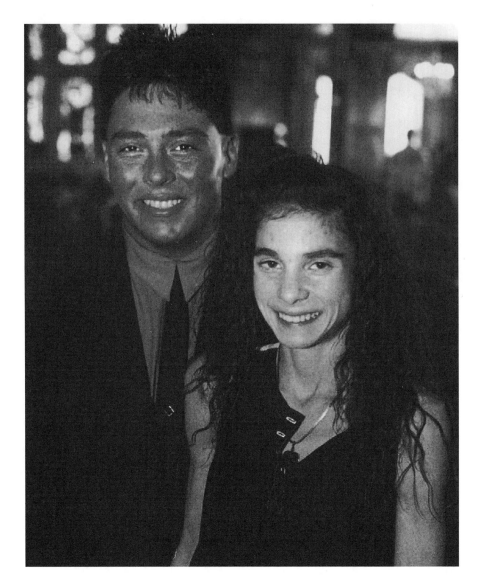

Inpatient hospitalization.

Inpatient hospitalization is indicated for patients whose eating disorder has reached life-threatening status. Criteria for admission to such programs are weight loss of 25 percent or more of ideal body weight or the presence of an eating disorder in a child or adolescent. It may also be necessary for individuals who are medically unstable. Usually, participants in inpatient programs are anorexic, although hospitalization for bulimia may be necessary if there is serious deterioration of vital signs, uncontrollable vomiting, or concurrent psychiatric illness.

The immediate goals of inpatient treatment are weight gain and stabilization of vital signs. In many cases, the patient is so fragile that complete bed rest is required. Eating is gently encouraged. In extreme medical situations refusal may be met with tube feeding or, in rare instances, intravenously.

Medication.

Medication is increasingly becoming a routine part of treatment for eating disorders. Antidepressants, particularly the selective serotonin reuptake inhibitors (SSRIs), are the most effective and most commonly used medication in treating this spectrum of illnesses. They are found to be of greatest benefit when used in combination with therapy, and are of little value if offered on their own. In the case of anorexia, these medications are most effective if employed after successful weight restoration is achieved, at which time they can be useful for relapse prevention and the treatment of coexisting psychiatric conditions. SSRIs are also used in preventing binge relapses among bulimics, although their effectiveness ceases once the medication is discontinued. Although antidepressants have also been employed in the treatment of binge eating disorder, outcomes have not been sufficiently positive to warrant recommendations for their use.

Outcomes

Individuals are usually considered to be ready to terminate therapy once they have achieved a healthy body weight and can eat all foods free of guilt or **anxiety**. For a complete recovery, extensive treatment may be required from six months to two years, and for as long as three to five years in cases where other psychiatric conditions are present. For some, eating disorders will be a lifelong struggle, with stressful or traumatic events triggering relapses that may require occasional check-in therapy to restore healthful eating patterns.

anxiety: nervousness

Of individuals with anorexia nervosa, 50 percent will have favorable outcomes, 30 percent will have intermediate results, and 20 percent will have poor outcomes. The prognosis for bulimics is slightly less favorable, with 45 percent achieving favorable outcomes, 18 percent having intermediate results, and 21 percent with poor results. Among both anorexics and bulimics, 5.6 percent will die of complications related to their illness. Those who receive treatment early in the course of their disease have a greater chance of full recovery on both a physical and an emotional level. A favorable prognosis is also likely with an early age at diagnosis, healthy parent-child relationships, and close supportive relationships with friends or therapists. With early identification and treatment, eating disorders can be prevented from becoming chronic and potentially lethal. SEE ALSO ADDICTION, FOOD; ANOREXIA NERVOSA; BULIMIA NERVOSA; EATING DISTURBANCES.

Karen Ansel

Bibliography

American Academy of Pediatrics (2003). "Policy Statement: Identifying and Treating Eating Disorders." *Pediatrics* 111(1):204–211.

American Psychiatric Association (2000). *Diagnostic and Statistical Manual of Mental Disorders*, 4th edition. Washington, DC: Author.

Berkow, Robert M., ed. (1997). *The Merck Manual of Medical Information Home Edition*. Whitehouse Station, NJ: Merck Research Laboratories.

Cassell, Dana, and Gleaves, David (2000). *The Encyclopedia of Eating Disorders*, 2nd edition. New York: Facts on File.

Costin, Carolyn (1996). *The Eating Disorder Sourcebook*. Los Angeles: Lowell House.

Pritts, Sarah D., and Susman, Jeffrey (2003). "Diagnosis of Eating Disorders in Primary Care." *American Family Physician* January 15.

Rome, Ellen S., et al. (2003). "Children and Adolescents with Eating Disorders: The State of the Art." Pediatrics 111:e98–e108.

Stice, Eric; Maxfield, Jennifer; and Wells, Tony (2003). "Adverse Effects of Social Pressure to Be Thin on Young Women: An Experimental Investigation of the Effects of 'Fat Talk.'" *International Journal of Eating Disorders* 34:108–117.

Woolsey, Monika M. (2002). *Eating Disorders: A Clinical Guide to Counseling and Treatment*. Chicago: American Dietetic Association.

Eating Disorders throughout History

Although eating disorders first came to widespread attention in the 1970s, self-starvation and other pathological eating practices are found throughout recorded history. Bulimia was widely known in both Greek and Roman societies and was recorded in France as early as the eighteenth century. Self-starvation for religious reasons became widespread in Europe during the Renaissance, as hundreds of women starved themselves, often to death, in hopes of attaining communion with Christ. During the nineteenth century, as corpulence stopped being viewed as a symbol of prosperity, self-starvation became common again. The incidence of eating disorders varies widely among cultures and time periods, suggesting that they can be encouraged or inhibited by social and economic factors. Eating disorders have most often been seen in affluent societies and are rarely reported during periods of famine, plague, and warfare.

—*Paula Kepos*

Internet Resources

American Psychiatric Association (2001). "Men Less Likely to Seek Help for Eating Disorders." Available from <http://www.nlm.nih.gov/medlineplus>

American Psychiatric Association. "Practice Guideline for the Treatment of Patients with Eating Disorders." Available from <http://www.psych.org>

Anorexia Nervosa and Related Eating Disorders, Inc. (2002). "Males with Eating Disorders." Available from <http://www.anred.com/males.html>

Devlin, Michael J., and Walsh, Timothy B. (2000) "Psychopharmacology of Anorexia Nervosa, Bulimia Nervosa, and Binge Eating." American College of Neuropsychopharmacology. Available from <http://www.acnp.org/g>

National Eating Disorders Association (2002). "Males and Eating Disorders." Available from <http://www.nationaleatingdisorders.org>

National Eating Disorders Association (2002). "What Causes Eating Disorders?" Available from <http://www.nationaleatingdisorders.org>

Renfrew Center Foundation (2002). "Eating Disorders: A Summary of Issues, Statistics and Resources." Available from <http://www.renfrew.org>

Eating Disturbances

An eating disturbance shares many similar characteristics with eating disorders, but is less severe in scope. As a result, many abnormal dietary patterns and behaviors, such as **binge** eating, excessive exercising, weight cycling, and **chronic** dieting may involve many of the same attitudes and impulses as eating disorders, though they do not meet the clinical criteria for diagnosis.

Eating disturbances usually develop during adolescence and early adulthood. While they occur in both males and females, they are far more prevalent among females. They are characterized by distorted eating patterns and usually occur in individuals of normal weight who have a history of dieting and a strong desire to become thin. As with eating disorders, body perception and self-esteem are closely intertwined. Many cases may start out innocently, with only small dietary changes such as eating smaller or larger portions of food, and eventually progress beyond the individual's control. For some, eating may become highly restrictive, accompanied by stringent elimination of certain high-calorie, high-fat foods. Others may consume these foods in excess, but only during episodes of gorging. Symptoms include obsession with food and calories, fear of specific **nutrients** (such as fat), rigid categorization of foods as "good" or "bad," irrational fear of weight gain, excessive weighing, avoidance of social situations where food is served, and denial of eating problems.

Binge Eating

Binge eating is a frequent precursor to **bulimia** nervosa and binge eating syndrome. Individuals who indulge in binge eating may eat tremendous quantities of food, well past the point of being comfortably full and possibly to the point of extreme discomfort or even pain. Bingeing may take place over a short period of time, or it may be prolonged—lasting for several hours, sometimes continuing from morning until nighttime. For individuals prone to binge eating, food becomes a focal point of life, with an obsession about what can or cannot be eaten. Eating may take place very quickly and is often unrelated to hunger. Although there may be variation in the types of food chosen, high-calorie, high-fat sweets are favored. Since bingeing is

binge: uncontrolled indulgence

chronic: over a long period

nutrient: dietary substance necessary for health

bulimia: uncontrolled episodes of eating (bingeing) usually followed by self-induced vomiting (purging)

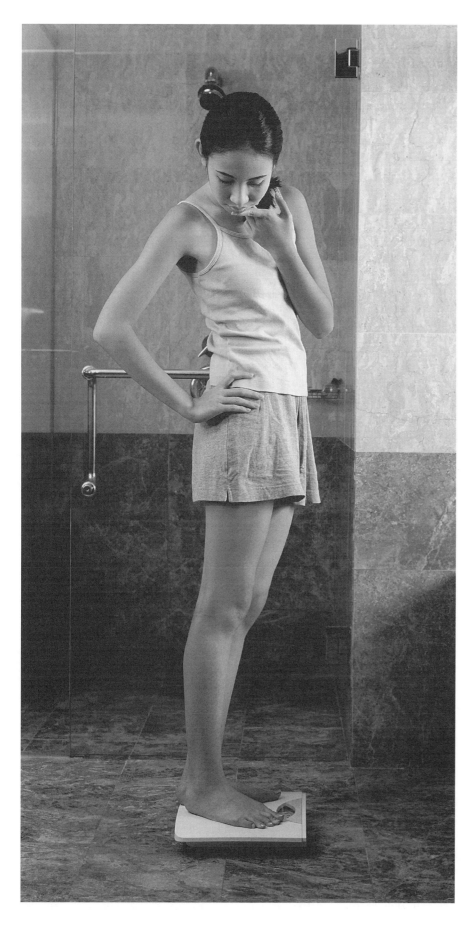

Eating disturbances are milder than eating disorders, but both are characterized by a preoccupation with food, weight, fitness, or body image. *[Eric K. K. Yu/Corbis. Reproduced by permission.]*

depression: mood disorder characterized by apathy, restlessness, and negative thoughts

obesity: the condition of being overweight, according to established norms based on sex, age, and height

eating disorder: behavioral disorder involving excess consumption, avoidance of consumption, self-induced vomiting, or other food-related aberrant behavior

amenorrhea: lack of menstruation

osteoporosis: weakening of the bone structure

electrolyte: salt dissolved in fluid

physiological: related to the biochemical processes of the body

neurological: related to the nervous system

neurotransmitter: molecule released by one nerve cell to stimulate or inhibit another

accompanied by a sense of shame, embarrassment, and lack of self-control, episodes usually take place alone, in secret.

Bingeing is frequently triggered by troubled relationships, extreme hunger subsequent to stringent dieting, or feelings of melancholy. While gorging on coveted foods may temporarily improve one's mood, it is usually followed by feelings of **depression** and low self-esteem. Although these incidents may contribute to **obesity**, they may also occur in individuals of normal body weight who compensate for binges with excessive exercising or even fasting.

Excessive Exercising

Also known as activity disorder, excessive exercising is an extreme method of weight control. Individuals suffering from this syndrome are compelled to exercise for prolonged periods on a daily basis and to indulge in constant activity to burn excess calories. Eventually they experience a loss of control over the desire to exercise, in the same way that a person with an **eating disorder** cannot control behaviors relative to eating.

Excessive exercisers suffer from the same obsession with body weight and shape as anorexics and bulimics, and exercise eventually becomes necessary not only for weight control, but also for mood stabilization and self-definition. Utterly powerless to restrain their urge to exercise, they will pursue daily activity in spite of injury or exhaustion, or in places and settings that are completely inappropriate. They are usually accomplished individuals, both professionally and academically, and they may appear to be vigorously fit and healthy. Despite their overtly sound appearance, however, over time they may suffer health consequences far more serious than routine athletic injuries. Drastic weight loss may lead to **amenorrhea**, which, in turn, may weaken bones and increase **osteoporosis** risk. Vitamin and mineral deficiencies may develop and **electrolyte** imbalances may occur, which may lead to cardiac arrest in extreme cases.

Cravings

Cravings for carbohydrate-rich foods cause many bulimics and binge eaters to center their binges around desserts and high-starch foods. Many individuals suffering from disordered eating commonly avoid foods low in carbohydrate and high in fat, and instead seek out excessive sugar, routinely using large quantities to sweeten foods and beverages. This may stem from a **physiological** and evolutionary need for ample carbohydrate to ensure proper **neurological** function. Large quantities of carbohydrate eaten in a short time frame are capable of altering **neurotransmitter** synthesis, producing a calming effect on the brain, and thus may be the impetus for such cravings in certain eating disorders and disturbances.

Weight Cycling

Also known as yo-yo dieting, weight cycling is common in Westernized nations, particularly among young women. Often observed among chronic dieters, weight cycling is an ongoing sequence of dieting, weight loss, cessation from dieting, and weight gain. This final stage of weight gain is particularly detrimental, as the amount regained often exceeds the quantity originally lost, resulting in an increase in overall body weight. As muscle mass accounts for a portion of the lost weight, weight cycling may ultimately slow overall **metabolism**, with every 5 percent of body weight lost resulting in a 15 percent decrease in resting metabolism. This compensatory mechanism, adapted to help prevent weight loss during times of starvation, eventually prompts further weight gain, frequently initiating a renewed cycle of dieting.

metabolism: the sum total of reactions in a cell or an organism

Chronic Dieting

Many individuals with eating disorders report habitual dieting prior to the onset of their illness. Repeated dieting during adolescence increases the risk of eating disorders, with some patients reporting attempts at weight loss as early as age nine. The **incidence** of eating disorders may be as much as eight times greater among girls with a history of dieting, with the initiation of a weight loss regimen often marking the onset of the eating disorder itself. Dietary restriction may result in alterations in brain chemistry that can further increase anorexic tendencies, while hunger resulting from caloric restriction can set off binge eating, thus establishing a pattern. While most healthy individuals who attempt to lose weight can stop at any given time, depression and major life stresses in combination with habitual dieting can predispose others to develop an eating disorder. SEE ALSO ADDICTION, FOOD; ANOREXIA NERVOSA; BULIMIA NERVOSA; EATING DISORDERS.

incidence: number of new cases reported each year

Karen Ansel

Bibliography

American Dietetic Association (1998). *Nutrition Intervention in the Treatment of Anorexia Nervosa, Bulimia Nervosa, and Eating Disorder Not Otherwise Specified (EDNOS).* Chicago: Author.

American Psychiatric Association (2000). *Diagnostic and Statistical Manual of Mental Disorders,* 4th edition. Washington, DC: Author.

Cassell, Dana, and Gleaves, David (2000). *The Encyclopedia of Eating Disorders,* 2nd edition. New York: Facts on File.

Cataldo, Corrine B.; Rolfes, Sharon R.; Whitney, Eleanor N. (1994). *Understanding Normal and Clinical Nutrition,* 4th edition. St. Paul, MN: West Publishing.

Costin, Carolyn (1996). *The Eating Disorder Sourcebook.* Los Angeles: Lowell House.

Dare, Chris; Szmukler, Georg; Treasure, Janet (1995). *Handbook of Eating Disorders: Theory, Treatment, and Research.* New York: Wiley.

Escott-Stump, Sylvia, and Mahan, L. Kathleen (1996). *Krause's Food, Nutrition, and Diet Therapy,* 9th edition. Philadelphia: W. B. Saunders.

Franseen, Lisa (1999). "Understanding and Identifying Eating Problems in Synchronized Swimmers, Part 1." *Synchro Swimming USA* (Winter).

Garfinkel, Paul E., and Garner, David M. (1997) *Handbook of Treatment for Eating Disorders,* 2nd edition. New York: Guilford Press.

Rosenbloom, Christine A., ed. (1999). *Sports Nutrition: A Guide for the Professional Working with Active People.* Chicago: American Dietetic Association.

Woolsey, Monika M. (2002). *Eating Disorders: A Clinical Guide to Counseling and Treatment.* Chicago: American Dietetic Association.

Internet Resources

McKinley Health Center, University of Illinois at Urbana. "Understanding Eating Disturbances and Disorders: A Guide for Helping Family and Friends." Available from <http://www.mckinley.uiuc.edu>

National Institute of Mental Health. "Eating Disorders: Facts about Eating Disorders and the Search for Solutions." Available from <http://www.nimh.nih.gov>

Eating Habits

The term *eating habits* (or *food habits*) refers to why and how people eat, which foods they eat, and with whom they eat, as well as the ways people obtain, store, use, and discard food. Individual, social, cultural, religious, economic, environmental, and political factors all influence people's eating habits.

Why and How People Eat

All humans eat to survive. They also eat to express appreciation, for a sense of belonging, as part of family customs, and for self-realization. For example, someone who is not hungry may eat a piece of cake that has been baked in his or her honor.

learned behaviors: actions that are acquired by training and observation, in contrast to innate behaviors

People eat according to **learned behaviors** regarding etiquette, meal and snack patterns, acceptable foods, food combinations, and portion sizes. *Etiquette* refers to acceptable behaviors. For example, for some groups it is acceptable to lick one's fingers while eating, while for other groups this is rude behavior. Etiquette and eating **rituals** also vary depending on whether the meal is formal, informal, or special (such as a meal on a birthday or religious holiday).

ritual: ceremony or frequently repeated behavior

A meal is usually defined as the consumption of two or more foods in a structured setting at a set time. Snacks consist of a small amount of food or beverage eaten between meals. A common eating pattern is three meals (breakfast, lunch, and dinner) per day, with snacks between meals. The components of a meal vary across cultures, but generally include grains, such as rice or noodles; meat or a meat substitute, such as fish, beans, or **tofu**; and accompaniments, such as vegetables. Various food guides provide suggestions on foods to eat, portion sizes, and daily intake. However, personal preferences, habits, family customs, and social setting largely determine what a person consumes.

tofu: soybean curd, similar in consistency to cottage cheese

What and how people eat is determined by a variety of factors, including economic circumstances, cultural norms, and religious restrictions. Here, an Iranian family sits on the floor and eats from a cloth laden with regional delicacies. *[Photograph by Earl and Nazima Kowall. Corbis. Reproduced by permission.]*

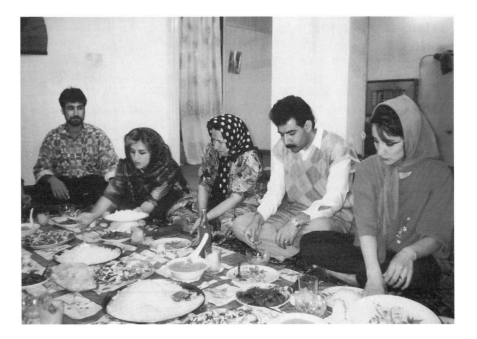

What People Eat

In each culture there are both acceptable and unacceptable foods, though this is not determined by whether or not something is edible. For example, alligators exist in many parts of the world, but they are unacceptable as food by many persons. Likewise, horses, turtles, and dogs are eaten (and even considered a delicacy) in some cultures, though they are unacceptable food sources in other cultures. There are also rules concerning with whom it is appropriate to eat. For example, doctors in a health facility may eat in areas separate from patients or clients.

Obtaining, Storing, Using, and Discarding Food

Humans acquire, store, and discard food using a variety of methods. People may grow, fish, or hunt some of their food, or they may purchase most of it from supermarkets or specialty stores. If there is limited access to energy sources, people may store small amounts of foods and get most of what they eat on a day-to-day basis. In homes with abundant space and energy, however, people purchase food in bulk and store it in freezers, refrigerators, and pantries. In either case there must also be proper disposal facilities to avoid environmental and health problems.

Exposure to Foods

There are innumerable flavors and food combinations. A liking for some flavors or food combinations is easily acceptable, but others must develop or be learned. Sweetness is a universally acceptable flavor, but a taste for salty, savory, spicy, tart, bitter, and hot flavors must be learned. The more a person is exposed to a food—and encouraged to eat it—the greater the chances that the food will be accepted. As the exposure to a food increases, the person becomes more familiar and less fearful of the food, and acceptance may develop. Some persons only eat specific foods and flavor combinations, while others like trying different foods and flavors.

Influences on Food Choices

There are many factors that determine what foods a person eats. In addition to personal preferences, there are cultural, social, religious, economic, environmental, and even political factors.

Individual Preferences. Every individual has unique likes and dislikes concerning foods. These preferences develop over time, and are influenced by personal experiences such as encouragement to eat, exposure to a food, family customs and rituals, advertising, and personal values. For example, one person may not like frankfurters, despite the fact that they are a family favorite.

Cultural Influences. A cultural group provides guidelines regarding acceptable foods, food combinations, eating patterns, and eating behaviors. Compliance with these guidelines creates a sense of identity and belonging for the individual. Within large cultural groups, subgroups exist that may practice variations of the group's eating behaviors, though they are still considered part of the larger group. For example, a hamburger, French fries, and a soda are considered a typical American meal. Vegetarians in the United

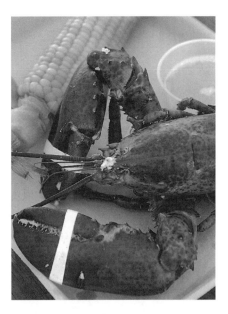

Someone who is repeatedly exposed to certain foods is less hesitant to eat them. For example, lobster traditionally was only available on the coasts, and is much more likely to be accepted as food by coastal dwellers. [AP/Wide World Photos. Reproduced by permission.]

States, however, eat "veggie-burgers" made from mashed beans, pureed vegetables, or soy, and people on diets may eat a burger made from lean turkey. In the United States these are appropriate cultural substitutions, but a burger made from horsemeat would be unacceptable.

social group: tribe, clique, family, or other group of individuals

Social Influences. Members of a **social group** depend on each other, share a common culture, and influence each other's behaviors and values. A person's membership in particular peer, work, or community groups impacts food behaviors. For example, a young person at a basketball game may eat certain foods when accompanied by friends and other foods when accompanied by his or her teacher.

proscription: prohibitions, rules against

Religious Influences. Religious **proscriptions** range from a few to many, from relaxed to highly restrictive. This will affect a follower's food choices and behaviors. For example, in some religions specific foods are prohibited, such as pork among Jewish and Muslim adherents. Within Christianity, the Seventh-day Adventists discourage "stimulating" beverages such as alcohol, which is not forbidden among Catholics.

Economic Influences. Money, values, and consumer skills all affect what a person purchases. The price of a food, however, is not an indicator of its nutritional value. Cost is a complex combination of a food's availability, status, and demand.

ecological: related to the environment and human interactions with it

Environmental Influences. The influence of the environment on food habits derives from a composite of **ecological** and social factors. Foods that are commonly and easily grown within a specific region frequently become a part of the local cuisine. However, modern technology, agricultural practices, and transportation methods have increased the year-round availability of many foods, and many foods that were previously available only at certain seasons or in specific areas are now available almost anywhere, at any time.

Political Influences. Political factors also influence food availability and trends. Food laws and trade agreements affect what is available within and across countries, and also affect food prices. Food labeling laws determine what consumers know about the food they purchase.

Eating habits are thus the result of both external factors, such as politics, and internal factors, such as values. These habits are formed, and may change, over a person's lifetime. SEE ALSO DIET; POPULAR CULTURE, FOOD AND.

Judith C. Rodriguez

Bibliography

Haviland, William A. (1990). *Cultural Anthropology*. Chicago: Holt, Rinehart and Winston.

Kittler, Pamela G., and Sucher, Kathryn P. (1998). *Food and Culture in America: A Nutrition Handbook*, 2nd edition. Belmont, CA: West/Wadsworth.

Klimis-Zacas, Dorothy J., ed. (2001). *Annual Editions: Nutrition 01/02*. Guilford, CT: McGraw Hill/Dushkin.

Lowenberg, Miriam Elizabeth; Todhunter, Elizabeth Neige; Wilson, E. D.; Savage, J. R.; and Lubawski, J. L. (1979). *Food and People*. New York: Wiley.

Schlosser, Eric (2001). *Fast Food Nation: The Darker Side of the All American Meal*. New York: Houghton Mifflin.

Emergency Nutrition Network

The Emergency Nutrition Network (ENN) is a network of humanitarian agencies and researchers that supports and facilitates activities that increase the effectiveness of emergency food and nutrition interventions. The planning for the ENN was done in 1995 at a meeting sponsored by the United Nations High Commissioner for Refugees (UNHCR), and the network began operating in November 1996.

Humanitarian agencies sometimes provide interventions and food that are not always logistically or culturally appropriate. In addition, many agencies have high staff turnover, inadequate record keeping, and limited resources, all of which can delay access to appropriate information at critical times. The goal of the ENN is to improve the effectiveness of emergency food and nutrition programs by:

- Providing a forum for relief workers to exchange ideas and experiences
- Helping network agencies work more efficiently and effectively
- Providing field staff and relief workers with knowledge of current and relevant research
- Helping researchers to identify priorities and constraints of the emergency sector

ENN primarily operates through a newsletter, *Field Exchange*. The institutional base for ENN is Trinity College, Dublin. Project staff includes a full-time coordinator and a part-time technical consultant. Representatives from key agencies are available for technical support. ENN is currently funded by the Irish Department of Foreign Affairs, MSF International, Concern Worldwide, the Canadian International Development Agency, the U.S. Agency for International Development, the World Health Organization, UNHCR, and other organizations. Partnership in the network is not dependent on any financial contributions. SEE ALSO DISASTER RELIEF ORGANIZATIONS; FAMINE.

Delores C. S. James

Internet Resources

Dublin Business Innovation Center. "Company Profile: Emergency Nutrition Network (ENN)." Available from <http://www.dbic.ie/ENN.htm>

Emergency Nutrition Network. "About the ENN." Available from <http://www.ennonline.net>

One World. "Emergency Nutrition Network." Available from <http://www.oneworld.org>

Ergogenic Aids

Ergogenic aids are dietary supplements intended to enhance athletic performance. Athletes often look for a "magic bullet" that can give them an advantage over their opponents. However, while they tend to be highly disciplined regarding training, they are not always careful in their use of dietary supplements. The important points about supplement usage include:

- Supplements are not one size fits all
- Natural and safe are not synonymous terms

- Supplements may be age- and gender-specific
- Supplements are sports-specific, and may be position-specific
- The **efficacy** of supplements is contingent upon the underlying **hydration**, **diet**, and training
- The issue of "stacking" (using many different supplements) may create safety problems
- Supplements may interact with both prescription and **over-the-counter** medications

efficacy: effectiveness

hydration: degree of water in the body

diet: the total daily food intake, or the types of foods eaten

over-the-counter: available without a prescription

Ergogenic aids are not a substitute for food, fluid, or activity. Athletes who are already at the peak of physical ability and consume an optimal diet will, for the most part, realize little if any benefit from supplement use. The most commonly used supplements are **anabolic** agents, ginseng, ephedra, and caffeine.

anabolic: promoting building up

Anabolic Agents

steroids: group of hormones that affect tissue build-up, sexual development, and a variety of metabolic processes

amino acid: building block of proteins, necessary dietary nutrient

The most frequently and widely used category of ergogenic aids is those with supposed anabolic effects; that is, they mimic the benefits of **steroids** (in a legal manner). Creatine is the most widely used supplement taken by both recreational and professional athletes. Creatine is synthesized in the kidneys, pancreas, and liver from **amino acid** precursors (methionine, arginine, and glycine), and is also found in meat, fish, and poultry. The ergogenic effect of supplemental creatine is attributed to its ability to increase tissue creatine levels beyond what the body can synthesize on its own, resulting in increased work capacity during intense activity requiring maximal or near maximal effort. It can also expedite the recovery rate following exercise. These benefits are most likely seen with a regimen of 20 to 25 grams of creatine over five to seven days, divided into four- or five-gram doses (this is called the *loading* phase). Creatine levels will fall to presupplementation levels six weeks later. For optimal effect, each dose of creatine should be consumed with a **carbohydrate** and without caffeine, which can counteract the ergogenic effect. Muscle **hypertrophy** and fluid retention can occur during the loading phase, causing a weight gain of four to seven pounds. This increase may be advantageous for the strength athlete, but less so for an athlete who relies on speed. Short-term studies have not shown an increase in muscle strains, cramps, or pulls with creatine, but it is critical for the athlete to maintain optimal hydration. There are some concerns with product contamination, as creatine supplements could be contaminated with herbs, or even with other anabolic agents not listed on the label.

carbohydrate: food molecule made of carbon, hydrogen, and oxygen, including sugars and starches

hypertrophy: excess increase in size

trace: very small amount

testosterone: male sex hormone

nausea: unpleasant sensation in the gut that precedes vomiting

blood pressure: measure of the pressure exerted by the blood against the walls of the blood vessels

Other anabolic agents include HMB (beta-hydroxy beta-methylbutyrate), which, in clinical studies, has resulted in an increase in muscle mass. The number of studies has been quite small, however. Boron is a **trace** mineral involved in cellular functions, but it does not increase **testosterone** levels as some claims would suggest. It can suppress appetite and impair digestion in doses higher than 50 mg per day. Yohimbe is a supplement derived from the tree bark of a South American plant that confers a stimulant effect, not an anabolic effect. Ingestion of this product can cause dizziness, nervousness, headaches, **nausea**, vomiting, and an elevated **blood pressure**. It can also interact with blood-pressure medication and increase the toxicity of

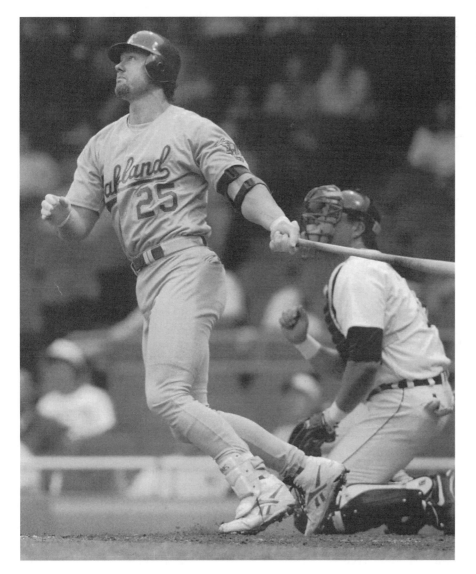

Mark McGwire astounded baseball fans when he hit 70 home runs in 1998. But his use of legal performance-enhancing supplements, such as androstenedione, raised tough questions for athletes and trainers. [*AP/Wide World Photos. Reproduced by permission.*]

psychotherapeutic medications, and it may be harmful to the kidneys. Chromium is an essential mineral involved in blood **glucose** control. It can be taken in a dosage of between 50 and 300 micrograms per day, but it does not have any anabolic effects.

glucose: a simple sugar; the most commonly used fuel in cells

Other supposed anabolic agents include dehydroepiandrosterone (DHEA), androstenedione, and *Tribulus terrestris* (tribestan). All of these are banned by the U.S. Olympic Committee, the National Collegiate Athletic Association (NCAA), the National Football League, and the American Tennis Federation. Studies have demonstrated the ineffectiveness of androstenedione as an anabolic substance or strength enhancer, but they have demonstrated potentially worrisome side effects, including a decrease in **serum HDL** level and an increase in serum estrone and **estradiol**, which increases the likelihood of gynecomastia (breast enlargement). In addition, several laboratory tests have shown that the amount of actual product in these supplements can vary dramatically, and some are contaminated with **nandrolone**, an anabolic steroid that can cause a positive result in a drug test.

serum: non-cellular portion of the blood

HDL: high density lipoprotein, a blood protein that carries cholesterol

estradiol: female hormone; a type of estrogen

nandrolone: hormone related to testosterone

Protein Supplements.

Protein is essential for muscle growth and development, but the maximum usable amount of protein is one gram per pound of body weight. Protein powders contain large quantities of protein, plus large doses of **vitamins**, **minerals**, and herbs. Amino acid supplementation has been associated with **gastrointestinal** side effects, such as nausea, diarrhea, or vomiting, that may negate any potential ergogenic benefits. In addition, selective amino acid supplementation is a very inefficient way to provide protein to the body and can create an amino-acid imbalance.

Energy Boosters

Many athletes take supplements to boost energy, particularly ginseng, ephedra, and caffeine. Ginseng functions as an adaptogen, or **immune system** stimulant, but it does not have an effect on athletic performance. (Athletes who choose to take ginseng should look for *Panax* ginseng standardized to 4–7 percent; ginsenosides, with the following dosing regimen: 100–200 milligrams per day for two–three weeks, then one–two weeks of no use before resuming).

Ephedra (also called Ma Huang, epitonin, and sida cordifolia) is a central **nervous system** stimulant that is sold as an energy booster or "fat-burning" supplement. Marketed as *Metabolife*, *Xenadrine*, *Herbal Rush*, *Energy Rush*, *Thermoburn*, or *Thermofuel* (among others), ephedra may delay **fatigue** by sparing the body's **glycogen** reserves during exercise. However, it can also increase blood pressure, respiration rate, heart rate, **anxiety**, migraines, and irregular heartbeat, and it can cause insomnia, psychosis, and nervousness. Ephedra and caffeine are often present in the same product, which can be detrimental to the heart. The maximum safe level of ephedra is 24 mg per day, but many products contain over 300 mg per dose. This supplement is **contraindicated** in those with a history of **heart disease** or **hypertension**, kidney or thyroid disease, seizure disorder, or **diabetes**.

Caffeine is a stimulant that in certain athletes may increase free fatty-acid availability to delay fatigue, improve reaction time, and reduce the perceived effort of exertion. It tends to be most effective in caffeine-naïve, trained endurance athletes with a dose of 200 to 300 milligrams one hour prior to a sporting event. The legal limit of caffeine is 800 milligrams, but this level can cause nervousness, anxiety, irritability, headaches, increased urination, and diarrhea. In addition to products such as Vivarin, No-Doz, and Excedrin, caffeine can be found in herbal form in guarana, maté, and kola nut. Caffeine also augments the stimulatory effects of ephedra.

Weight Loss Agents

Weight loss agents contain ingredients such as L-carnitine, which may prevent **lactic acid** accumulation but does not promote fat loss; quercetin, an **antioxidant** that is important for the heart but does not aid the loss of body fat; hydroxycitrate (a diuretic); ephedra; caffeine, and senna and/or cascara (herbal laxatives). Chitin, or chitosan (advertised as a "fat trapper" or "fat blocker"), is made from the shells of insects and shellfish and may lower **cholesterol**, but it also does not lower body fat levels. It can bind with **calcium**, **iron**, and magnesium and interfere with the **absorption** of Vitamins A, D, E, and K. Any weight loss experienced with the use of these products is primarily due to water loss associated with the laxative/diuretic components.

vitamin: necessary complex nutrient used to aid enzymes or other metabolic processes in the cell

mineral: an inorganic (non-carbon-containing) element, ion, or compound

gastrointestinal: related to the stomach and intestines

immune system: the set of organs and cells, including white blood cells, that protect the body from infection

nervous system: the brain, spinal cord, and nerves that extend throughout the body

fatigue: tiredness

glycogen: storage form of sugar

anxiety: nervousness

contraindicated: not recommended

heart disease: any disorder of the heart or its blood supply, including heart attack, atherosclerosis, and coronary artery disease

hypertension: high blood pressure

diabetes: inability to regulate level of sugar in the blood

lactic acid: breakdown product of sugar in the muscles in the absence of oxygen

antioxidant: substance that prevents oxidation, a damaging reaction with oxygen

cholesterol: multi-ringed molecule found in animal cell membranes; a type of lipid

calcium: mineral essential for bones and teeth

iron: nutrient needed for red blood cell formation

absorption: uptake by the digestive tract

Dangerous Supplements

One of the more dangerous supplements is GBL/GHB (Gamma butyro-lactone and gamma hydroxy butryric acid), which is marketed as *Rest-Eze*, *Blue Nitro*, *Revivarant G*, *Ecstasy*, *GH Revitalizer*, *GHR*, *Remforce*, *Renewtrient*, and *Gamma G*. As of December 2002, use of these products has resulted in three deaths and one hundred adverse reactions, including coma and breathing difficulties.

The potential harmful effects of yohimbe, ephedra, and excessive caffeine intake have already been mentioned. Kava is an herb used to treat anxiety, but it may cause liver failure. In addition, individuals on prescription or over-the-counter medications should be wary of supplements, as there may be adverse interactions.

Athletes at all levels should have their supplement use carefully monitored. Coaches, parents, or others working with athletes should ask what they take and in what dosage and frequency. Labels should be examined, and all information should be documented in the medical record. It is best if athletes try only one product at a time, and supplement use should be discontinued if any unusual dizziness, stomach upset, or headaches occur. All coaches should be familiar with the available supplements and their dangers.
SEE ALSO DIETARY SUPPLEMENTS; SPORTS NUTRITION.

Leslie Bonci

Bibliography

Medical Economics Company (2001). *PDR for Nutritional Supplements*. Montvale, NJ: Medical Economics.

Williams, Melvin. *The Ergogenics Edge: Pushing the Limits of Sports Performance*. Champaign, IL: Human Kinetics.

Internet Resources

Alternative Medical Foundation. "Electronic Herbal Database." Available from <http://www.herbmed.org>

ConsumerLab.com. "Product Reviews" and "Natural Product Encyclopedia." Available from <http://www.consumerlab.com>

Gatorade Sports Science Institute. "Dietary Supplements." Available from <http://www.gssiweb.com>

National Center for Drug Free Sport. "Drug and Supplement Education." Available from <http://www.drugfreesport.com>

National Institutes of Health, Office of Dietary Supplements. "What Are Dietary Supplements." Available from <http://dietary-supplements.info.nih.gov>

Exchange System

Prior to the development of exchange lists in 1950, meal planning for persons in the United States with **diabetes** was chaotic, with no agreement among the major organizations involved with diabetes and **nutrition**. To solve this problem, the concept of "exchange," or "substitution," of similar foods was developed by the American Dietetic Association, the American Diabetes Association, and the U.S. Public Health Service. The goal was to develop an educational tool for persons with diabetes that would provide uniformity in meal planning and allow for the inclusion of a wider variety of foods.

diabetes: inability to regulate level of sugar in the blood

nutrition: the maintenance of health through proper eating, or the study of same

calorie: unit of food energy

carbohydrate: food molecule made of carbon, hydrogen, and oxygen, including sugars and starches

protein: complex molecule composed of amino acids that performs vital functions in the cell; necessary part of the diet

fat: type of food molecule rich in carbon and hydrogen, with high energy content

metabolic: related to processing of nutrients and building of necessary molecules within the cell

polyunsaturated: having multiple double bonds within the chemical structure, thus increasing the body's ability to metabolize it

nutrient: dietary substance necessary for health

Definition

The word *exchange* refers to the fact that each item on a particular list in the portion listed may be interchanged with any other food item on the same list. An exchange can be explained as a substitution, choice, or serving. Each list is a group of measured or weighed foods of approximately the same nutritional value. Within each food list, one exchange is approximately equal to another in **calories**, **carbohydrate**, **protein**, and **fat**. To use the exchange lists, an individual needs an individualized meal plan that outlines the number of exchanges from each list for each meal and for snacks. The American Diabetes Association recommends that because of the complexity of nutrition issues, a registered dietitian, knowledgeable and skilled in implementing nutrition therapy into diabetes management and education, be the team member developing and implementing meal plans. The meal plan is developed in cooperation with the person with diabetes and is based on an assessment of eating changes that would assist the individual in achieving his or her target **metabolic** goals and of changes the individual is willing and able to make. Because of the accuracy and convenience of the exchange system, the exchange lists are used for weight management as well for diabetes management.

The exchange system categorizes foods into three main groups: Carbohydrates, Meat and Meat Substitutes, and Fats. Foods are further subdivided in these three groups into specific exchange lists. The Carbohydrate Group contains the Starch, Fruit, Milk, Sweets and desserts (other carbohydrates), and Vegetable lists. Foods from the Starch, Fruit, Milk, and Sweets lists can be interchanged in the meal plan, as they each contain foods with 60 to 90 calories and approximately 15 grams of carbohydrate. The Meat and Meat Substitute Group contains food sources of protein and fat. The group is divided into four lists: Very Lean Meats, Lean Meats, Medium-Fat Meats, and High-Fat Meats, allowing the user to see at a glance which meats are low-fat and which meats are high-fat. The lists have foods containing 35, 55, 75, and 100 calories, and 1, 3, 5, and 8 grams of fat, respectively. The Fat Group contains three lists: Monounsaturated Fats, **Polyunsaturated** Fats, and Saturated Fats. Each food source contains an average of 45 calories and 5 grams of fat. The exchange lists also identify foods that contribute significant amounts of sodium. A sodium symbol is shown next to foods that contain 400 mg or more of sodium per exchange serving.

Advantages and Disadvantages

An advantage of the food exchange system is that it provides a system in which a wide selection of foods can be included, thereby offering variety and versatility to the person with diabetes. Other advantages of the lists are: (1) they provide a framework to group foods with similar carbohydrate, protein, fat, and calorie contents; (2) they emphasize important management concepts, such as carbohydrate amounts, fat modification, calorie control, and awareness of high-sodium foods; (3) by making food choices from each of the different lists a variety of healthful food choices can be assured; and (4) they provide a system that allows individuals to be accountable for what they eat. Furthermore, with an understanding of the **nutrient** composition of the exchange lists, nutrient values from food labels can be used and a wider variety of foods can be incorporated accurately into a meal plan.

Helpful Hints for Using the Exchange Lists

- Cereals, grains, pasta, breads, crackers, snacks, starchy vegetables, and cooked beans, peas, and lentils are on the starch list. In general, one starch exchange is ½ cup cereal, grain, or starchy vegetable; one ounce of a bread product, such as one slice of bread; one-third cup rice or pasta; or three-fourths to one ounce of most snack foods.

- Fresh, frozen, canned, and dried fruits and fruit juices are on the fruit list. In general, one fruit exchange is: one small to medium fresh fruit, one-half cup of canned or fresh fruit or fruit juice, or one-fourth cup of dried fruit.

- Different types of milk and milk products, such as yogurt, are on the milk list. One cup (eight fluid ounces) or two-thirds cup (six ounces) of fat-free or low-fat flavored yogurt sweetened with a non-nutritive sweetener are examples of one exchange.

- Vegetables are included in the Carbohydrate Group and are important components of a healthful diet. However, since three servings of vegetables are the equivalent of one carbohydrate serving, one or two servings per meal need not be counted. This was done to encourage consumption of vegetables and to simplify meal planning.

- Meat and meat substitutes that contain both protein and fat are on the meat list. In general, one exchange is: one ounce meat, fish, poultry, or cheese; or one-half cup beans, peas, lentils.

- In general, one fat exchange is: one teaspoon of regular margarine, mayonnaise, or vegetable oil; one tablespoon of regular salad dressings or reduced-fat mayonnaise; or two tablespoons of reduced-fat salad dressings.

- A *free food* is any food or drink that contains less than 20 calories or less than five grams of carbohydrate per serving. Foods with approximately 20 calories should be limited to three servings per day and spread throughout the day.

- Some foods are in one list, but they may fit just as appropriately in another list. For example, foods in the Starch, Fruit, and Milk lists of the Carbohydrate Group each contribute similar amounts of carbohydrates and calories and may be interchanged. If fruits or starches are regularly substituted for milk, calcium intake may be decreased. Conversely, regularly choosing milk instead of fruits or starches may result in inadequate fiber intake. Foods from the Other Carbohydrate list of the Carbohydrate Group, the Combination Foods list, and the fast foods list are also interchangeable with the Starch, Fruit, and Milk lists. However, most of the dessert-type foods on the Other Carbohydrate list are higher in sugars and fat and need to be eaten within the context of a healthful meal plan.

- Beans, peas, and lentils are included in the Starch list of the Carbohydrate Group. The serving size (usually one-half cup) is counted as one starch and one very lean meat for vegetarian meal planning. If individuals are not practicing vegetarians, or use these foods less frequently and often as side dishes rather than main dishes, the very lean meat exchange does not need to be counted— one-half cup is equivalent to one starch.

- Skim and reduced-fat milks are recommended for adults and children over two years of age, rather than whole milk.

- Meat choices from the Very Lean or Lean Meat lists are encouraged. However, it is not necessary to add or subtract fat exchanges when using meat lists that differ from those ordinarily consumed.

- Whenever possible, monounsaturated or polyunsaturated fats should be substituted for saturated fats.

The exchange lists are updated periodically and a database is kept of the **macronutrient** composition of each food, thus assuring the accuracy of the lists. For health professionals, the macronutrient and calorie values of the exchange lists provide a useful and efficient tool for evaluating food records and for assessing nutrition adequacy.

macronutrient: nutrient needed in large quantities

Despite the many advantages the exchange lists offer, they may not be the most appropriate meal-planning tool for many persons. For instance, they are not appropriate for those who cannot understand the concept of "exchanging" foods. Because the exchange booklets are written at a ninth- to tenth-grade reading level, individuals must be able to either read at this level or understand the concept of exchanging foods. For an individual to use them effectively, several educational sessions, and practice, may be required.

Historical Background

In 1950, the following problems that had led to inconsistencies in food recommendations for persons with diabetes were identified: (1) methods used to estimate the composition of a **diet** were prolonged and needlessly precise; (2) there were many inconsistencies in the inclusion or restriction of foods; and (3) sizes of recommended portions were often stated in impractical amounts that were difficult to measure. Recognizing these facts, the food values given in table 1 were established. By combining foods of similar composition into food exchange lists, long and extensive lists of foods could be greatly abbreviated.

The first major revision of the exchange lists was published in 1976. The goals at that time were: to be more accurate in the caloric content of listed foods, to emphasize fat modification, and to provide for individualized meal plans to be used with the exchange lists.

The next revision of the exchange lists occurred in 1986. The goals of this revision were to ensure the exchange lists would reflect the principles of nutrition and to develop a database of the nutrient composition of the foods listed. Using the data from the database, revisions in the nutrient values assigned to some exchanges were made. For example, the Fruit list was changed from 10 grams of carbohydrate to 15 grams, with a subsequent increase in calories from 40 to 60 per exchange serving, to reflect the content of typical fruit portions.

The goals of the 1995 revision were: (1) to group carbohydrate food sources into one section to provide more flexibility in food choices; (2) to update the lists of foods and the database, primarily to add fat-modified foods, vegetarian food items, and fast foods; and (3) to allow for more accurate calculation of exchanges from nutrient information on labels, recipes, and prepared foods. The most significant revision in the 1995 revision was in the order and grouping of the lists. The Carbohydrate Group was listed

diet: the total daily food intake, or the types of foods eaten

1950 FOOD VALUES FOR CALCULATING DIABETIC DIETS

Group	Amount	Weight (grams)	Carbohydrate (grams)	Protein (grams)	Fat (grams)	Energy (calories)
Milk, whole	½ pt	240	12	8	10	170
Vegetable, Group A	as desired	—	—	—	—	—
Vegetable, Group B	½ cup	100	7	2	—	36
Fruit	varies	—	10	—	—	40
Bread exchanges	varies	—	15	2	—	68
Meat exchanges	1 oz	30	—	7	5	73
Fat exchanges	1 tsp	5	—	—	5	45

SOURCE: Caso, E. K., *Journal of the American Dietetic Association.*

NUTRIENT VALUES IN ONE SERVING FROM EACH EXCHANGE LIST

Groups/Lists	Carbohydrate (grams)	Protein (grams)	Fat (grams)	Calories
Carbohydrate Group				
Starch	15	3	0–1	80
Fruit	15	—	—	60
Milk				
Fat-Free	12	8	0–3	90
Reduced-Fat	12	8	5	129
Whole	12	8	8	150
Sweets, Desserts, and Other Carbohydrates	15	varies	varies	varies
Vegetables	5	2	—	25
Meat and Meat Substitute Group				
Very Lean	—	7	0–1	35
Lean	—	7	3	55
Medium-Fat	—	7	5	75
High-Fat	—	7	8	100
Fat Group	—	—	5	45

SOURCE: American Dietetic Association and American Diabetes Association, 2003.

first and included the Other Carbohydrates list, which lists foods containing carbohydrate and fat, such as sweets, pie, cake, and ice cream. Foods on the Other Carbohydrate list usually provide 1 to 2 carbohydrate choices and 1 to 2 fat exchanges, and they may be interchanged with items on the Starch, Fruit, or Milk lists and the Fat list, if appropriate.

The American Diabetes Association and the American Dietetic Association published the latest version of the *Exchange Lists for Meal Planning* in January 2003. Food lists were updated and the Other Carbohydrate list was renamed the Sweets, Desserts, and Other Carbohydrates list. Each list begins with generalized servings of exchange. The nutrient values from the 1995 and 2003 exchange lists are the same and are listed in table 2. Also included in the booklet are a listing of free foods (foods containing less than 20 calories and 5 grams of carbohydrate); combination foods (entrees, frozen entrees, soups), and fast foods. SEE ALSO Diabetes.

Marion J. Franz

Bibliography

American Diabetes Association, and American Dietetic Association (2003). *Exchange Lists for Meal Planning*. Chicago and Alexandria, VA: American Dietetic Association and American Diabetes Association.

American Dietetic Association (2003). "Evidence-Based Nutrition Principles and Recommendations for the Treatment and Prevention of Diabetes and Related Complications." *Diabetes Care* 26(suppl. 1):S51–S61.

Caso, E. K. (1950). "Calculation of Diabetic Diets. Report of the Committee on Diabetic Diet Calculations, American Dietetic Association. Prepared Cooperatively with the Committee on Education, American Diabetes Association and Diabetes Branch, U.S. Public Health Service." *Journal of the American Dietetic Association* 26:575–582.

Franz, M. J.; Barr, P.; Holler, H.; Powers, M. A.; Wheeler, M. L.; Wylie-Rosett, J. (1987). "Exchange Lists, Revised 1985." *Journal of the American Dietetic Association* 87:28–34.

Wheeler, M. L.; Franz, M.; Barrier, P.; Holler, H.; Cronmiller, N.; Delahanty, L. (1996). "Macronutrient and Kilocalorie Database for the 1995 Exchange Lists for Meal Planning: A Rationale for Clinical Practice Decisions." *Journal of the American Dietetic Association* 96:1167–1171.

Exercise

sedentary: not active

More than 28 percent of Americans are completely **sedentary** (they engage in no physical activity), with an additional 60 percent being inadequately active (engaging in less than 30 minutes of activity per day). For those who strive to achieve and maintain a high quality of health, it must be recognized that physical activity is vital to optimal health. This is reaffirmed by numerous studies that have found an association between physical activity, health, longevity, and an improved quality of life. In addition, the number of deaths related to sedentary living or **obesity** is approximately a half-million per year. Physical activity may impact quality of life in several ways: it can be used to improve self-image and self-esteem, physical **wellness**, and health.

obesity: the condition of being overweight, according to established norms based on sex, age, and height

wellness: related to health promotion

Participation in physical activity can be beneficial for anyone and can be started during any stage of life. One goal of *Healthy People 2010*, a set of national health objectives established by the U.S. Department of Health and Human Services, is to increase the number of people who participate in daily physical activity. This activity can take many forms, ranging from a regimented exercise program to daily life activities such as house or yard work, walking a pet, or walking around town to complete errands.

Definition of Terms

Physical activity is a broad term that encompasses all forms of muscle movements. These movements can range from sports to lifestyle activities. Furthermore, exercise can be defined as physical activity that is a planned, structured movement of the body designed to enhance physical fitness. Regimented or purposeful exercise consists of a program that includes twenty to sixty minutes of activity at least three to five days a week. Some examples of this type of activity include walking, running, cycling, or swimming.

anaerobic: without air, or oxygen

aerobic: designed to maintain adequate oxygen in the bloodstream

energy: technically, the ability to perform work; the content of a substance that allows it to be useful as a fuel

oxygen: O$_2$, atmospheric gas required by all animals

Exercise may be classified in one of two categories, **anaerobic** and **aerobic**, depending on where **energy** is derived from. There is a distinct difference between the two, and specific training techniques are used to enhance both. Anaerobic exercise does not require **oxygen** for energy. This is due to the intensity and duration of anaerobic events, which typically are high intensity and last only a few seconds to a minute or two. These activities range from a tennis serve to an eight-hundred-meter run.

Aerobic exercise does require oxygen for energy. This is observed during exercise that is less intense but of longer duration. This energy system is primarily used during events lasting longer than several minutes, such as a two-mile run or the Tour de France bicycle race. The potential does exist that one can use both systems, as in soccer, where a match requires ninety minutes of continual activity with short intense bursts of effort.

Benefits of Exercise

The American College of Sports Medicine (ACSM), the Centers for Disease Control and Prevention (CDC), and the Surgeon General have all issued statements that recommend placing an emphasis on adopting physical activity into one's lifestyle. Their intention is to make the public more aware of the health benefits associated with increased physical activity, as well as to

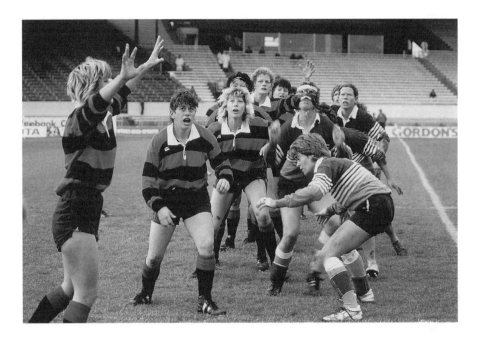

Female rugby players form a lineout, waiting for the ball to be thrown. Rugby can improve both aerobic and anaerobic fitness because, like many sports, it requires steady activity as well as frequent bursts of exertion. *[© Kevin Fleming/Corbis. Reproduced by permission.]*

highlight the amount and intensity of activity necessary to achieve optimal benefits.

There are numerous benefits associated with regular participation in an aerobic exercise program, including improved **cardiovascular** and respiratory functioning, reduced coronary **artery** disease (CAD) risk, and increased quality of life. Beneficial improvements in cardiovascular and respiratory function include an increased ability of exercising muscles to consume oxygen, lowered resting and exercise heart rates, increased stamina, resistance to **fatigue**, more effective management of **diabetes**, reduced bone-mineral loss, decreased **blood pressure**, and increased efficiency of the heart. Although it is recognized that specific exercises can be used for the purpose of increasing strength, muscular endurance, and flexibility, it is important to recognize that cardiovascular exercise has the most dramatic effect on the body. This is because cardiovascular exercise engages large muscle groups in an aerobic manner.

Role of Exercise in Disease Prevention

Studies have shown that exercise can have a direct effect on preventing **heart disease**, **cancer**, and other causes of premature death. Furthermore, participation in regular physical activity may reduce the rate of occurrence of these maladies. An inverse relationship exists between disease and exercise, meaning that with increased levels of physical activity there is a decreased **prevalence** for certain diseases. Currently, there is strong evidence that exercise has powerful effects on mortality, CAD (including blood lipid profiles), and colon cancer. Research has also confirmed that aerobic exercise can reduce **high blood pressure**, obesity, **type II diabetes,** and **osteoporosis**. In addition, **stroke** and several types of cancer (such as breast, **prostate**, and lung cancer) can also be reduced with regular physical activity.

Even more important, several of these factors are interrelated. For example, when an individual lowers his or her high blood pressure, the risk for heart disease, stroke, and kidney disease is also reduced. Another example is that exercise favorably alters blood lipid profiles. These profiles include

cardiovascular: related to the heart and circulatory system

artery: blood vessel that carries blood away from the heart toward the body tissues

fatigue: tiredness

diabetes: inability to regulate level of sugar in the blood

blood pressure: measure of the pressure exerted by the blood against the walls of the blood vessels

heart disease: any disorder of the heart or its blood supply, including heart attack, atherosclerosis, and coronary artery disease

cancer: uncontrolled cell growth

prevalence: describing the number of cases in a population at any one time

high blood pressure: elevation of the pressure in the bloodstream maintained by the heart

type II diabetes: inability to regulate the level of sugar in the blood due to a reduction in the number of insulin receptors on the body's cells

osteoporosis: weakening of the bone structure

stroke: loss of blood supply to part of the brain, due to a blocked or burst artery in the brain

prostate: male gland surrounding the urethra that contributes fluid to the semen

Components of Physical Fitness

Cardiovascular Fitness

The ability of the body to perform prolonged, large-muscle, dynamic exercise at moderate to high levels of intensity. This is dependent on the ability of the heart and lungs to deliver oxygen to the working muscles. As fitness levels improve, the body functions more efficiently and the heart can better withstand the strains of everyday stress.

Muscular Strength

The maximal amount of force a muscle can exert with a single maximal effort. Strong muscles are important for carrying out everyday tasks, such as carrying groceries, doing yard work, and climbing stairs. Muscular strength can help to keep the body in proper alignment, prevent back and leg pain, and provide support for good posture.

Muscular Endurance

The ability of a muscle or group of muscles to perform repetitive contractions over a period of time. Endurance is a key for everyday life activities and operates with muscular endurance to help maintain good posture and prevent back and leg pain. In addition, endurance can en-

hance performance during sporting events, as well as help an individual cope with everyday stress.

Flexibility

This refers to the range of motion in a joint or group of joints, correlated with muscle length. This component becomes more important as people age and their joints stiffen up, preventing them from doing everyday tasks. Additionally, good range of motion will allow the body to assume more nautral positions to help maintain good posture. Stretching is therefore an important habit to start, as well as continue, as one ages.

Body Composition

The relative proportion of fat-free mass to fat mass in the body. Fat-free mass is composed of muscle, bone, organs, and water, whereas fat is the underlying adipose tissue. Excessive fat is a good predictor of health problems because it is associated with cardiovascular disease, high cholesterol, and high blood pressure. Higher proportions of fat-free mass indicate an increase in muscle, and thus an increased ability to adapt to everyday stress.

---

cholesterol: multi-ringed molecule found in animal cell membranes; a type of lipid

triglyceride: a type of fat

measurements of total **cholesterol** (TC, complete count of all cholesterol in the blood), high-density lipoprotein cholesterol (HDL-C, the "good" cholesterol), low-density lipoprotein cholesterol (LDL-C, the "bad" cholesterol), and **triglycerides** (TRG, storage form of energy), which reduce the risk of plaque buildup in the coronary arteries, a sign of CAD.

Exercise Prescription

Adequate physical activity is dependent on having a well-rounded program that encompasses all aspects of improving health and preventing disease. A well-rounded program includes cardiovascular fitness, muscular strength and endurance, flexibility, posture, and maintenance of body composition.

The most effective way to participate in a well-rounded program is by following a simple mnemonic device called FITT (Frequency, Intensity, Time, Type). The FITT principle includes how many times a week one should exercise (frequency), how intense the workout should be (intensity), how long the workout is (time), and what modality to use (type of exercise). Modality is dependent primarily on what an individual prefers. This exercise prescription in based on an individual's fitness level when entering the exercise program, and ultimately upon the goals of the individual. For example, an untrained individual who wants to lose weight and likes to walk would be placed on a program of treadmill or outdoor walking (type), for thirty minutes a day (time), three to five times per week (frequency), and of light to moderate intensity (intensity).

A good example of an exercise program would include three stages. The first stage is a warm-up, where one should complete light calisthenics to activate and warm the muscles, immediately followed by stretching, which helps to maintain flexibility. The second stage is the conditioning stage, which consists of cardiovascular work to enhance the function of the heart and lungs and a resistance-training regimen to strengthen and tone major muscle groups, such as the quadriceps, hamstrings, chest, biceps, triceps, back, and abdominals. The final stage consists of a cool down, or reduction in heart rate to resting levels, as well as stretching again, since the greatest modification in flexibility comes from post-exercise stretching.

Maintenance of physical activity is important to maintain a healthy lifestyle. In addition, it is important to follow an exercise regime that will start slow and gradually increase as fitness level and exercise tolerance increases. The key is to complete at least thirty minutes of activity most days of the week in the form of activities that one enjoys, such as walking, jogging, swimming, aerobic dance, biking, skateboarding, or participating in a sport. This will enable an individual to reach the goals of *Healthy People 2010*, which include improving the quality of life through fitness with the adoption and maintenance of regular exercise and physical activity programs.
SEE ALSO SPORTS NUTRITION.

Robert J. Moffatt
Sara A. Chelland

Bibliography

American College of Sports Medicine (2000). *ACSM's Guidelines for Exercise Testing and Prescription*, 6th edition. Philadelphia: Lippincott, Williams & Wilkins.

Corbin, Charles B.; Lindsey, Ruth; and Welk, Greg (2000). *Concepts of Physical Fitness and Wellness: A Comprehensive Lifestyle Approach*, 3rd edition. Boston: McGraw-Hill.

McArdle, William D.; Katch, Frank I.; and Katch, Victor L. (2001). *Essentials of Exercise Physiology*. Philadelphia: Lea & Faber.

Robbins, Gwen; Powers, Debbie; and Burgess, Sharon (2002). *A Wellness Way of Life*, 5th edition. Boston: McGraw-Hill.

United States Department of Health and Human Services (1996). *Physical Activity and Health: A Report of the Surgeon General*. Atlanta: U.S. Department of Health and Human Services, Centers for Disease Control and Prevention.

Wallace, Janet P. (2001). "Health Benefits of Exercise and Fitness." In *Foundations of Exercise Science*, ed. Gary Kamen. Philadelphia: Lippincott, Williams & Wilkins.

Exercise Addiction

Individuals with an exercise addiction are characterized by their compulsive exercise behaviors, an overinvolvement in exercise, and the presence of an activity disorder—meaning they exercise at a duration, intensity, and frequency beyond that required for sport. A rigid schedule of intense exercise is maintained, accompanied by strong feelings of guilt when this schedule is violated. These individuals resist the temptation to lapse into nonexercise, and if they do lapse, the amount of exercise they partake in increases after

Exercise addicts may be driven to work out despite exhaustion or injury. Intense exercise addiction can lead to permanent physical damage, as the body is not allowed to recuperate between workouts. *[Photo Researchers, Inc. Reproduced by permission.]*

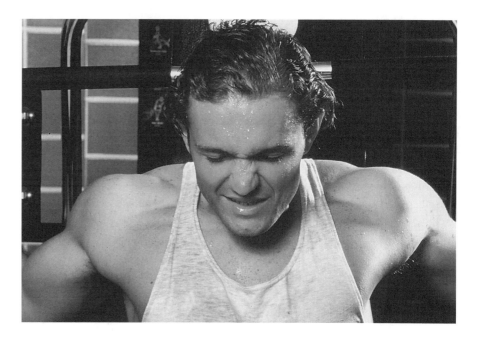

fatigue: tiredness

testosterone: male sex hormone

hormone: molecules produced by one set of cells that influence the function of another set of cells

stress: heightened state of nervousness or unease

osteoporosis: weakening of the bone structure

muscle wasting: loss of muscle bulk

anxiety: nervousness

the lapse. Exercise addicts will skip school or work to exercise, forgo social events to exercise, exercise even when they are ill or tired, and keep detailed journals of their workouts. In addition, exercise addiction can lead to disordered eating behaviors.

Physical signs of exercise addiction include **fatigue**, soreness and stiffness, and hormonal changes, including decreased **testosterone** in males and increased production of cortisol, a **hormone** produced in response to **stress** that can cause the breakdown of bone, leading to an increased risk of stress fractures and **osteoporosis**. Exercise addiction can also lead to **muscle wasting**. Behavioral signs include increased **anxiety** and discomfort with rest or relaxation, and an inability to stop exercising. SEE ALSO EATING DISORDERS; EATING DISTURBANCES; SPORTS NUTRITION.

Leslie Bonci

Expanded Food Nutrition and Education Program

diet: the total daily food intake, or the types of foods eaten

The Expanded Food Nutrition and Education Program (EFNEP), established in 1968, is funded by the United States Department of Agriculture. By providing grants to local communities, the program assists U.S. counties in developing programs to improve home and family life. EFNEP's purpose is to help economically and socially disadvantaged families improve their food practices and their **diet**. This may include advice on planning meals; selecting, purchasing, and preparing foods; and solving housekeeping problems (especially those involving storage and sanitation) that may interfere with proper food and nutrition management. EFNEP trains homemakers living in the community to be education and training facilitators, thereby advancing women and improving neighborhood networks.

Susan Himburg

Bibliography

Owen, Anita Y.; Splett, Patricia L.; and Owen, George M. (1999). *Nutrition in the Community: The Art of Delivering Services*, 4th edition. Boston: McGraw-Hill.

Internet Resource

United States Department of Agriculture. "Expanded Food and Nutrition Education Program." Available from <http://www.reeusda.gov>

Fad Diets

F

Americans are obsessed with dieting. They willingly try the latest **diet** appearing in popular magazines, discussed on talk shows, and displayed on the shelves of their local bookstore. Many fad diets defy logic, basic biochemistry, and even appetite appeal. They are popular because they promise quick results, are relatively easy to implement, and claim remarkable improvements in how their followers will look or feel. Unfortunately, the one thing most fad diets have in common is that they seldom promote sound weight loss. More important, they only work short-term. As many as 95 percent of people who lose weight gain it back within five years. It is not surprising that nearly 25 percent of Americans are confused when it comes to information about dieting.

diet: the total daily food intake, or the types of foods eaten

Despite the popularity of dieting, the **prevalence** of **overweight** and **obesity** has increased steadily since the 1970s. In 1980, 25 percent of adults in the United States were overweight. By 1991, this figure had risen to 33 percent, and by 2001, over 66 percent of the adult population were classified as overweight or **obese**. Each year, Americans spend more than $30 billion fighting fat—often for gimmicks that do not work. Most people who are trying to lose weight are not using the recommended combination of reducing caloric intake and increasing physical activity. Fad diets provide

prevalence: describing the number of cases in a population at any one time

overweight: weight above the accepted norm based on height, sex, and age

obesity: the condition of being overweight, according to established norms based on sex, age, and height

obese: above accepted standards of weight for sex, height, and age

COMMON FAD DIETS: SUMMARY OF INFORMATION

Diet	Philosophy	Foods to Eat	Foods to Avoid	Practicality	Lose and Maintain Weight?
Dr. Atkins' New Diet Revolution	Eating too many carbohydrates (CHO) causes obesity and other health problems; elimination of CHO solves problems.	Meat, fish, poultry, eggs, cheese, low-CHO vegetables, butter, oil; no alcohol.	Carbohydrates, specifically bread, pasta, milk, most fruits and vegetables	Limited food choices.	Yes, but initial weight loss is mostly water. Difficult to maintain long-term due to food restrictions.
The Zone	Eating the right combination of foods leads to metabolic state at which body functions at peak level, and results in weight loss and increased energy.	Most foods, so long as they are consumed in the exact proportion (40/30/30) at each meal.	Carbohydrates, specifically bread, pasta, some fruits, and saturated fats	Difficult to calculate portions and follow.	Yes, because of lower caloric intake. Could result in weight maintenance if followed long-term. However, diet rigid and difficult to maintain long-term.
Protein Power	Eating CHO releases insulin that contributes to obesity and other health problems.	Meat, fish, poultry, eggs, cheese, low-CHO vegetables, butter, oil, salad dressings, alcohol in moderation.	Carbohydrates	Rigid rules. Not practical long-term.	Yes, via caloric restriction. Could result in weight maintenance if followed long-term. However, diet rigid and difficult to maintain long-term.
Sugar Busters!	Sugar is toxic, leads to insulin resistance, which then makes you overweight.	Protein and fat. Low-glycemic-index foods. Alcohol in moderation.	Potatoes, white rice, corn, carrots, beets, white bread, all refined white flour products	Eliminates many carbohydrates; discourages eating fruit with meals.	Yes, via caloric restriction. Difficult to maintain long-term due to food restrictions.

Dr. Robert Atkins, 1931–2003. Atkins's books promote a low-carbohydrate diet that is proven to cause weight loss, but which may cause dangerous side effects and malnutrition. *[AP/Wide World Photos. Reproduced by permission.]*

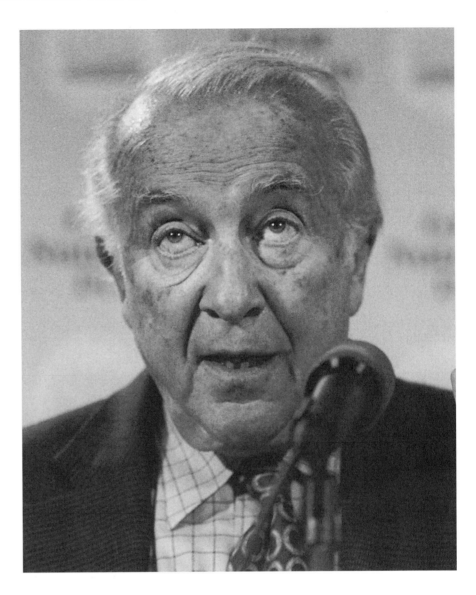

carbohydrate: food molecule made of carbon, hydrogen, and oxygen, including sugars and starches

advice counter to that provided by science-based governmental and non-governmental organizations. Is it any wonder that such diets fail to achieve long-term results, so needed by the majority of Americans?

Fad diets take many forms. Over the years, they have promoted consumption of specific foods (e.g., the Cabbage Soup Diet, the Drinking Man's Diet, the Grapefruit Diet), specific combinations of foods (e.g., the Zone) and specific times that foods must be eaten (e.g., the Rotation Diet). Some popular diets recommend elimination of certain foods (e.g., **carbohydrates** in the Atkins Diet, Protein Power, the Carbohydrate Addicts Diet, Life without Bread, and Sugar Busters!). Others recommend eating based on a person's blood type (e.g., Eat Right for Your Type), or eating like a caveman (e.g., Neanderthin). Celebrities promote diets (e.g., Suzanne Somers' Get Skinny on Fabulous Food), and fad diets have taken the name of well-known places associated with wealth, fame, and thinness (e.g., the Beverly Hills Diet, the South Beach Diet). If any one of these fad diets worked, the problem of obesity would likely have been solved long ago.

Some fad diets have been popular for many years (e.g., Atkins' Diet Revolution). Books appear as "new, revised" editions and continue to sell

Letter on Corpulence

The excerpt below is from the first low-carbohydrate diet to come to public attention, in William Banting's *Letter on Corpulence* of 1864. After many fruitless attempts to lose weight, Banting, an English casket maker, began the diet on the advice of Dr. William Harvey and lost 45 pounds. Harvey advised Banting to abstain from bread, butter, milk, sugar, beer, and potatoes because they contain "starch and saccharine matter, tending to create fat." The first three editions of the *Letter* sold 63,000 copies in the United Kingdom alone.

- For breakfast, at 9.0 A.M., I take five to six ounces of either beef mutton, kidneys, broiled fish, bacon, or cold meat of any kind except pork or veal; a large cup of tea or coffee (without milk or sugar), a little biscuit, or one ounce of dry toast; making together six ounces solid, nine liquid.

- For dinner, at 2.0 P.M., Five or six ounces of any fish except salmon, herrings, or eels, any meat except pork or veal, any vegetable except potato, parsnip, beetroot, turnip, or carrot, one ounce of dry toast, fruit out of a pudding not sweetened; any kind of poultry or game, and two or three glasses of good claret, sherry, or Madeira—Champagne, port, and beer forbidden; making together ten to twelve ounces solid, and ten liquid.

- For tea, at 6.0 P.M., Two or three ounces of cooked fruit, a rusk or two, and a cup of tea without milk or sugar; making two to four ounces solid, nine liquid.

- For supper, at 9.0 P.M. Three or four ounces of meat or fish, similar to dinner, with a glass or two of claret or sherry and water; making four ounces solid and seven liquid.

- For nightcap, if required, A tumbler of grog—(gin, whisky, or brandy, without sugar)—or a glass or two of claret or sherry.

—Paula Kepos

millions of copies. Unfortunately, there is nothing new or revised about the diets; they simply appeal to a new generation of overweight, frustrated dieters. The underlying reason why diets (including fad diets) work is that they result in decreased caloric intake. When **energy** intake is less than energy expenditure, people lose weight. Fad diets that lead to decreased caloric intake, whether by eliminating carbohydrates, eating cabbage soup all day, or adding grapefruit to every meal, will result in weight loss. If a person followed such a diet long-term, he or she would keep the weight off. Of course, no one wants to live on cabbage soup forever, or eliminate carbohydrates forever, so people break the "diet" and gain back the weight they lost—and often even more. The accompanying table provides information about some common fad diets.

energy: technically, the ability to perform work; the content of a substance that allows it to be useful as a fuel

The American Heart Association provides some tips that can be used to recognize a fad diet. First, does the diet contain magic or miracle foods or proprietary ingredients? There are no "super foods" or "magic ingredients" that can undo the long-term effects of overeating and lack of activity. Next, beware of fad diets that claim rapid weight loss (e.g., "lose 10 pounds this weekend!"). Though quite appealing, weight loss occurring this quickly is due to loss of fluid, not fat. Studies show that gradual weight loss increases a person's success at keeping it off permanently. Sound weight loss plans aim for losing no more than one to two pounds per week.

Another sign of a fad diet is losing weight without exercise. Studies consistently show that the single most important variable that predicts long-term success at weight loss and maintenance (not gaining back the weight that was lost) is physical activity. Simple activities like walking or riding a bike (to and from school, for example) should be incorporated into one's

binge: uncontrolled indulgence

nutrient: dietary substance necessary for health

folate: one of the B vitamins, also called folic acid

calcium: mineral essential for bones and teeth

iron: nutrient needed for red blood cell formation

zinc: mineral necessary for many enzyme processes

fiber: indigestible plant material that aids digestion by providing bulk

saturated fat: a fat with the maximum possible number of hydrogens; more difficult to break down that unsaturated fats

cholesterol: multi-ringed molecule found in animal cell membranes; a type of lipid

legumes: beans, peas, and related plants

chronic: over a long period

life. Also, beware of the promotion of bizarre quantities of foods or the elimination of other types of foods (e.g., cabbage soup for breakfast, lunch, and dinner; avoiding dairy foods; and eliminating carbohydrates). Forbidding certain foods or entire food groups, in addition to being unhealthy, may increase the likelihood that one will cheat, **binge**, or just give up on the diet. Finally a rigid menu or rigid schedule of eating is a good sign that one should avoid the diet. Limiting food choices and adhering to specific eating times is a daunting task. Rather, one should look for a plan that can be followed not for a week or a month, but for an entire lifetime.

Knowledgeable practitioners do not recommend fad diets because such diets do not work long-term. Even though they might work in the short run, there is little value in losing weight if one is only going to regain it after the diet ends. With repeated dieting, weight loss becomes more difficult and results in frustration, feelings of failure, and loss of self-esteem.

From a nutritional standpoint, many fad diets lack important **nutrients**. For example, high-fat, low-carbohydrate diets (such as the Atkins Diet) are low in vitamins E, A, thiamin, B_6, **folate**, **calcium**, magnesium, **iron**, **zinc**, potassium, and dietary **fiber**, and they also require supplementation. In addition, they are high in **saturated fat** and **cholesterol**. On the other hand, when individuals are allowed to choose foods from all food groups, their diet is likely to be nutritionally adequate and healthful long-term.

In conclusion, fad diets do not result in long-term weight loss, are nutritionally inadequate, and should be avoided. The optimal diet for weight loss is one that reduces overall caloric intake and promotes physical activity. It is a diet high in vegetables, fruits, complex carbohydrates (grains and **legumes**), and low-fat dairy products. It is associated with fullness and satiety and reduces the risk of **chronic** disease. It is also convenient and inexpensive to follow. SEE ALSO WEIGHT LOSS DIETS; WEIGHT MANAGEMENT.

Marjorie R. Freedman

Bibliography

Freedman, M. R.; King, J.; and Kennedy, E. (2001). *Popular Diets: A Scientific Review. Obesity Research* 9 (Suppl. 1):1S-40S.

Thomas, P. R., ed. (1995). *Weighing the Options*. Washington, DC: National Academy Press.

Internet Resouces

American Heart Association. <http://www.americanheart.gov>

National Center for Chronic Disease Prevention and Health Promotion. "Healthy Eating Tips" and "Obesity and Overweight." Available from <http://www.cdc.gov>

National Heart, Lung, and Blood Institute. <http:www.nhlbi.nih.gov>

Shape Up America. <http://www.shapeupamerica.org>

failure to thrive: lack of normal developmental progress or maintenance of health

malnutrition: chronic lack of sufficient nutrients to maintain health

Failure to Thrive

Failure to thrive is a term used to describe infants and young children who are not growing or are losing weight due to **malnutrition**, neglect, abuse, or medical conditions. In failure to thrive, the child may have a low body weight (below the third percentile for the child's age), a low height for age, or a small head circumference. A child with failure to thrive is not eating or being offered enough **calories** to meet his or her nutritional needs. Besides impaired growth, other symptoms include tiredness, sleeplessness, irritability, lethargy, resistance to eating, vomiting, and problems with elimination. The child may be suffering from an illness, medical condition, or recurring infections; taking medications; or come from a poor, distressed, or socially isolated family. To attain normal growth levels, a child with this condition requires from 1.5 to 2 times the normal amount of calories. SEE ALSO INFANT NUTRITION.

Heidi J. Silver

calorie: unit of food energy

Bibliography

Bithoney, W. G.; Dubowitz, H.; and Egan, H. (1992). "Failure to Thrive/Growth Deficiency." *Pediatrics in Review* 13:453–460.

Schwartz, D. (2000). "Failure to Thrive: An Old Nemesis in the New Millennium." *Pediatrics in Review* 21:257–264.

Internet Resource

American Academy of Pediatrics. "Failure To Thrive." <http://www.medem.com>

Famine

Famine is the culmination of a long process, typically covering two or more crop seasons, in which increasing numbers of people lose their access to food. Although early detection seems highly possible, the origins of famine are unclear, and early response is therefore rare. Famine is distinct from generalized **chronic** hunger, **malnutrition**, or undernourishment. It is a more dramatic and exceptional event that triggers institutional responses.

chronic: over a long period

malnutrition: chronic lack of sufficient nutrients to maintain health

Famine has been defined as the regional failure of food production or distribution systems leading to sharply increased mortality due to starvation and associated disease. Excessive mortality—deaths that would not have occurred otherwise—are a core feature of famine. Other important determinants of famine are regional issues, shifting market demand for different foods, and changes in the food aggregate supply. Famine also leads to extensive social disintegration, hoarding of food, smuggling, black-market food sales, and crime. Many people in distress sell their only assets such as their jewelry, animals, or land. Families often divide in search of work or succor—wives may even be cast adrift and children sold. Out-migration also increases as people abandon their lands, homes, and communities in desperation.

Famine is generally accompanied by a recession in the entire rural economy, affecting production and exchange, employment, and the income of farm and nonfarm households alike. Landless laborers, artisans, and traders are among those most vulnerable to famine because of shrinking demand for their labor, goods, and services. Fishermen and those who raise livestock are also vulnerable because they rely on the exchange of meat and marine products to obtain the cheaper grain **calories** they require. Amartya Sen, a Nobel Prize–winning economist, has argued that famine is more than just severe food shortage. His economic theory of famine is based on evidence

calorie: unit of food energy

When inadequate food supply in a region causes excessive mortality, the region is in a state of famine. Economic, political, and social forces contribute to the situation. *[AP/Wide World Photos. Reproduced by permission.]*

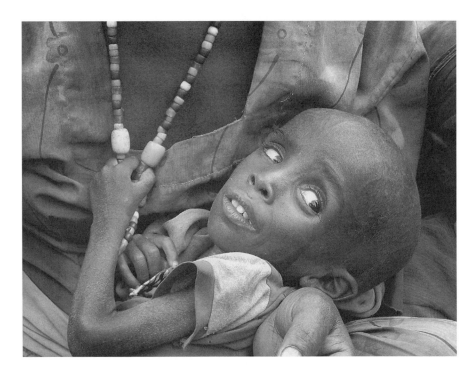

that even with relatively small changes in the food supply, famine has been caused by other economic factors. Each person has an economic "entitlement," a range of different goods that can be acquired with an individual's resources, according to Sen. People starve when their entitlement is not enough to procure the food required to survive. How much the food is available to people depends on income distribution and the ability to provide services that others are willing to pay for. However, this does not mean that the supply of food is irrelevant in the cause of famine. A scarcity of food will usually increase the competition among people to acquire it, and thereby increase its price. For those already close to the margin of hunger and poverty, this may drive them to the point of starvation.

The twentieth century saw four major famines: the great Bengal famine in colonial India under British rule in 1943–1944, in which more than three million people died; the famine in several provinces of Ethiopia between 1972 and 1974; the drought and famine in the Sahel region of Africa between 1968 and 1973; and the famine in Bangladesh in 1974 (the same region as the 1943–1944 famine, but now under a different government). It has been argued that the only way certain parts of the world can become less prone to famine is through economic development. SEE ALSO DISASTER RELIEF ORGANIZATIONS; EMERGENCY NUTRITION NETWORK; FOOD AID FOR DEVELOPMENT; FOOD AND AGRICULTURE ORGANIZATION; FOOD INSECURITY; HUNGER; MALNUTRITION; UNITED NATIONS CHILDREN'S FUND (UNICEF).

Nilesh Chatterjee

Bibliography

Field, John O. (1993). *The Challenge of Famine: Recent Experience, Lessons Learned.* West Hartford, CT: Kumarian Press.

Sen, Amartya (1981). *Poverty and Famines: An Essay on Entitlement and Deprivation.* New York: Oxford University Press.

Young, E. M. (1997). *World Hunger.* London: Routledge.

Fast Foods

Fast foods are relatively inexpensive foods that are prepared and served quickly. The **fast-food** industry had its beginnings around the mid-twentieth century, and it grew tremendously during the last three decades of the twentieth century. Growth of the fast-food industry is projected to be even greater outside the United States during the twenty-first century.

The most common type of U.S. fast-food restaurant specializes in a meal consisting of a hamburger, French fries, and a beverage. Examples include McDonald's, Burger King, and Wendy's. Some, such as Kentucky Fried Chicken, specialize in chicken; some, such as Subway, provide sandwiches; and others, such as Taco Bell, provide **Americanized** ethnic foods. Outside of the United States, these fast-food eateries serve some of the standard American dishes, such as hamburgers, but they may also serve regionally popular items. There are also fast-food restaurants in other countries that specialize in providing ethnic foods, such as soups in Japan or crepes in France.

Nutritional Issues

Many fast foods are fried (which facilitates quick preparation), high in **fat** and sodium, and low in **fiber**, **vitamins**, and some **minerals**. The "added value" option, whereby customers can order larger sizes for a minimal additional charge, adds to the total **calorie** and fat intake. Many of these eateries now offer salads, low-calorie or fat-free dressings, low-fat ice cream, and plain, broiled chicken sandwiches or other foods low in fat and/or calories. Menu options will probably continue to increase in response to health concerns and changing demographics. SEE ALSO CONVENIENCE FOODS; DIETARY TRENDS, AMERICAN; DIETARY TRENDS, INTERNATIONAL.

Judith C. Rodriguez

fast food: food requiring minimal preparation before eating, or food delivered very quickly after ordering in a restaurant

Americanized: having adopted more American habits or characteristics

fat: type of food molecule rich in carbon and hydrogen, with high energy content

fiber: indigestible plant material that aids digestion by providing bulk

vitamin: necessary complex nutrient used to aid enzymes or other metabolic processes in the cell

mineral: an inorganic (non-carbon-containing) element, ion, or compound

calorie: unit of food energy

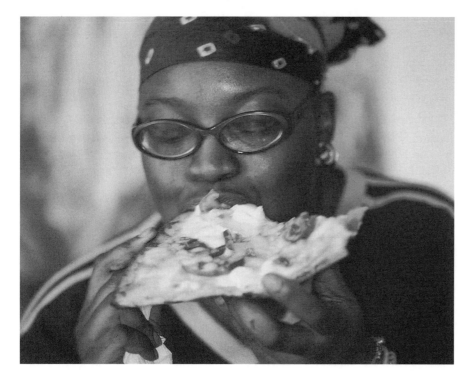

Extra-large portions of fast food may seem like a bargain, but such items add excessive empty calories to the diet. A "supersized combo meal" may provide a person's entire daily recommended intake of calories, but will probably include very few essential nutrients. *[Photograph by Steve Prezant. Corbis. Reproduced by permission.]*

Bibliography

Price, Charlene (1996). "The U.S. Foodservice Industry Looks Abroad." *Food Review* 19(2):13–17.

Schlosser, Eric (2001). *Fast Food Nation: The Darker Side of the All-American Meal.* New York: Houghton Mifflin.

Fasting

eating disorder: behavioral disorder involving excess consumption, avoidance of consumption, self-induced vomiting, or other food-related aberrant behavior

proscription: prohibitions, rules against

ketones: chemicals produced by fat breakdown; molecule containing a double-bonded oxygen linked to two carbons

carbohydrate: food molecule made of carbon, hydrogen, and oxygen, including sugars and starches

The term *fasting* refers to voluntarily or involuntarily going without food. A person may fast voluntarily because of an **eating disorder**, as a dietary practice related to religious **proscriptions**, or for health reasons, such as weight loss or internal cleansing. There are, however, no nutritional benefits to fasting.

During a full fast a person abstains from all foods except water or other liquids. A person may also engage in a partial fast, during which particular foods are avoided. Extended fasts lasting longer than a few days can be dangerous because intake is not supporting growth and maintenance. Fasting also promotes the development of **ketones**, which can be harmful to body organs if they accumulate in the body. Ketones are acidic compounds produced from the incomplete breakdown of fats when there is insufficient **carbohydrate** intake, and they can disturb the body's acid-base balance. SEE ALSO DIETING; RELIGION AND DIETARY PRACTICES.

Judith C. Rodriguez

Bibliography

Anderson, J., and Deskins, B. (1995). *The Nutrition Bible.* New York: William Morrow.

Fat Substitutes

nutrient: dietary substance necessary for health

essential fatty acids: particular molecules made of carbon, hydrogen, and oxygen that the human body must have but cannot make itself

vitamin: necessary complex nutrient used to aid enzymes or other metabolic processes in the cell

energy: technically, the ability to perform work; the content of a substance that allows it to be useful as a fuel

hormone: molecules produced by one set of cells that influence the function of another set of cells

Since the late 1980s, fat-free and reduced-fat foods have become widely available. While not all new products survive the competitive marketplace, thousands of new reduced-fat and fat-free products have been introduced each year since 1990.

In part, these new reduced-fat food products are the result of consumer demand. But they are also a response to public health concerns and initiatives. In 1990, Healthy People 2000 asked food manufacturers to double the availability of reduced-fat food products by the year 2000, a goal that was easily met.

Dietary Fat: A Good Thing in Moderation

Despite fat's bad reputation, it is a very important **nutrient**. Dietary fat plays many critical roles in the body, such as providing **essential fatty acids**, fat-soluble **vitamins**, and **energy**. It also serves structural functions in **hormones** and in cells.

Fat is also a key factor in how foods taste. Fat absorbs the essence of spices and flavors and allows people to experience their full aroma. Not only does fat carry flavor, it also determines whether a cookie crunches or a muf-

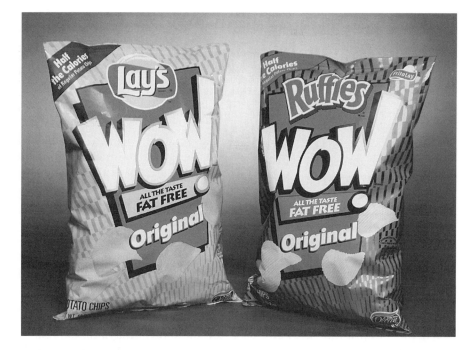

Fat substitutes come in several varieties, including carbohydrate-based substitutes and protein-based substitutes. A more recent innovation is the fat-based substitute called olestra, which is an indigestible molecule that cannot be absorbed by the body. *[Octane Photographic. Reproduced by permission.]*

fin crumbles. In other words, fat is one of the main reasons people enjoy food.

Since the 1970s, **nutrition** scientists have researched the effects of **diet** on **chronic** diseases. Eating a diet lower in fat, **saturated fat**, and **cholesterol** appears to help prevent or delay the development of some serious illnesses, such as certain cancers and **heart disease**.

Most government health agencies and professional health organizations encourage people five years old and older to eat a diet with less than 30 percent of total **calories** from fat, and less than 10 percent of that from saturated fat.

Consumers are concerned about nutrition, and they want to moderate the fat in their diet but there are challenges to overcome. Nutrition, price, convenience, and product safety are important, but taste is the key driver behind food selection for most people. And many consumers still think that less fat means less taste. Fat substitutes were developed to help meet consumers' expectations about taste while providing fewer calories from fat.

What Are Fat Substitutes?

Substitutes, or fat replacers, provide the sensory and functional qualities normally provided by fat. For example, fat provides moistness in baked goods, texture in ice cream, and crispiness in potato chips. Because fat has so many diverse functions in foods, it is virtually impossible to replace it with a single compound or process. The ingredients used in place of fat depend on how a food product will be eaten or prepared. For instance, not all fat-substitute ingredients are stable when heated, so the type of fat substitute used in a fat-free salad dressing may not work well in a muffin mix.

Many fat substitutes are simply old ingredients used in new ways. For example, the Food and Drug Administration (FDA) approved polydextrose for use as a moisture-binding agent in the early 1980s, but more recently it

nutrition: the maintenance of health through proper eating, or the study of same

diet: the total daily food intake, or the types of foods eaten

chronic: over a long period

saturated fat: a fat with the maximum possible number of hydrogens; more difficult to break down that unsaturated fats

cholesterol: multi-ringed molecule found in animal cell membranes; a type of lipid

heart disease: any disorder of the heart or its blood supply, including heart attack, atherosclerosis, and coronary artery disease

calorie: unit of food energy

COMMON FAT SUBSTITUTES

Carbohydrate-based	Protein-based	Fat-based
Cellulose	Microparticulated protein	Caprenin
Dextrins	Modified whey protein	Salatrim
Fiber	concentrate	Emulsifiers (mono- and
Gums		diglycerides)
Inulin		Sucrose polyester (olestra)
Maltodextrins		
Oatrim		
Polydextrose		
Polyols		
Starch/modified		
food starch		
Z-Trim		

carrageenan: a thickener derived from red seaweed

guar gum: a thickener made from a tropical bean

protein: complex molecule composed of amino acids that performs vital functions in the cell; necessary part of the diet

molecule: combination of atoms that form stable particles

food additive: substance added to foods to improve nutrition, taste, appearance or shelf-life

has been used as a fat substitute. **Carrageenan** has been used since the early 1960s as an emulsifier, stabilizer, and thickener, but is now commonly used to replace fat in foods, as is **guar gum**, which has been used as a thickener for nearly a hundred years.

Some fat substitutes are newer to the food supply, though they are made from familiar ingredients. For example, microparticulated **protein** is made from milk, egg, or whey protein. Other fat substitutes are new ingredients made from combinations of basic **molecules**.

In some cases, the FDA has approved fat-reduction ingredients as **food additives**. To be approved, food additives are tested extensively to assess their safety and level of use among different population groups. Examples of fat substitutes approved as food additives include carrageenan, olestra, and polydextrose.

In other instances, fat-reduction ingredients are "generally recognized as safe" (GRAS). GRAS ingredients are made from common food components and are considered by experts to be safe. For example, many spices and flavoring agents, such as sugar and salt, are GRAS ingredients. Examples of GRAS fat substitutes include guar gum and maltodextrin.

Categories of Fat Substitutes

Fat-substitute ingredients fall into three categories: carbohydrate-based, protein-based, and fat-based. Carbohydrate-based fat substitutes are the most common. They are very versatile and found in many types of food products. Carbohydrate-based fat substitutes provide between zero and four calories per gram. When used to replace fat, they may significantly lower the calorie content of a food. Most carbohydrate-based fat substitutes are GRAS substances. Some of these ingredients are only partially digestible. However, when consumed at expected levels, most carbohydrate-based fat substitutes have no digestive effects. Guar gum is an example of a carbohydrate-based fat substitute.

Protein-based fat substitutes are not as numerous as carbohydrate-based ingredients, but they have many applications and can be used in many products, including cheese, yogurt, sour cream, ice cream, mayonnaise, and salad dressing. Protein-based fat substitutes cannot be used for deep-frying. Whey protein concentrate is a protein-based fat substitute.

THE EFFECTS OF FAT SUBSTITUTES ON A TYPICAL AMERICAN MEAL						
Regular lunch	**Calories**	**Fat (g)**	**Lunch with fat substitutes**	**Calories**	**Fat (g)**
2 slices bread	130	2	2 slices bread	130	2
1 oz. cheese	105	9	1 oz. reduced-fat cheese	75	4
2 oz. bologna	180	17	2 oz. fat-free bologna	40	0
1 tbsp. mayonnaise	100	11	1 tbsp. low-fat mayonnaise	25	1
banana	105	0	banana	105	0
2 cookies	140	6	2 reduced-fat cookies	120	3
Total:	**760**	**45**	**Total:**	**495**	**10**

The last category of fat substitutes includes those that are fat-based. Because they are made from fat, they often come closest to providing fat's taste and cooking properties. Most Americans have heard of olestra, which is a fat-based fat substitute made from sucrose (table sugar) and **fatty acids** from vegetable oils. However, unlike sugar and vegetable oils, the body does not absorb olestra because the human digestive **enzymes** cannot break down such a large molecule. Olestra has the potential to inhibit **absorption** of some fat-soluble nutrients in the digestive tract, and, to offset any possible effects, products made with olestra have appropriate amounts of vitamins A, D, E, and K added.

fatty acids: molecules rich in carbon and hydrogen; a component of fats

enzyme: protein responsible for carrying out reactions in a cell

absorption: uptake by the digestive tract

Ensuring Safety

Most fat substitutes are not new to the food supply. Ingredients that are new, or used in new ways, must meet the FDA's strict criteria to be either classified as GRAS or approved as food additives. Whether they are GRAS or food additives, those ingredients approved for use in foods are considered safe for people of all ages.

Can Fat Substitutes Help to Reduce Dietary Fat?

Several studies have shown that using reduced-fat versions of food products can significantly reduce the amount of fat that people eat. For some people, eating less fat may lead to eating fewer calories and, eventually, to weight loss. As illustrated in the table above, by using reduced-fat foods, a typical lunch can be trimmed of one-third of its calories and three-fourths of its fat.

A common misconception about reduced-fat foods is that they also are low in calories. For many products, however, this is not the case. Most reduced-fat foods have had other ingredients added to replace the texture or flavor provided by fat, so that while the calories may be slightly lower in a fat-reduced product, the difference between it and a full-fat product may not be significant. With fat-modified products, as with all foods, portion size and calories still count.

Fat-modified foods can fit into a healthy eating plan. According to the American Dietetic Association, they offer a safe, feasible, and effective means to maintain the palatability of diets that are controlled in fat or calories. But they are only one of the many tools that can be used to achieve nutrition goals. Foods with fat substitutes should be consumed as part of an overall healthful eating plan, such as that outlined in the Dietary Guidelines for Americans. SEE ALSO ARTIFICIAL SWEETENERS; DIETARY GUIDELINES FOR AMERICANS; FATS.

Susan T. Borra

Bibliography

Diamond, L. (1997). "The Dietary Guidelines Alliance: Reaching Consumers with Meaningful Health Messages." *Journal of the American Dietetic Association* 97(3):247.

Hahn, N. I. (1997). "Replacing Fat with Food Technology." *Journal of the American Dietetic Association* 3:15–16.

Heimbach, James T.; Van Der Riet, Brooke E.; and Egan, S. Kathleen. "Impact of the Use of Reduced-Fat Foods on Nutrient Adequacy" (1997). *Annals of the New York Academy of Sciences: Nutritional Implications of Macronutrient Substitutes* 819:108–114.

Kurtzweil, Paula (1996). "Taking the Fat Out of Food." *FDA Consumer* 30(6).

Morgan, Rebecca; Sigman-Grant, Madeleine; Taylor, Dennis S.; Moriarty, Kristen; Fishell, Valerie; and Kris-Etherton, Penny (1997). "Impact of Macronutrient Substitutes on the Composition of the Diet and U.S. Food Supply." *Annals of the New York Academy of Sciences: Nutritional Implications of Macronutrient Substitutes* 819:70–95.

Internet Resources

American Dietetic Association (1998). "Position of the American Dietetic Association: Fat Replacers." Available from <http://www.eatright.com>

U.S. Department of Health and Human Services (1999). *Healthy People 2000.* Available from <http://www.health.gov/healthypeople>

U.S. Department of Health and Human Services, and U.S. Department of Agriculture (2000). *Nutrition and Your Health: Dietary Guidelines for Americans,* 5th ed. Available from <http://www.health.gov/dietaryguidelines>

Fats

atoms: fundamental particles of matter

Lipids are organic substances consisting mostly of carbons and hydrogen **atoms.** They are hydrophobic, which means that they have little or no affinity to water. All lipids are soluble (or dissolvable) in nonpolar solvents, such as ether, alcohol, and gasoline. There are three families of lipids: (1) fats, (2) phospholipids, and (3) steroids.

Fatty acids and glycerol make up the larger molecule of fats. A fatty acid consists of a long carbon skeleton of 16 or 18 carbon atoms, though some are even longer. The carbonyl group, which is a carbon atom double-bonded to an oxygen atom and single-bonded to an oxygen attached to a hydrogen (OH-C=O), is the acidic group of the fatty acids. The acidic property is determined by the ability of the hydrogen to dissociate, or break away, from the oxygen atom. The carbonyl group is followed by a long chain of carbon atoms bonded to hydrogen, which is referred to as the hydrocarbon "tail." The long hydrocarbon tail gives fatty acids their hydrophobic, or "water-fearing" property. Fats cannot be dissolved in water because fats are nonpolar (an equal distribution of electrons) and water is polar (an unequal distribution of electrons). The polarity of water is unable to form bonds and break down the nonpolar fatty acid molecule.

There are different types of fatty acids, which vary in length and the number of bonds. Saturated fatty acids have single bonds between the carbon atoms that make up the tail. The carbon atoms are "full" or saturated, and therefore cannot take up any more hydrogen. Most animal fat, such as butter, milk, cheese, and coconut oil, are saturated. Unsaturated fatty acids have one or more double bonds between carbon atoms. A double bond is the sharing of four electrons between atoms, while a single bond is the sharing of two electrons. The double bond has the ability to lend its extra two electrons to another atom, thereby forming another bond. Monounsaturated fatty acids contain only one double bond, such that each of the carbon atoms of the double bond can bond with a hydrogen atom. An example of monounsaturated fatty acids is oleic acid, which is found in olive oil. **Polyunsaturated** fatty acids contain two or more double bonds, such that four or more carbon atoms can bond with hydrogen atoms. Most vegetable fats are polyunsaturated fatty acids. The double bonds change the structure of the fatty acid, in that there is a slight bend where the double bond is located.

polyunsaturated: having multiple double bonds within the chemical structure, thus increasing the body's ability to metabolize it

Foods high in saturated fatty acids include whole milk, cream, cheese, egg yolk, fatty meats (e.g., beef, lamb, pork, ham), coconut oil, regular margarine, and chocolate. Foods high in polyunsaturated fatty acids include vegetable oils (e.g., safflower, corn, cottonseed, soybean, sesame, sunflower), salad dressing made from vegetable oils, and fish such as salmon, tuna, and herring.

Triglycerides are the basic unit of fat and are composed of three ("tri-") fatty acids individually bonded to each of the three carbons of glycerol. Fatty acids rarely exist in a free form in nature because they are highly reactive, and therefore make bonds spontaneously.

Fat Function, Metabolism, and Storage

Fats and lipids play critical roles in the overall functioning of the body, such as in digestion and **energy** metabolism. Usually, 95 percent of the fat in food is digested and absorbed into adipose, or fatty, tissue. Fats are the body's energy provider and energy reserve, which helps the body maintain a constant temperature. Fats and lipids are also involved in the production and regulation of steroid **hormones**, which are hydrophobic (or "water-fearing") **molecules** made from **cholesterol** in the smooth endoplasmic reticulum, a compartment within a cell in which lipids, hormones, and **proteins** are made. Steroid hormones are essential in regulating sexuality, reproduction, and development of the human sex organs, as well as in regulating the water balance in the body. Steroid hormones can also freely flow in and out of cells, and they modify the transcription process, which is the first step in protein synthesis, where segments of the cell's **DNA**, or the **genetic** code, is copied.

energy: technically, the ability to perform work; the content of a substance that allows it to be useful as a fuel

hormone: molecules produced by one set of cells that influence the function of another set of cells

molecule: combination of atoms that form stable particles

cholesterol: multi-ringed molecule found in animal cell membranes; a type of lipid

protein: complex molecule composed of amino acids that performs vital functions in the cell; necessary part of the diet

DNA: deoxyribonucleic acid; the molecule that makes up genes, and is therefore responsible for heredity

genetic: inherited or related to the genes

Fats and lipids also have important structural roles in maintaining nerve impulse transmission, memory storage, and tissue structure. Lipids are the major component of cell membranes. The three most common lipids in the membranes of eukaryots, or nucleus-containing cells, are phospholipids, glycolipids, and cholesterol. A phospholipid has two parts: (1) the hydrophilic ("water-loving") head, which consists of choline, phosphate, and glycerol, and (2) the hydrophobic ("water-fearing") fatty acid tail, which consists of carbon and hydrogen. The hydrophilic head is the part of the phospholipids that is in contact with water, since it shares similar chemical properties with water molecules. The hydrophobic tail of the phospholipids faces inward, and therefore is able to avoid any contact with water. In this particular arrangement, the phospholipids arrange themselves in a bilayer (double layer) alignment in **aqueous** solution.

Fats are metabolized primarily in the small **intestines** because the **enzymes** of the stomach cannot break down fat molecules due to their hydrophobicity. In the small intestines, fat molecules stimulate the release of cholecystokinin (CCK), a small-intestine hormone, into the bloodstream. The CCK in the blood triggers the pancreas to release digestive enzymes that can break down lipids. The gallbladder is also stimulated to secrete **bile** into the small intestines. Bile acids coat the fat molecules, which results in the formation of small fat globules, which are called *micelles*. The coating prevents the small fat globules from fusing together to form larger fat molecules, and therefore the small fat globules are more easily absorbed. The pancreatic enzymes can also break down triglycerides into monoglycerides and fatty acids. Once this occurs, the broken-down fat molecules are able to diffuse into the intestinal cells, in which they are converted back to triglycerides, and finally into chylomicrons.

Chylomicrons, which are composed of fat and protein, are macromolecules that travel through the bloodstream into the lymphatic capillaries called *lacteals*. The **lymphatic system** is a special system of vessels that carries a clear fluid called *lymph*, in which lost fluid and proteins are returned to the blood. The lacteals absorb the fat molecules and transport them from the digestive tract to the circulatory system, dumping chylomicrons in the bloodstream. The adipose and liver tissues, which release enzymes called lipoprotein lipase, break down chylomicrons into monoglycerides and fatty acids. These molecules diffuse into the adipose and liver cells, where they are converted back to triglycerides and stored as the body's supply of energy.

Fat Nutrition

The energy value of fats is 9 kcal/gram (kilocalories per gram), which supplies the body with important sources of calories. Calories are units of energy. The breaking of bonds within fat molecules releases energy that the body uses. A kilocalorie is the unit used to measure the energy in foods. It is the equivalent of "calories" listed on Nutrition Facts labels on food packaging.

Some of the foods known to contain large amounts of fat include the obvious examples, such as butter on toast, fried foods, and hamburgers. But many of the foods that people consume on a daily basis have hidden sources of fat that may not be obvious to the person eating them. These foods include cookies and cakes, cheese, ice cream, potato chips, and hot dogs. One way to avoid foods that contain high amounts of fat is to look at the Nutrition Facts label located on the packages of most foods, where the total fat content of the food is listed.

Actual intake of fat can vary from 10 percent to 40 percent of the calories consumed daily, depending on personal or cultural regimens. Limiting one's daily fat intake to less than 30 percent of total calorie intake and increasing consumption of polyunsaturated fatty acids have been shown to be beneficial in maintaining a healthful **diet**.

New food-labeling regulations scheduled to take effect in 2006 require manufacturers to list trans fat content on their products' Nutrition Facts panel. According to the U.S. Food and Drug Administration, consumption of foods high in cholesterol, saturated fat, or trans fat should be avoided. *[Photograph by Akira Ono. AP/Wide World Photos. Reproduced by permission.]*

Effects of Excess Dietary-Fat Intake

The recommended intake of fats in the American diet is to limit fats to below 30 percent of the total daily caloric intake. One-third of fats should come from saturated fats, with the other two-thirds split evenly between monounsaturated and polyunsaturated fat. It is estimated that in the average American diet (as of 2002), fats make up 42 percent of calories, with **saturated fat** making up between a third and a half of that amount.

The effects of this excess intake of dietary fat has some well-established implications for the health of **overweight** Americans. For instance, the consumption of excess amounts of saturated fats has been recognized as the most important dietary factor to increase levels of cholesterol. A high cholesterol level is detrimental to health and leads to a condition known as *atherosclerosis*. Atherosclerosis is the build-up of cholesterol on the walls of **arteries**, which may eventually result in the blocking of blood flow. When this occurs in the arteries of the heart, it is called *coronary artery disease*. When this process occurs in the heart, a myocardial infarction, or **heart attack**, may occur.

Besides the cholesterol implications due to high fat intake, **obesity** is a factor in the causation of disease. Being overweight or **obese** is highly associated with increasing the risk of **type II diabetes**, gallbladder disease, **cardiovascular** disease, **hypertension**, and **osteoarthritis**.

Fat-Replacement Strategies

The purpose of fat-replacement strategies is to reduce the percentage of fat in various foods, without taking away the appealing taste of the food. There are three broad categories of fat-replacement strategies: (1) adding water, starch derivatives, and gums to foods, (2) using protein-derived fat replacements, and (3) using engineered fats.

The addition of water to foods lowers the quantity of fat per serving in the selected food item. When starch derivatives are added to food, they bind

saturated fat: a fat with the maximum possible number of hydrogens; more difficult to break down that unsaturated fats

overweight: weight above the accepted norm based on height, sex, and age

artery: blood vessel that carry blood away from the heart toward the body tissues

heart attack: loss of blood supply to part of the heart, resulting in death of heart muscle

obesity: the condition of being overweight, according to established norms based on sex, age, and height

obese: above accepted standards of weight for sex, height, and age

type II diabetes: inability to regulate the level of sugar in the blood due to a reduction in the number of insulin receptors on the body's cells

cardiovascular: related to the heart and circulatory system

hypertension: high blood pressure

osteoarthritis: inflammation of the joints

Americans get an average of 14 to 21 percent of their calories from saturated fats, in fatty meats, fried foods, and dairy products such as ice cream. The recommended daily intake of saturated fat is 10 percent of total calories consumed. *[Photograph by Georgio Borgia. AP/Wide World Photos. Reproduced by permission.]*

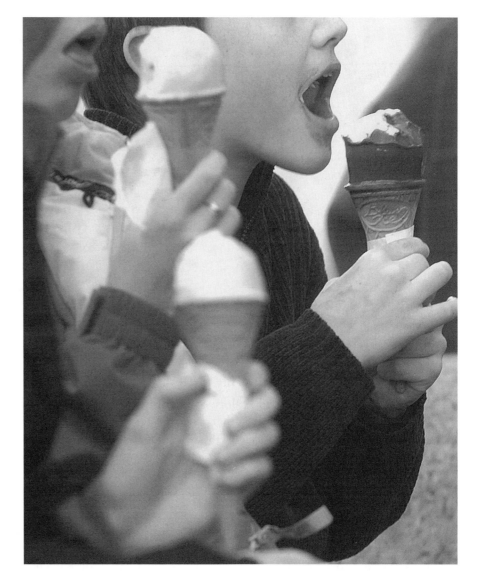

cellulose: carbohydrate made by plants; indigestible by humans

to the water in the food, thus providing a thicker product that simulates the taste and texture of fat in the mouth. Examples of specific starch derivatives include **cellulose**, Z-trim, maltrin, stellar, and oatrim. The problem with starch derivatives, however, is their limitations as a fat replacement in foods that require frying.

Protein-derived fat replacements are made from egg and milk proteins, which are made into a microscopic globule of protein. They give the sensation of fat in the mouth, although they contain no fatty acids. One such product is Simplesse, which is used mostly in frozen desserts. Because its chemical structure is easily destroyed by cooking or frying, its use is limited in most other foods.

The third fat-replacement strategy includes the use of engineered fats, which are made by putting together various food substances. One popular engineered fat is olestra, which is made by adding fatty acids to regular table sugar molecules (sucrose). This process results in a product that can neither be broken down in the digestive tract nor absorbed. It therefore cannot provide energy, in terms of **carbohydrates** or fatty acids, to the body. Olestra

carbohydrate: food molecule made of carbon, hydrogen, and oxygen, including sugars and starches

is the first engineered fat to be used in fried foods. It does have its drawbacks, however. Olestra can cause abdominal cramping, loose stools, and it can bind beneficial substances that are normally absorbed, such as the fat-soluble **vitamins** (vitamins A, D, E, and K) and **carotenoids**.

In addition to fat-replacement strategies, there are low-fat or fat-free versions of many foods on the market. Some products made to be low-fat or fat-free include milk, yogurt, some cheeses, and deli meats. As a general rule, products that claim to have reduced amounts of fat should conform to the following stipulations: (1) a product labeled "reduced-fat" must have at least 25 percent less fat than the normal product, (2) a "low-fat" product can have no more than three grams of fat per serving, and (3) a "fat-free" product most have less than 0.5 grams of fat per serving. But one does not always need to look for foods made to contain less fat than normal, as there are plenty of natural foods that contain very little fat, or no fat at all, including most fruits and vegetables. Other foods that fit into the category of low-fat or nonfat foods include egg whites, tuna in water, skinless chicken, and pasta.

Foods that are low in fat are important for a healthful diet. While fats are essential components for bodily function, excess consumption of fats can lead to health problems such as obesity and **heart disease**. A healthful diet therefore consists of balanced proportions of proteins, fats, and carbohydrates. SEE ALSO FAT SUBSTITUTES; LIPID PROFILE; OMEGA-3 AND OMEGA-6 FATTY ACIDS.

Jeffrey Radecki
Susan Kim

vitamin: necessary complex nutrient used to aid enzymes or other metabolic processes in the cell

carotenoid: plant-derived molecules used as pigments

heart disease: any disorder of the heart or its blood supply, including heart attack, atherosclerosis, and coronary artery disease

Bibliography

Campbell, Neil A., et al. (2000). *Biology*, 4th edition. San Francisco: Benjamin/Cummings.

Must, A., et al. (1999). "The Disease Burden Associated with Overweight and Obesity." *Journal of the American Medical Association* 282: 1523.

Robinson, Corinne H.; Weigley, Emma S.; and Mueller, Donna H. (1993). *Basic Nutrition and Diet Therapy*, 7th edition. New York: Macmillan.

Wardlaw, Gordon M., and Kessel, Margaret (2002). *Perspectives in Nutrition*, 5th edition. Boston: McGraw-Hill.

Female Athlete Triad

The female athlete triad is a common nutritional disorder among female athletes caused by the drive of girls and women to be unrealistically thin in an attempt to improve performance. The disorder is most common in sports judged by build (e.g., gymnastics, diving, figure skating), sports with a weight classification (e.g., light-weight crew), and endurance sports (e.g., distance running). It is characterized by three interrelated conditions: (1) disordered eating, such as bingeing, purging, or severe **calorie** restriction; (2) amenorrhea, or the absence of normal menstrual periods; and (3) osteoporosis, a condition marked by reduced bone density.

Physical signs of the female athlete triad include: amenorrhea for more than three months, irregular or slow pulse, skipped heartbeats, fainting, loss of greater than 10 percent of ideal body weight, and recurrent stress

calorie: unit of food energy

depression: mood disorder characterized by apathy, restlessness, and negative thoughts

anxiety: nervousness

fractures. The condition is also marked by **depression, anxiety**, low self-esteem, excessive exercise, and a preoccupation with food and weight management.

Treatment for those with the female athlete triad is multidisciplinary and includes medical care, counseling and nutritional services, and an adjustment in exercise. Some athletes require hospitalization if there are coexisting medical problems, and counseling is done on an individual basis and in support groups. SEE ALSO EATING DISORDERS; EATING DISTURBANCES; OSTEOPOROSIS; SPORTS NUTRITION.

Leslie Bonci

Bibliography

Otis, Carol, and Goldingay, Roger (2000). *The Athletic Woman's Survival Guide.* Champaign, IL: Human Kinetics.

Fetal Alcohol Syndrome

Fetal alcohol syndrome (FAS) is a birth defect caused by a mother's alcohol intake during pregnancy. The symptoms of FAS are mental retardation, poor growth, facial defects, and behavioral problems. It is one of the leading causes of mental retardation in children. The effects are lifelong. Fetal alcohol effects (FAE) is a less severe set of the same symptoms. FAS is found in infants of all races and ethnic groups. Since it is not known how much

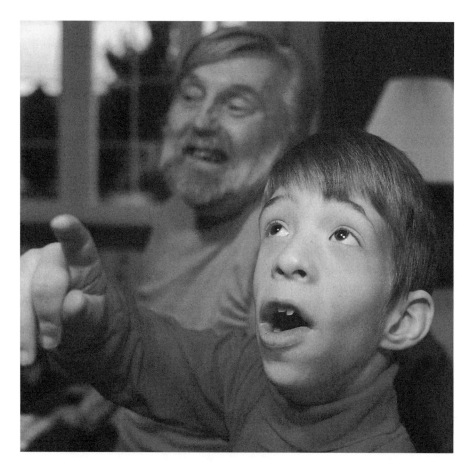

The Centers for Disease Control estimate that up to three children of every 2,000 are born with fetal alcohol syndrome. The condition causes physical and mental disabilities, but it is 100 percent preventable. *[Photograph by David H. Wells. Corbis. Reproduced by permission.]*

alcohol a pregnant woman must drink to cause the syndrome, it is recommended that women not drink alcohol at all during pregnancy. SEE ALSO ALCOHOL AND HEALTH; PREGNANCY.

Sheah Rarback

Internet Resource

National Organization on Fetal Alcohol Syndrome. <http://www.nofas.org>

Fiber

Fiber, which is found in all plant-based foods, is composed of a group of compounds that makes up the framework of plants. Although fiber cannot be digested, it is an essential **nutrient** for good health. The health benefits of a **diet** rich in fiber include lower **cholesterol** and a reduced risk of **heart disease** and certain cancers. Also referred to as roughage, fiber is made up of many compounds, mostly **carbohydrates**. It can be found in a variety of foods, including wheat, potatoes, and certain fruits and vegetables. Although the recommended amount of fiber is 20 to 35 grams a day, the average American consumes only 12 to 15 grams on a daily basis. Asians, on average, consume three times as much fiber as Americans do.

Types of Fiber

Complex carbohydrates, which are a major source of **energy** for the body, are comprised of two main classes: starch, which is digestible, and fiber, which is generally not digestible. There are also two kinds of fiber: insoluble and soluble. Insoluble fiber, found in wheat bran and some fruits and vegetables, cannot be dissolved in water. This type of fiber is made up of cellulose and hemicellulose, substances that offer rigidity to plant material (e.g., the peels and skins of fruits and vegetables, wood, stems, and the outer coverings of nuts, seeds, and grains). Insoluble fiber acts as a natural laxative, giving stool the bulk necessary to move quickly through the **gastrointestinal** tract. In addition to preventing **constipation** and **hemorrhoids**, insoluble fiber may also reduce the risk of colon **cancer** by speeding the passage of food through the digestive tract.

Soluble fiber, found in beans, oats, and some fruits and vegetables, is fiber that can be dissolved in water. This type of fiber is made up of pectins, gums, and mucilages. Marie Boyle notes that, because it reduces the level of cholesterol in the blood, soluble fiber can reduce the risks of heart and **artery** disease and **atherosclerosis**. When consumed in large amounts, soluble fiber also slows **glucose absorption** from the small intestine, which can be helpful in treating **diabetes**. Finally, a diet high in fiber may also promote weight control and reduce the risk of developing **obesity**.

How Much Fiber Is Necessary?

According to the American Dietetic Association, the daily goal for fiber intake is between 20 and 35 grams. However, the average intake in the United States is only 12 to 15 grams. In contrast, people in China consume as much as 77 grams of fiber per day. Children also need fiber, although in different

nutrient: dietary substance necessary for health

diet: the total daily food intake, or the types of foods eaten

cholesterol: multi-ringed molecule found in animal cell membranes; a type of lipid

heart disease: any disorder of the heart or its blood supply, including heart attack, atherosclerosis, and coronary artery disease

carbohydrate: food molecule made of carbon, hydrogen, and oxygen, including sugars and starches

energy: technically, the ability to perform work; the content of a substance that allows it to be useful as a fuel

gastrointestinal: related to the stomach and intestines

constipation: difficulty passing feces

hemorrhoids: swollen blood vessels in the rectum

cancer: uncontrolled cell growth

artery: blood vessel that carry blood away from the heart toward the body tissues

atherosclerosis: build-up of deposits within the blood vessels

glucose: a simple sugar; the most commonly used fuel in cells

absorption: uptake by the digestive tract

diabetes: inability to regulate level of sugar in the blood

obesity: the condition of being overweight, according to established norms based on sex, age, and height

FIBER CONTENT OF VARIOUS FOODS

Food	Amount	Fiber (g)
Whole-wheat bread	1 slice	1.6
Rye bread	1 slice	1.0
White bread	1 slice	0.6
Brown rice (cooked)	½ cup	2.4
White rice (cooked)	½ cup	0.1
Spaghetti (cooked)	½ cup	0.8
Kidney beans (cooked)	½ cup	5.8
Lima beans (cooked)	½ cup	4.9
Potato (baked)	Medium	3.8
Corn	½ cup	3.9
Spinach	½ cup	2.0
Lettuce	½ cup	0.3
Strawberries	¾ cup	2.0
Banana	Medium	2.0
Apple (with skin)	Medium	2.6
Orange	Small	1.2

SOURCE: Adapted from Edlin et al., 2002.

amounts than adults. For children up to age 18, the recommended daily dose (in grams) is determined by adding five to a child's age. For example, a seven-year-old child would need 12 grams of fiber a day.

The recommended daily amount of fiber can be consumed by eating a diet high in fiber-rich fruits, vegetables, and whole grains. There are several ways to ensure one consumes enough fiber. First, it is important to read food labels. Although they do not distinguish between the two types of fiber, the labels of almost all foods will provide the amount of dietary fiber in each serving. Raw or slightly cooked vegetables will also provide an excellent source of fiber. However, overcooking vegetables may reduce the fiber content. Whole-grain cereals, whole-wheat bread, fresh or dried fruit, beans, rice, and salad are all good sources of fiber. The table presents the fiber content of various foods.

Problem with High-Fiber Diets

Including fiber in one's daily diet has definite benefits. However, although very uncommon, fiber has the potential to cause harm if taken in excess of 60 or 70 grams daily. "Since fiber carries water out of the body, taking too much can cause **dehydration** and intestinal discomfort or gas," (Boyle, p. 84). Large amounts of fiber require a high fluid intake. Therefore, as one increases fiber in the diet, water intake must also be increased. If one does not consume enough fluid, then one's stool could become very hard, resulting in difficult and painful elimination.

Fiber speeds the movement of foods through the digestive system. Since **iron** is mainly absorbed early during digestion, high amounts of fiber may limit the opportunity for the absorption of iron, **calcium**, and other nutrients. Finally, large amounts of fiber can also cause deficiencies of nutrients and energy by causing one to feel full before enough nutrients have been consumed. Children and elderly persons are especially vulnerable to these concerns, since they eat smaller portion sizes.

In conclusion, fiber is an important element of the diet and provides several health benefits. Eating balanced meals containing whole grain and

dehydration: loss of water

iron: nutrient needed for red blood cell formation

calcium: mineral essential for bones and teeth

fresh fruits and vegetables will ensure meeting the proper recommended allowances. SEE ALSO CANCER; CARBOHYDRATES; HEART DISEASE; NUTRIENTS.

Elissa M. Howard-Barr

Bibliography

Boyle, Marie, A. (2001). *Personal Nutrition*, 4th edition. Belmont, CA: Wadsworth/Thomson Learning.

Edlin, Gordon; Golanty, Eric; and McCormick Brown, Kelli, eds. (2002). *Health and Wellness*, 7th edition. Sudbury, MA: Jones and Bartlett.

Wardlaw, Gordon M. (2000). *Contemporary Nutrition, Issues and Insights*, 4th edition. Boston: McGraw Hill.

Internet Resources

American Dietetic Association. "Health Implications of Dietary Fiber—Position of ADA." Available from <http://www.eatright.com>

Food and Drug Administration. "Why Is Fiber Important to Your Diet?"Available from <http://www.cfsan.fda.gov>

Nutrition Newsletter (1997). "China Project Monograph Named China's Best Scientific Publication." Available from <http://www.nutrition.cornell.edu/news>

Food Aid for Development and the World Food Programme

Food aid has been a key to global agricultural development and trade policy since the end of World War II. Food aid creates agricultural development and income growth in poor nations, and thus creates future markets for donor countries, according to Christopher Barrett. However, food aid may be inflationary because it increases demand and costs for nonfood items in the recipient countries.

The World Food Programme (WFP), the food-assistance agency of the United Nations, was established in 1963 to fight global hunger. WFP has many partners, including the Food Aid for Development (FAD) Office of the World Health Organization. The goal of this combined effort is to ensure that everyone has access to nutritious foods at all times.

Since its inception, WFP has invested $27.8 billion and more than 43 million metric tons of food to combat hunger, promote economic and social development, and provide relief assistance in emergencies to eighty-three countries. In 2000, WFP fed 83 million people. WFP has three main programs:

- *Food-for-Life*. Eighty percent of WFP resources are used by this program for emergency relief activities for refugees and displaced individuals.

- *Food-for-Growth*. Projects in this program aim to prevent nutritional problems among pregnant and breastfeeding women, infants, school children, and the elderly. Literacy and **nutrition** classes are also offered.

- *Food-for-Work*. Chronically hungry individuals are paid with food through the Food-for-Work program. Workers assist with projects to improve local infrastructure, such as building roads and ports, re-

nutrition: the maintenance of health through proper eating, or the study of same

The Food-for-Work program offers food to hungry people in exchange for work they do to improve vital infrastructure. Here, Somalis gather around water tanks, which were built to stabilize the water supply for drinking and irrigation in the drought-afflicted country. *[© Kevin Fleming/Corbis. Reproduced by permission.]*

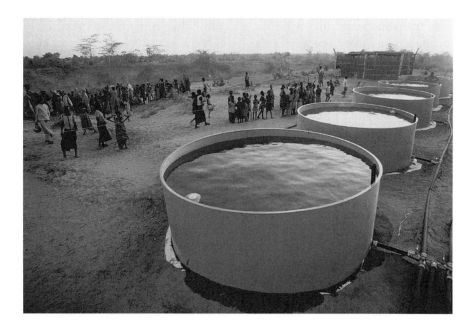

pairing dykes, terracing hillsides, replanting forests, and repairing irrigation systems. SEE ALSO FAMINE; FOOD INSECURITY; UNITED NATIONS CHILDREN'S FUND (UNICEF).

Delores C. S. James

Bibliography

Barrett, Christopher B. (1998). "Food Aid: Is It Development Assistance, Trade Promotion, Both, or Neither?" *American Journal of Agricultural Economics* 80(3):566–582.

Internet Resources

World Health Organization. "Food Aid for Development." Available from <http://www.who.int>

World Food Programme. "Fighting the Global War on Hunger from the Frontline." Available from <http://www.wfp.org>

Food and Agricultural Organization

nutrition: the maintenance of health through proper eating, or the study of same

The Food and Agricultural Organization (FAO) is one of the largest specialized agencies of the United Nations. Founded in 1945, it is responsible for raising levels of **nutrition** and standards of living, increasing agricultural productivity, and improving rural living conditions throughout the world. The FAO is an international organization that has 183 member countries, plus one member organization, the European Community. The FAO Conference, which meets every two years, is the governing body of the FAO.

The FAO is comprised of eight departments: Administration and Finance, Agriculture, Economic and Social, Fisheries, Forestry, General Affairs and Information, Sustainable Development, and Technical Cooperation. Funding for the FAO's work falls into two categories: the Regular Program, which covers internal operations, and the Field Program, which implements projects that are usually undertaken in cooperation with national governments and other agencies.

Special programs and activities of the FAO include: (1) the World Food Summit, which strives to reduce worldwide hunger; (2) the Special Program for Food Security, a program for advancing food technologies; (3) Tele-Food, an annual campaign to help poor families produce more food; (4) the Technical Cooperation Program, which promotes the sharing of technical expertise between countries; and (5) EMPRES (Emergency Prevention System for Transboundary Animal and Plant Pests and Diseases) which strives to eradicate pests and diseases. SEE ALSO FAMINE; FOOD AID FOR DEVELOPMENT; FOOD INSECURITY; UNITED NATIONS CHILDREN'S FUND (UNICEF).

Karen Bryla

Internet Resource

Food and Agricultural Organization of the United Nations. <http://www.fao.org>

Food Guide Pyramid

The Food Guide Pyramid is a graphic representation of *A Pattern for Daily Food Choices*, a food guide that was developed by the U.S. Department of Agriculture (USDA) in the 1980s. Food guides are tools designed to help people select healthful diets. The USDA has been developing food guides since 1916, and recommendations have changed over the years due to emerging knowledge about **nutrient** needs and the relationships between **diet** and health, changing economic conditions (such as the Great Depression in the 1930s), and changing lifestyles.

nutrient: dietary substance necessary for health

diet: the total daily food intake, or the types of foods eaten

nutrition: the maintenance of health through proper eating, or the study of same

A Pattern for Daily Food Choices replaced the *Basic Four* food guide which was the centerpiece of **nutrition** education in the United States for over twenty years. The new food guide was not widely used in nutrition education until the USDA released The Food Guide Pyramid in 1992. Since that time, nutrition educators, dietitians, and teachers have used the Pyramid and accompanying educational materials to teach people how to select foods to build healthful diets. The Pyramid is also a familiar feature on food labels, where it is used by food manufacturers to show where foods fit into the food groups that make up the Pyramid.

Design and Recommendations of The Food Guide Pyramid

USDA nutritionists spent many years designing, testing, and refining the Food Guide Pyramid. The goal was to have an easy-to-use graphic that would help people select a diet that promoted nutritional health and decreased the risk of disease. They designed the Pyramid to be flexible enough to be used by most healthy Americans over the age of two. However, they also recognized that people with substantially different eating habits, such as vegetarians, may need a different food guidance system.

The Pyramid includes five major food groups, each of which provides nutrients needed for good health. By making healthful choices within these food groups, like selecting low-fat and high-fiber foods, people can promote good health and reduce their risk of disease. The placement of foods within the Pyramid shows that foods of plant origin should supply most of the servings of food in the daily diet.

The Breads, Cereals, Rice, and Pasta Group forms the base of the Pyramid, with the largest number of servings recommended (six to eleven servings recommended daily). The next layer up includes the Fruit Group (two to four servings) and the Vegetable Group (three to five servings). At the third level are the Milk, Yogurt, and Cheese Group (two to three servings) and the Meat, Poultry, Fish, Dry Beans, Eggs, and Nuts Group (two to three servings). At the tip of the Pyramid are Fats, Oils, and Sweets. These foods and food ingredients should be used "sparingly" to avoid excess **calories** and/or fat. It is not necessary to completely avoid foods such as salad dressing, butter, margarine, candy, soft drinks, and sweet desserts, but they should be consumed infrequently.

The Pyramid includes symbols that represent the fats and added sugars found in foods. These are most concentrated at the tip of the Pyramid, but are also found in foods from the five major food groups. This reveals that some foods within the five food groups are high in fat and/or sugar. People can limit their fat and sugar intake, as suggested by the Dietary Guidelines for Americans, by selecting foods low in fat and added sugars most of the time.

Uses of the Food Guide Pyramid

Individuals can use the Pyramid educational materials to plan a diet that contains all needed nutrients and is moderate in fat and **saturated fat**. This is important in the United States, where the major causes of death, such as **heart disease**, are related to diets high in fat, especially saturated fat. **Obesity** is also a major health concern in the United States. Although physical activity is a critical component of weight management, food intake also plays a role in **energy** balance. The Food Guide Pyramid educational materials provide serving sizes and a recommended number of servings for people of different ages and activity levels. This guide can help people learn to eat reasonable amounts of food in a country where large portion sizes are the norm.

Development of Alternative Pyramids

Some nutrition and health professionals disagree with the dietary recommendations of the USDA's Food Guide Pyramid. Critics of the Pyramid have expressed various concerns. Some believe that the food guide does not go far enough in emphasizing plant-food consumption, and that there is an overemphasis on foods of animal origin. Another concern is the inclusion of foods that are high in fats and/or sugars within the basic five food groups, which may lead people to maintain high fat and calorie intake. Others have indicated that the Pyramid is not appropriate for use with various ethnic and cultural groups, although this fact was recognized by the nutritionists who developed the Pyramid.

One alternative pyramid is the Traditional Healthy Mediterranean Diet Pyramid, developed by the Oldways Preservation and Exchange Trust in cooperation with Harvard School of Public Health and the World Health

calorie: unit of food energy

saturated fat: a fat with the maximum possible number of hydrogens; more difficult to break down than unsaturated fats

heart disease: any disorder of the heart or its blood supply, including heart attack, atherosclerosis, and coronary artery disease

obesity: the condition of being overweight, according to established norms based on sex, age, and height

energy: technically, the ability to perform work; the content of a substance that allows it to be useful as a fuel

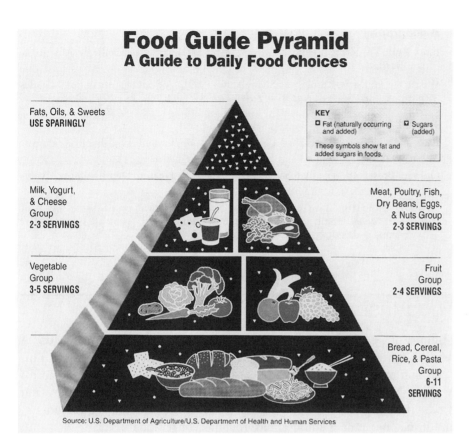

Food Guide Pyramid
A Guide to Daily Food Choices

Fats, Oils, & Sweets
USE SPARINGLY

KEY
☐ Fat (naturally occurring and added) ☐ Sugars (added)
These symbols show fat and added sugars in foods.

Milk, Yogurt, & Cheese Group
2-3 SERVINGS

Meat, Poultry, Fish, Dry Beans, Eggs, & Nuts Group
2-3 SERVINGS

Vegetable Group
3-5 SERVINGS

Fruit Group
2-4 SERVINGS

Bread, Cereal, Rice, & Pasta Group
6-11 SERVINGS

Source: U.S. Department of Agriculture/U.S. Department of Health and Human Services

The Food Guide Pyramid, last updated in 1992, could be revised for release in 2005. Proposed changes would include more recent nutritional recommendations and may be tailored to specific ages and activity levels to help reverse the nation's trend toward obesity. *[EPD Photos. The Gale Group.]*

Organization. This Pyramid has an increased emphasis on foods of plant origin and limits red meat consumption to a monthly serving. It recommends daily olive oil consumption, wine "in moderation," and daily consumption of six glasses of water. The Mediterranean Pyramid is based on a diet that has long been associated with reduced risk for heart disease, though some Americans might find it difficult adapting to such a different eating plan.

Pyramids targeting specific ethnic groups have been developed by a variety of organizations. They include Latin American, Puerto Rican, Asian, Vietnamese, soul food, and vegetarian pyramids, among others. As information emerged about the nutritional needs of older people, the need for a food guide targeted to this growing population became clear. In 1999, nutritionists at Tufts University developed a prototype of a pyramid targeted to persons seventy years of age and older. Several other pyramids for older adults have been developed at other universities since that time. To meet the needs of children, the USDA released the Food Pyramid Guide for Young Children in 1999.

The USDA Food Guide Pyramid reflects a food guide that was designed to meet the nutritional needs, and to promote long-term health, of Americans over the age of two. It supports the goals of the Dietary Guidelines for Americans, which are designed to promote healthy lifestyles and to reduce health risks. The messages of the Food Guide Pyramid are most effective when accompanied by nutrition education to help people make healthful choices from the five food groups. SEE ALSO DIETARY ASSESSMENT; DIETARY GUIDELINES; HEALTHY EATING INDEX.

Linda Benjamin Bobroff

Bibliography

Insel, Paul; Turner, R. Elaine; and Ross, Don (2001). *Nutrition.* Sudbury, MA: Jones and Bartlett.

Welsh, Susan; Davis, Carole; and Shaw, Anne (1992). "A Brief History of Food Guides in the United States." *Nutrition Today* 27:6–11.

Internet Resources

Food and Nutrition Information Center. *Food Guide Pyramid.* Available from <http://www.nal.usda.gov/fnic>

Oldways Preservation and Exchange Trust. "Oldways Healthy Diet Pyramids." Available from <http://www.oldwayspt.org>

U.S. Department of Agriculture, Human Nutrition Information Service. *The Food Guide Pyramid.* Home and Garden Bulletin Number 252. Available from <http://www.cnpp.usda.gov>

Food Insecurity

undernutrition: food intake too low to maintain adequate energy expenditure without weight loss

chronic: over a long period

Millions of people worldwide suffer from hunger and **undernutrition**. A major factor contributing to this international problem is *food insecurity*. This condition exists when people lack sustainable physical or economic access to enough safe, nutritious, and socially acceptable food for a healthy and productive life. Food insecurity may be **chronic**, seasonal, or temporary, and it may occur at the household, regional, or national level.

The United Nations estimates there are 840 million undernourished people in the world. The majority of undernourished people (799 million) reside in developing countries, most of which are on the continents of Africa and Asia. This figure also includes 11 million people located in developed countries and 30 million people located in countries in transition (e.g., the former Soviet Union). The U.S. Department of Agriculture estimates that nearly 11 percent of U.S. households are food insecure, with approximately one-third of these households experiencing moderate to severe hunger.

In developing countries, the root causes of food insecurity include: poverty, war and civil conflict, corruption, national policies that do not promote equal access to food for all, environmental degradation, barriers to trade, insufficient agricultural development, population growth, low levels of education, social and gender inequality, poor health status, cultural insensitivity, and natural disasters. In the United States, the primary cause of food insecurity is poverty. Low levels of education, poor health status, and certain disabilities also increase the risk of food insecurity for individuals and households in the United States.

Globally, certain groups of people are more vulnerable to food insecurity than others. Vulnerable groups include: victims of conflict (e.g., refugees and internally displaced people); migrant workers; marginal populations (e.g., school dropouts, unemployed people, homeless people, and orphans); dependent populations (e.g., elderly people, children under five, and disabled and ill people); women of reproductive age; ethnic minorities; and low literacy households.

For food security to exist at the national, regional, and local levels, food must be available, accessible, and properly utilized. Availability of food means

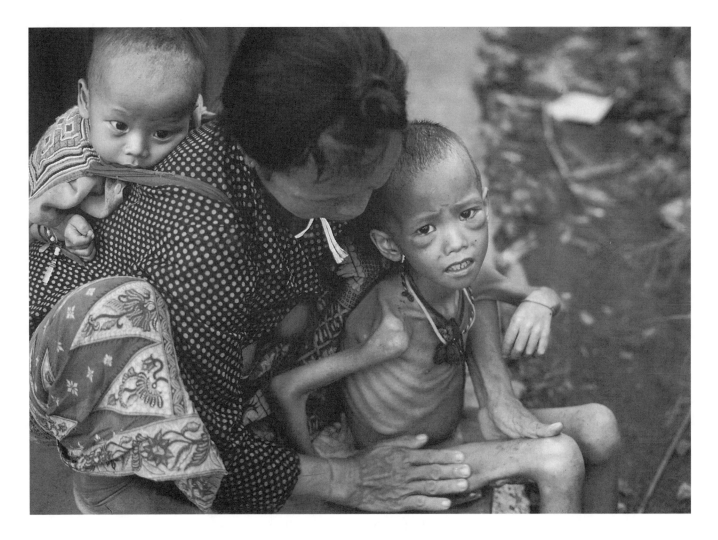

Food insecurity affects millions of people around the world, including these children in Thailand. The situation in that country and a handful of others has improved slightly, but progress is slow. [© Bettmann/ Corbis. Reproduced by permission.]

that enough safe and nutritious food is either domestically produced or imported from the international market. However, food availability does not ensure food accessibility. Government policies must also contribute to equal distribution of food within nations, regions, and communities. In addition, for food to be accessible, individuals and families must be able to afford the food prices on the market. Finally, food must be properly utilized. Proper utilization depends on proper food storage to guard against spoilage, appropriate handling to avoid disease transmission, and proper preparation to ensure nutritiously balanced meals.

Individuals need adequate amounts of a variety of quality, safe foods to be healthy and well-nourished. Undernutrition results from an insufficient intake or an improper balance of **protein**, **energy**, and micronutrients. Nutritional consequences of insufficient food or undernutrition include protein energy **malnutrition**, **anemia**, vitamin A deficiency, iodine deficiency, and **iron** deficiency.

Food insecurity and malnutrition result in catastrophic amounts of human suffering. The World Health Organization estimates that approximately 60 percent of all childhood deaths in the developing world are associated with chronic hunger and malnutrition. In developing countries, persistent malnutrition leaves children weak, vulnerable, and less able to fight such common childhood illnesses as diarrhea, **acute** respiratory infections, **malaria**,

protein: complex molecule composed of amino acids that performs vital functions in the cell; necessary part of the diet

energy: technically, the ability to perform work; the content of a substance that allows it to be useful as a fuel

malnutrition: chronic lack of sufficient nutrients to maintain health

anemia: low level of red blood cells in the blood

iron: nutrient needed for red blood cell formation

acute: rapid-onset and short-lived

malaria: disease caused by infection with Plasmodium, a single-celled protozoon, transmitted by mosquitoes

fatigue: tiredness

psychological: related to thoughts, feelings, and personal experiences

stress: heightened state of nervousness or unease

anxiety: nervousness

depression: mood disorder characterized by apathy, restlessness, and negative thoughts

and measles. Even children who are mildly to moderately malnourished are at greater risk of dying from these common diseases. Malnourished children in the United States suffer from poorer health status, compromised immune systems, and higher rates of illnesses such as colds, headaches, and **fatigue**.

Adolescents and adults also suffer adverse consequences of food insecurity and malnutrition. Malnutrition can lead to decreased energy levels, delayed maturation, growth failure, impaired cognitive ability, diminished capacity to learn, decreased ability to resist infections and illnesses, shortened life expectancy, increased maternal mortality, and low birth weight.

Food insecurity may also result in severe social, **psychological**, and behavioral consequences. Food-insecure individuals may manifest feelings of alienation, powerlessness, **stress**, and **anxiety**, and they may experience reduced productivity, reduced work and school performance, and reduced income earnings. Household dynamics may become disrupted because of a preoccupation with obtaining food, which may lead to anger, pessimism, and irritability. Adverse consequences for children include: higher levels of aggressive or destructive behavior, hyperactivity, anxiety, difficulty with social interactions (e.g., more withdrawn or socially disruptive), increased passivity, poorer overall school performance, increased school absences, and a greater need for mental health care services (e.g., for **depression** or suicidal behaviors).

To understand the magnitude of food insecurity, hunger, and malnutrition, one must consider both the continued rapid growth in world population and the number of individuals below the poverty line. In 1999 the world population reached 6 billion. The United Nations estimates the world population will exceed 8 billion by 2025. In terms of poverty, the World Bank estimates that nearly 1.2 billion people live on less than one dollar a day, which is the internationally recognized standard for measuring poverty. Another 2.8 billion live on less than two dollars a day.

In addition to these progress-slowing conditions, the number of undernourished people is actually growing in most developing regions. A few large countries have made significant gains, making the global picture appear more promising than it really is. China, Indonesia, Vietnam, Thailand, Nigeria, Ghana, and Peru have all made important gains in reducing food insecurity and hunger. However, in nearly fifty other countries, the number of undernourished people increased by almost 100 million between 1993 and 2003. The absolute numbers continue to rise as a result of rapid population growth, even though the proportion of undernourished people in most developing countries is actually decreasing.

Worldwide commitment to improve global food insecurity was demonstrated at the 1996 World Food Summit, where 186 countries pledged to reduce the number of hungry, food-insecure people in the world by 50 percent (to 400 million) by the year 2015. Progress toward this goal has been slow, with a decrease of only 2.5 million people a year since 1992. At the current pace, the goal will be reached more than one hundred years late. Despite slow progress, some innovative programs have been implemented around the globe to combat food insecurity and undernutrition. Examples of innovative program include: community gardens, farmers markets, community-supported sustainable agricultural programs, food for work exchange programs, farm to school initiatives, credit to poor households, income transfer schemes, and agricultural diversification programs.

Food insecurity remains a significant international problem, with developing regions of the world enduring most of the burden. Food insecurity results in considerable health, social, psychological, and behavioral consequences and is undeniably linked to poverty. Despite international commitment, the number of food insecure individuals remains unacceptably high.

SEE ALSO Famine; Food Aid for Development and the World Food Programme; Food and Agricultural Organization; Food Safety; Hunger; Malnutrition; United Nations Children's Fund (UNICEF).

Lori Keeling Buhi

Internet Resources

Bellamy, Carol (1998). *The State of the World's Children 1998: Focus on Nutrition.* United Nations Children's Fund. Available from <http://www.unicef.org>

Brandeis University (2002). "The Consequences of Hunger and Food Insecurity for Children, Evidence from Recent Scientific Studies." Center on Hunger and Poverty, Heller School for Social Policy and Management. Available from <http://www.centeronhunger.org>

Food and Agriculture Organization of the United Nations (2002). *The State of Food Security in the World,* 4th edition. Available from <http://www.fao.org>

Nord, Mark; Andrews, Margaret; and Carlson, Steve (2002). *Household Food Security in the United States, 2001.* Food Assistance and Nutrition Research Report No. 29. Economic Research Service, U.S. Department of Agriculture. Available from <http://www.ers.usda.gov>

United Nations Food and Agriculture Organization. "Rome Declaration on World Food Security." Proceedings from the World Food Summit, November 13–17, 1996. Rome, Italy. Available from <http://www.fao.org>

U.S. Department of Agriculture (1999). *U.S. Action Plan on Food Security, Solutions to Hunger.* U.S. Department of Agriculture. Available from <http://www.fas.usda.gov>

World Bank Group. "Income Poverty: The Latest Global Numbers." Updated August 2, 2002. Available from <http://www.worldbank.org>

World Health Organization. "Nutrition Research: Pursuing Sustainable Solutions." Updated September 16, 2002. Available from <http://www.who.int/en>

Food Labels

The quality and safety of foods are a worldwide concern and have been a societal issue since the beginning of civilization. In the United States, very complex laws and regulations have been developed to address food safety concerns. These laws and regulations are designed not only to insure that food is safe to eat, but also to insure that the product label provides information consumers need to make educated food-purchasing decisions.

Overview of Food Labeling

Food labels on products sold in the United States must have the product name (product identity statement); the manufacturer's name and address; the net contents in terms of weight, measure, or count; a list of ingredients; and, in most cases, a Nutrition Facts statement. To insure consistent presentation of information so consumers can easily compare food products, each component of the label is defined by regulations in terms of placement, terminology, and type size. Regulation of food labeling falls primarily under the jurisdiction of two federal agencies: the Food and Drug Administration (FDA) and the United States Department of Agriculture (USDA). Both the FDA and the USDA publish regulations governing food labeling in the *Federal Register* (FR), which is published daily. Each year, all federal regulations are updated and compiled in the *Code of Federal Regulations* (CFR); FDA labeling regulations appear in Title 21 and USDA regulations in Title 9 of the CFR.

nutrient: dietary substance necessary for health

The regulations define two categories of claims: **nutrient** content claims and health claims. Nutrient content claims are statements about the level of a nutrient in a food. Health claims, on the other hand, link the nutrient profile of a food to a health or disease condition. Food products made by very small businesses and foods with insignificant amounts of nutrients may be exempt from labeling regulations.

Product Identity Statement

Food labeling regulations require food products to be labeled prominently with a product identity statement to ensure consumers obtain important information about both the type and form of food contained in the package. The product identity statement should be a standard name or a common or usual name that is familiar to consumers. If it is marketed in various forms (e.g., whole, sliced, diced), the form of the food needs to be included. If it is an imitation food, the statement must include the word "imitation." Any information that is important to describe the food product must be included as part of Product Identity statement.

Net Quantity of Contents

The purpose of the "net quantity of contents" statement is to inform the consumer of the amount of product contained in the package. Regulations require specific wording, type size, and placement. Federal and state agencies monitor food products to ensure products contain the amount of the food stated on the food label.

Ingredient List

A list of the ingredients must be included on all foods that have more than one ingredient. Ingredients must be listed in descending order of predominance and in defined terminology. Ingredients that are present in amounts of less than 2 percent of the product do not necessarily need to appear in order of predominance.

Nutrition Labeling

FDA's voluntary nutrition labeling program was initiated in 1976. Under this program, unless the product bore a nutrition claim or nutrients were added to the product, food manufacturers had the option of providing nutrition information on their products. On November 8, 1990, President George Bush signed into law the Nutrition Labeling and Education Act of 1990 (NLEA), requiring nutrition labeling for most foods (except meat and poultry) and outlining the appropriate use of nutrient content and health claims. Regulations implementing NLEA became effective January 6, 1993. Since then, the Food and Drug Administration (FDA) has issued over forty

NUTRIENTS AND DAILY VALUES USED FOR LABELING

Nutrient	Daily Value
Calories*	—
Calories from fat	—
Calories from Saturated Fat	—
Total Fat*	65g
Saturated Fat	20g
Stearic Acid (USDA only)	—
Polyunsaturated Fat	—
Monounsaturated Fat	—
Cholesterol	300mg
Sodium*	2,400mg
Potassium	3,500mg
Total Carbohydrate*	300mg
Dietary Fiber	25g
Soluble Fiber	—
Insoluble Fiber	—
Sugars	—
Sugar Alcohol	—
Other Carbohydrate	—
Protein*	59g**
Vitamin A	5,000 IU
Beta-carotene	—
Vitamin C	60mg
Calcium	1,000mg
Iron	18mg
Vitamin D	400 IU
Vitamin E	30 IU
Thiamin	1.5mg
Riboflavin	1.7m
Niacin	20mg
Vitamin B$_6$	2.0mg
Folate	400mg
Vitamin B$_{12}$	6.0mg
Biotin	0.3mg
Pantothenic Acid	10mg
Phosphorus	1,000mg
Iodine	150mg
Magnesium	400mg
Zinc	15mg
Copper	2.0mg

Mandatory Nutrients are in **bold**
*Core nutrients
**%DV is not required for protein. If included, special rules apply.

major regulations for NLEA and many more minor regulations to revise existing regulations. As a result of these regulations, nutrition labeling is now virtually universal on packaged foods, the nutrition label format is easy to recognize, nutrient reference values have been standardized, nutrient claims have been defined, and disease-specific claims are now authorized.

Nutrition Facts Statement. In order to ensure consistency of information, both FDA and USDA regulations are very explicit about the layout of the Nutrition Facts panel. The type of information that may be included, as well as the format and order, is detailed in the CFR.

Required Nutrients. Manufacturers are required to provide information on fourteen nutrients, but they may omit some of these if they are present at insignificant levels. Food manufacturers determine the nutrient content either by laboratory analyses on the product as packaged, or by calculation using standardized nutrient databases. Of the fourteen nutrients, five are considered core nutrients and must always be included on the Nutrition Facts panel, even if they are present at insignificant levels. In addition to mandatory nutrients, other nutrients may be required in some circumstances, or manufacturers may include them on a voluntary basis. The nonmandatory

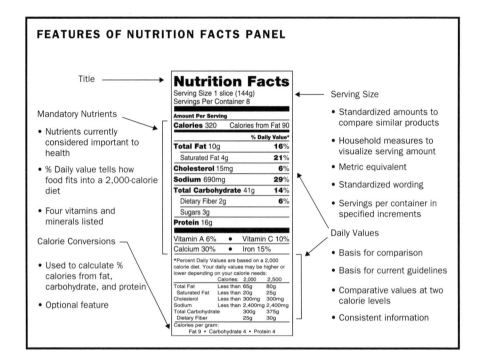

FEATURES OF NUTRITION FACTS PANEL

nutrients are defined by the regulations. All nutrients must appear in a specified order.

Percent Daily Value. In addition to declaring the gram or milligram amounts for macronutrients (such as **fat**, **cholesterol**, sodium, **carbohydrates**, and **protein**), the "Percent Daily Value" is also declared (with the exception of sugars and protein). All **vitamins** and **minerals** are presented as percentages of the Daily Value (based on a daily intake of 2,000 **calories**). Declaring nutrients as a percentage of the Daily Values provides a standard that is easy to use by individuals who are not familiar with the wide range of levels of different nutrients. For example, a food with 100 IU (international units) of Vitamin A may appear to contain a significant amount of this nutrient, but it is actually only 2 percent of the Daily Value (5,000 IU) for Vitamin A. Alternatively, a food with 6 grams of **saturated fat** may be thought of as low in Saturated Fat, when it actually contains 30 percent of the Daily Value (20 grams).

Serving Size. A serving size is the amount of food upon which the nutrient content is based. In order to ensure consistent serving sizes between similar products, NLEA defines serving size as the amount of food customarily eaten at one time. The serving size included on the Nutrition Facts panel may vary slightly between similar products, but it is based on the Reference Amounts Customarily Consumed Per Eating Occasion (RACC), as established by the FDA. The serving size is the household measure (e.g., cups, tablespoon, piece, slice, fraction, or container) closest to the RACC, followed by the metric equivalent. For a package of crackers where each cracker weighs 7 grams and the RACC is 15 grams, the serving size would read "2 crackers (14g)."

As a result of NLEA and other United States food labeling laws, health-conscious consumers are afforded a world of information on food labels. Food-labeling regulations provide the consistent standards consumers need

fat: type of food molecule rich in carbon and hydrogen, with high energy content

cholesterol: multi-ringed molecule found in animal cell membranes; a type of lipid

carbohydrate: food molecule made of carbon, hydrogen, and oxygen, including sugars and starches

protein: complex molecule composed of amino acids that performs vital functions in the cell; necessary part of the diet

vitamin: necessary complex nutrient used to aid enzymes or other metabolic processes in the cell

mineral: an inorganic (non-carbon-containing) element, ion, or compound

calorie: unit of food energy

saturated fat: a fat with the maximum possible number of hydrogens; more difficult to break down than unsaturated fats

to make food choices in an ever-changing food industry. SEE ALSO DAILY REFERENCE VALUES; DIETARY GUIDELINES; FUNCTIONAL FOODS; HEALTH CLAIMS; NUTRIENTS; REGULATORY AGENCIES.

Karen Hare

Food Safety

One of the many luxuries Americans enjoy is access to the safest and most abundant food supply in the world. This stems from many advances and improvements in food safety, sanitation, and crop production that reduce the chance of food-safety problems, including food-borne illness, pesticide contamination, or infectious disease. There are many reasons why food safety has become an issue. First, medical advances have made it possible for people to live longer, creating an aging population more susceptible to disease. Second, labor in the food industry is more diverse and less skilled. Learning barriers, personnel turnover, and limited food-preparation skills create challenges in training. Third, the U.S. food supply has expanded globally, and many types of food come from areas where food safety standards are less stringent than those in the United States. Other concerns for food safety stem from terrorist threats, food irradiation, and genetically modified foods.

Concerns exist about the use of radioactivity in food irradiation, the presence of possible subsequent toxicity, and the development of more virulent **bacteria**. These concerns, however, are unfounded and the benefits outweigh the risks. Evidence from over four decades of research in the United States shows the benefits to include a decrease in food-borne **pathogens**, an increase in the shelf life of some fruits and vegetables, and less fumigant use for controlling insect pests.

bacteria: single-celled organisms without nuclei, some of which are infectious

pathogen: organism that causes disease

Control and Oversight

The Food and Drug Administration (FDA) ensures that injury, such as disease or illness, will not result from substances in food by closely monitoring the food supply. This differs from monitoring for food hazards (the responsibility of the food handler), where harm is possible under normal conditions. Potential food hazards could include improper storage conditions and serving food at unsafe temperatures. The food handler is directly involved in controlling these potential hazards during receiving, storage, preparation, cooking, and service.

The primary agencies that monitor the safety of the U.S. food supply are the FDA, the U.S. Department of Agriculture (USDA), the Environmental Protection Agency, and the U.S. Fish and Wildlife Service. When monitoring the food supply, the FDA focuses first on microbial food-borne illness, followed by natural **toxins** in food, and residues in food, including environmental contaminants, pesticides, and animal drugs. Nutritional composition and intentional **food additives** are monitored more closely as artificial food products enter the market. The FDA *Food Code*, which is published every two years, provides guidance for restaurants, grocery stores, and institutions such as nursing homes on how to prevent food-borne illness. Managers and supervisors of these institutions are now required to be certified

toxins: poison

food additive: substance added to foods to improve nutrition, taste, appearance, or shelf-life

in food safety and sanitation. Local, state, and federal regulators use the *Food Code* as a model to develop their own food safety rules.

Food-Borne Illness

Each year, millions of people become ill from food-borne illness, the most common food safety-issue, although many cases are not reported. Food-borne illness is caused when toxic levels of pathogens or bacteria are present in food. Microbial food-borne illness, commonly called **food poisoning**, is monitored closely because the cases of food poisoning far outweigh any other type of food contamination. In the case of an infection from a pathogen such as *Salmonella*, contamination and food-borne illness results when a pathogen in a food product multiplies and infects the human body after ingestion. These **microorganisms** can multiply in food during agricultural production, transportation, preparation, and storage, or within the digestive tract after a person eats the contaminated food. Factors that contribute to food toxicity include the amount of the initial contamination, the time held in unsafe conditions, and the use of processes to inactivate or remove toxins and pathogens. The Centers for Disease Control and Prevention (CDC) reports that most food-borne illness outbreaks occur from improper handling of food in the retail area of the food industry (e.g., schools, restaurants). Equally important is safe food-handling by consumers who purchase food and consume it at home, since most cases of food poisoning are a result of improper handling or cooking after purchase.

For many victims, food-borne illness results only in discomfort or lost time from the job. Those at higher risk—pre-school-age children, older adults in health care facilities, and those with impaired immune systems—food-borne illness is more serious and may be life threatening. Symptoms of food-borne illness vary, but can include **nausea**, vomiting, abdominal cramps, headache, and in some cases difficulty speaking and swallowing. Some instances could result in **paralysis** or death. Fever **fatigue** and jaundice occur after several days in **hepatitis** cases.

To protect consumers from food-borne disease, efforts must focus on each point in the farm-to-table chain to better predict and prevent food-borne hazards, and to monitor and rapidly react to outbreaks of food-borne diseases. A food-service establishment should have an effective food-safety program to prevent hazards before they occur. For example, the Hazard Analysis Critical Control Point (HACCP) program is a proactive program initiated by the FDA to ensure food safety for the astronauts in the space program. The process starts by reviewing a food service's standard operating procedures to be sure that food hazards are controlled during receiving, storage, preparation, service, and cooling of foods for later use. An examination of sanitation, as well as food handlers' personal **hygiene** and work practices are important as well.

Pesticides and Biotechnology

The use of pesticides to control damage of food crops and enhance production has created a controversy related to potential hazards to consumers. While pesticides can be part of a safe food-protection program, they can be hazardous when handled or used inappropriately. High doses of pesticides applied to laboratory animals cause birth defects, sterility, tumors, organ

food poisoning: illness caused by consumption of spoiled food, usually containing bacteria

microorganisms: bacteria and protists; single-celled organisms

nausea: unpleasant sensation in the gut that precedes vomiting

paralysis: inability to move

fatigue: tiredness

hepatitis: liver inflammation

hygiene: cleanliness

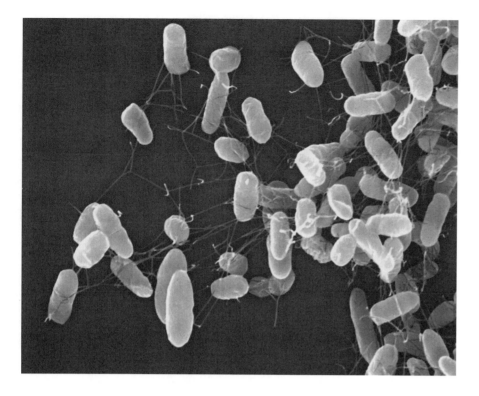

Salmonella enteritidis bacteria annually infect between two and four million people in the United States. Most outbreaks of food-borne illness are due to improper food handling or storage. *[USDA/Science Source/Photo Researchers, Inc. Reproduced by permission.]*

damage, and central **nervous system** impairment. As with **antibiotics**, the targeted insects become resistant and can survive exposure, emerging with increased vigor to again attack the crop. The same effects arise from herbicides and fungicides used on crops. New labeling laws introduced by the FDA in October 2002 have caused some organic producers to drop the term *organic* from their label, finding the requirements too restrictive.

Genetically modified foods have been a cause of concern in many parts of the world since their introduction, particularly in Europe. Campaigns have been launched by many groups opposing the practice of genetically altering **enzymes**, **amino acids**, and **genes** in foods for the purposes of increasing crop yields, nutritional quality, and profits while decreasing food waste. Whether it is about changing the degree of saturation in oils or adding amino acids to corn to make it a more complete **protein** source, food technologists are working hard to change the chemical make-up of food.

Organic farming groups and others will likely continue to fight against the use of pesticides and **genetic** modification in food production for years. When trying to feed the world, one must weigh the risks and benefits of both when establishing food-safety regulations.

Bioterrorism

With the advent of **vaccines** and antibiotics, many people in developed countries had become complacent about **infectious diseases**. However, the increase in acts of worldwide terrorism has caused food security to become a major concern for the food industry and for public health officials. Deliberate biological or chemical contamination of food or water remains the easiest method for widespread terrorism, according to the CDC, and since everyone eats, all are open to an attack. Bioterrorism and the emergence of strains of diseases that have become resistant to antibiotic therapy (such as

nervous system: the brain, spinal cord, and nerves that extend throughout the body

antibiotic: substance that kills or prevents the growth of microorganisms

enzyme: protein responsible for carrying out reactions in a cell

amino acid: building block of proteins, necessary dietary nutrient

gene: DNA sequence that codes for proteins, and thus controls inheritance

protein: complex molecule composed of amino acids that performs vital functions in the cell; necessary part of the diet

genetic: inherited or related to the genes

vaccine: medicine that promotes immune system resistance by stimulating pre-existing cells to become active

infectious diseases: diseases caused by viruses, bacteria, fungi, or protozoa, which replicate inside the body

237

FOOD SAFETY REGULATIONS AND LAWS

1897 Tea Importation Act—Customs inspection for purity
1890 First U.S. Legislation on Meat Inspection
1906 Certified Color Regulations—listed 7 artificial colors found suitable for foods
1907 Federal Meat Inspection Act—arose out of unsanitary conditions in meatpacking plants, use of poisonous preservatives and dyes in food, and cure-all claims for worthless and dangerous medicines
1923 Filled Milk Act
1938 Federal Food, Drug, and Cosmetic Act
1939 First Food Standards for canned tomatoes, tomato puree, tomato paste for consistency
1944 Public Health Service Act—covered a broad spectrum of health concerns including regulation of biological products and control of communicable disease
1954 Pesticide Amendment Act—followed recall of cranberries found with pesticide that can cause cancer
1954 Radiological Examination of Food—brought on by reports that tuna suspected of being radioactive were being imported from Japan following atomic blasts in the Pacific
1957 Poultry Products Inspection
1958 Food Additives Amendment—required manufactures of new additives to establish safety
1960 Color Additive Amendments—similar to food additives, identified safe colors
1966 Fair Packaging and Labeling Act—required honest labels
1967 Wholesome Meat Act—state (intrastate) inspections to match the federal inspection guidelines and closed loopholes in the 1906 act which required only interstate inspection
1968 Wholesome Poultry Products—included interstate and intrastate inspection guidelines for poultry
1970 Egg Products Inspection Act
1980 Swine Health Protection Act
1990 Sanitary Food Transportation Act

tuberculosis and some food-borne infections) constitute growing threats to health and life around the globe. An attack through plant or animal disease would have significant economic impact.

Current systems that detect food-borne illness outbreaks and link them to their source need to be enhanced for defense against food bioterrorism. However, the potential for an undetected contamination in industrialized countries is relatively low. Once food has been processed and readied for distribution, quick identification of any contamination and isolation from distribution is required. Imported food products may be more likely to be contaminated with a pathogen by terrorist groups. Another concern is deliberate infection of crops and herds.

Citizens must rely on government security and public health measures such as emergency preparedness, secure food and disinfected water supplies, and good medical care to reduce the likelihood of contamination. In response to an increased risk of terrorism, the Alliance for Food Security has partnered with the FDA and the National Food Processors Association to provide domestic food and water security. In addition, the FDA has published a guide that outlines strategies to minimize contamination, providing guidance in seven areas of food service, from management to operations.

History and Purpose of Food Safety Regulations

The U.S. Public Health Service Commissioned Corp (PHS) is a uniformed service of the United States comprised of health professionals and led by the Office of the Surgeon General. The origins of the agency can be traced to a 1798 act that was passed to provide care for sick and injured merchant seamen. Formalized in 1889, it oversaw quarantines and medical examinations of immigrants. The agency commissioned officers to control the spread of contagious diseases such as **smallpox** and yellow fever through the 1900s.

smallpox: deadly viral disease

It also conducted biomedical research, provided health care to deprived groups, and supplied medical assistance to victims of natural disasters.

The PHS began its food-protection activities in the early 1900s with studies on the role of milk in the spread of disease. Model food codes and other regulations soon evolved to ensure food quality and safety. These include sanitary practices at processing plants, safety standards for ingredients, and labeling laws to assist state and local governments in initiating and maintaining effective programs for the prevention of food-borne illness. SEE ALSO ADDITIVES AND PRESERVATIVES; BIOTECHNOLOGY; GENETICALLY MODIFIED FOODS; IRRADIATION; ORGANISMS, FOOD-BORNE; PESTICIDES; REGULATORY AGENCIES.

Marilyn K. Dahl

Bibliography

Jackson, R. (1997). *Nutrition and Food Services for Integrated Health Care.* Gaithersburg, MD: Aspen.

National Restaurant Association Foundation (2002). *ServSafe Essentials,* 2nd edition. Chicago: Author.

Sizer, Francis, and Whitney, Eleanor (2003). *Nutrition Concepts and Controversies,* 9th edition. Belmont, CA: Wadsworth/Thomson.

Internet Resources

U.S. Food and Drug Administration, Center for Food Safety and Applied Nutrition. *FDA Food Code.* Available from <http://www.dfsan.fda.gov>

U.S. Food and Drug Administration, Center for Food Safety and Applied Nutrition. "Retail Food Stores and Food Service Establishments: Food Security Preventative Measures Guidance." Available from <http://www.dfsan.fda.gov>

Fortification

Fortification is the addition of **nutrients** to foods to enhance their nutritional value. **Enrichment**, on the other hand, is the addition of nutrients to foods to restore nutrients lost during processing. Examples of fortification include the addition of **folate** and **iron** to grain products, **calcium** to juices, iodine to salt, and iron to infant formulas.

Decisions to fortify foods are often population-based to address geographical inadequacies, such as lack of iodine in the soil, or to increase the intake of key nutrients, such as calcium, vitamin A, and **vitamin D**. Challenges involved in fortification include identifying suitable foods to deliver the nutrients, selecting appropriate forms of the nutrients, designing appropriate processing techniques, and implementing systems to monitor the **efficacy** of the fortification. SEE ALSO ADDITIVES AND PRESERVATIVES; FUNCTIONAL FOODS.

M. Elizabeth Kunkel
Barbara H. D. Luccia

fortification: addition of vitamins and minerals to improve the nutritional content of a food

nutrient: dietary substance necessary for health

enrichment: addition of vitamins and minerals to improve the nutritional content of a food

folate: one of the B vitamins, also called folic acid

iron: nutrient needed for red blood cell formation

calcium: mineral essential for bones and teeth

vitamin D: nutrient needed for calcium uptake and therefore proper bone formation

efficacy: effectiveness

French Paradox

The term *French paradox* refers to the observation that although the French eat similar amounts of high-fat foods, exercise less, and smoke more than

heart disease: any disorder of the heart or its blood supply, including heart attack, atherosclerosis, and coronary artery disease

diet: the total daily food intake, or the types of foods eaten

antioxidant: substance that prevents oxidation, a damaging reaction with oxygen

blood pressure: measure of the pressure exerted by the blood against the walls of the blood vessels

incidence: number of new cases reported each year

Americans, they appear to have a markedly lower mortality rate from **heart disease**. Medical experts generally agree that a low-fat **diet**, exercise, and not smoking minimize the risk of heart attacks, which makes this paradox difficult to understand. Studies suggest that one of the reasons the French have a lower rate of heart disease may be their regular consumption of red wine.

The specific mechanism by which the French paradox operates has not yet been identified. Some research suggests that **antioxidants** called flavonoids, natural chemical compounds found in red wine, may confer important health benefits to the heart and blood vessels. Red grapes are one of the richest sources of flavonoids, which may make red wine more heart-healthy than white wine, beer, or other spirits. Other research suggests that pigments in red wine called polyphenols are responsible for explaining the French paradox. Polyphenols, found in red grape skins, are believed to act as antioxidants, control **blood pressure**, and reduce blood clots. Some research indicates that red grape juice is markedly less potent than wine in conferring health benefits. Researchers suggest that something in the wine-making process changes the polyphenols' properties.

Not all scientists believe in the French paradox. Some believe that it is a health myth caused by errors in health-data reporting on the **incidence** of heart disease in France. Also, some scientists argue that there is no scientific consensus over the protective effect of any alcoholic beverage on heart disease.

Dr. Serge Renaud, a scientist from Bordeaux University in France, coined the term *French paradox* after completing his 1992 landmark report that indicated France's low incidence of heart disease might be caused by wine consumption. SEE ALSO GREEKS AND MIDDLE EASTERNERS, DIET OF; HEART DISEASE; NORTHERN EUROPEANS, DIET OF.

Karen Bryla

Bibliography

Hackman, Robert M. (1998, September). "Flavonoids and the French Paradox." *USA Today*, v. 127, no. 2640, 58–59.

Internet Resources

MSNBC News. "Study May Explain French Paradox." Available from <http://www.msnbc.com/news>

Functional Foods

functional food: food whose health benefits are claimed to be higher than those traditionally assumed for similar types of foods

nutrition: the maintenance of health through proper eating, or the study of same

fiber: indigestible plant material that aids digestion by providing bulk

calcium: mineral essential for bones and teeth

Functional foods are foods that provide health benefits beyond basic **nutrition** due to certain physiologically active components, which may or may not have been manipulated or modified to enhance their bioactivity. These foods may help prevent disease, reduce the risk of developing disease, or enhance health. Consumer interest in functional foods increased during the late twentieth century as people's interest in achieving and maintaining good health increased. Health-conscious consumers have become aware of the health benefits associated with specific foods and are incorporating elements such as **fiber, calcium,** and soy into their diets. Rapid advances in food science and technology, an aging population, the rapid rise in health care costs,

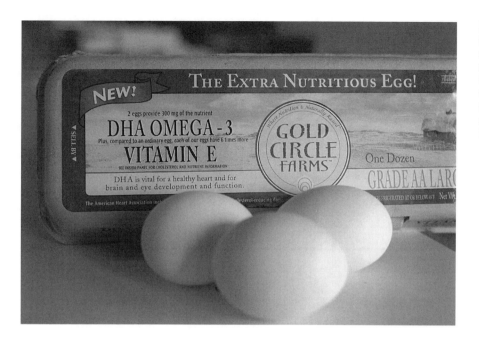

By feeding their hens a modified diet, some farms have increased the amount of omega-3 in the eggs they sell. These eggs are considered to be functional food because their higher omega-3 content can improve the health of consumers whose diets are deficient in that fatty acid. *[Photograph by Eric Risberg. AP/Wide World Photos. Reproduced by permission.]*

and changing government marketing and labeling regulations have also had an impact on the functional foods market.

There is a difference between the Western and Eastern perspective on functional foods. In the West, functional foods are considered revolutionary and represent a rapidly growing segment of the food industry. Food and pharmaceutical companies alike are competing to bring functional foods into the mass market. On the other hand, functional foods have been a part of Eastern cultures for centuries. Foods were used for medicinal purposes in traditional Chinese medicine as early as 1000 B.C.E. From ancient times, the Chinese have used foods for both preventive and therapeutic health effects, a view that is now being increasingly recognized around the world.

Clearly, most foods are functional in some way. What makes a "functional food," however, is its potential ability to positively affect health. Functional foods range from fruits, vegetables, and whole grains, which are naturally high in **phytochemicals**, to products in which a specific ingredient is added, removed, increased, or decreased. Examples of functional foods include soy, oats, flaxseed, grape juice, broccoli and other cruciferous vegetables, phytosterol/stanol-enriched margarine, eggs enhanced with omega-3 **fatty acids**, foods **fortified** with **herbal** preparations, and **psyllium**.

Regulations Related to Functional Foods

Functional foods are regulated by the United States Food and Drug Administration (FDA) under the authority of two laws. The Federal Food, Drug, and Cosmetic Act (FD&C) of 1938 provides for the regulation of all foods and **food additives**. The Dietary Supplement Health and Education Act (DSHEA) of 1994 amended the FD&C Act to cover dietary supplements and ingredients of dietary supplements. Functional foods may be categorized as whole foods, enriched foods, fortified foods, or enhanced foods. Labeling claims that are used on functional foods are of two types: (1) Structure and function claims, which describe effects on normal functioning of the body, but not claims that the food can treat, diagnose, prevent, or cure a disease

phytochemical: chemical produced by plants

fatty acids: molecules rich in carbon and hydrogen; a component of fats

fortified: altered by addition of vitamins or minerals

herbal: related to plants

psyllium: bulk-forming laxative derived from the Plantago psyllium seeds

food additive: substance added to foods to improve nutrition, taste, appearance, or shelf-life

cardiovascular: related to the heart and circulatory system

immune system: the set of organs and cells, including white blood cells, that protect the body from infection

(claims such as "promotes regularity," "helps maintain **cardiovascular** health," and "supports the **immune system**" fit into this category); and (2) Disease-risk reduction claims, which imply a relationship between dietary components and a disease or health condition.

Structure and function claims do not require preapproval by the FDA, and they require much less stringent scientific consensus than disease-risk reduction claims. Under the FD&C Act, structure and function claims cannot be false or misleading. However, the law does not define the nature or extent of evidence necessary to support these claims. To complicate matters, the evidence available to support structure and function claims varies widely

TYPES OF FUNCTIONAL FOODS

Functional food	Potential health benefit	Labeling claim
Whole foods		
Oats	Reduces cholesterol and constipation, reduces risk of heart disease	May reduce the risk of heart disease
Soy	Reduces cholesterol, reduces risk of osteoporosis, certain cancers, and heart disease	May reduce the risk of heart disease
Fruits and vegetables	Reduces risk of certain cancers and heart disease; reduces hypertension	May reduce the risk of some cancers; May reduce the risk of heart disease
Fish	Reduces cholesterol and triglycerides	None
Garlic	Reduces risk of heart disease and certain cancers, reduces cholesterol	None
Grapes/grape juice	Reduces risk of heart disease	Structure/function claim
Flaxseed	Reduces risk of heart disease and certain cancers; reduces triglycerides; increases blood-glucose control	None
Nuts	Reduces risk of heart disease	None
Enriched foods		
Grains	Reduces risk of certain cancers, heart disease, and nutrient deficiencies	May reduce the risk of some cancers; May reduce the risk of heart disease
Fortified foods		
Juices with calcium	Reduces risk of osteoporosis, reduces hypertension	Helps maintain healthy bones and may reduce risk of osteoporosis
Grains with folic acid	Reduces risk of heart disease and neural tube birth defects	May reduce risk of brain and spinal cord birth defects
Infant formulas with iron	Reduces risk of iron deficiency	None
Grains with added fiber	Reduces risk of certain cancers and heart disease; reduces cholesterol and constipation; increases blood-glucose control	May reduce the risk of some cancers; May reduce the risk of heart disease
Milk with vitamin D	Reduces risk of osteomalacia and osteoporosis	Helps maintain healthy bones and may reduce risk of osteoporosis
Juices with added fiber	Reduces risk of certain cancers and heart disease; reduces cholesterol, hypertension, and constipation	May reduce risk of some cancers
Enhanced foods		
Dairy products with probiotics	Reduces risk of colon cancer and candidal vaginitis; controls inflammation; treatment of respiratory allergies, diarrheal disorders, and eczema	Structure/function claim
Beverages and salad dressings with antioxidants	May support overall health	Structure/function claim
Foods and beverages containing herbal preparations	Varies with ingredients	Structure/function claim
Sports bars	Varies with ingredients	Structure/function claim
Spreads with stanol esters	Reduces cholesterol	Structure/function claim
Foods containing sugar alcohols in place of sugar	Reduces risk of tooth decay	May reduce risk of tooth decay
Eggs with omega-3 fatty acids	Reduces risk of heart disease	Structure/function claim

because some ingredients have been studied extensively, some have not been studied very much, and some ingredients are backed by mixed results.

Disease-risk reduction claims, typically called *health claims*, do require FDA approval before they can be used on products and must reflect scientific consensus. For example, the health claim for soy **protein** and its relation to cardiovascular disease reads: "Diets low in **saturated fat** and **cholesterol** that include 25 grams of soy protein a day may reduce the risk of **heart disease**. One serving of (name of food) provides _____ grams of soy protein." This claim may appear only on soy products that provide at least 6.25 grams of soy protein per serving. Other FDA-approved health claims include those related to fruits and vegetables and a reduced risk of **cancer**; saturated fat and an increased risk of heart disease; sodium and increased risk for **hypertension**, and folic acid–fortified foods and reduced risk of **neural** tube defects.

Many developed functional foods seem to have benefits for human health. For example, calcium-fortified orange juice provides approximately the same amount of calcium as milk. With more than half of all children under the age of five and nearly 85 percent of females age twelve to nineteen not meeting the Dietary Reference Intake (DRI) for calcium, calcium-fortified orange juice may contribute significantly to calcium intake. On the other hand, a positive impact on health is more difficult to establish for other developed functional foods. These include prepared foods spiked with herbal preparations, which may contain little of the herbal ingredients listed on the label, or insufficient quantities of these ingredients to produce the claimed effect. Additionally, some herbal ingredients can be harmful, such as kava, which has been associated with liver damage, and belladonna, which is toxic.

The Future

The future of functional foods will undoubtedly involve a continuation of the labeling and safety debates. As consumers become more health conscious, the demand and market value for health-promoting foods and food components is expected to grow. Before the full market potential can be realized, however, consumers need to be assured of the safety and **efficacy** of functional foods. Future research will focus on mechanisms by which food components such as phytochemicals positively affect health, and whether these components work independently or synergistically. According to the American Dietetic Association, dietetics professionals will be increasingly called upon to develop preventive meal plans, to recommend changes in food intake, to enhance phytochemical and functional food intake, and to evaluate the appropriateness of functional foods and dietary supplements to meet preventive (and therapeutic) intake levels for both healthy persons and those diagnosed with disease. SEE ALSO ANTIOXIDANTS; PHYTOCHEMICALS.

M. Elizabeth Kunkel
Barbara H. D. Luccia

protein: complex molecule composed of amino acids that performs vital functions in the cell; necessary part of the diet

saturated fat: a fat with the maximum possible number of hydrogens; more difficult to break down than unsaturated fats

cholesterol: multi-ringed molecule found in animal cell membranes; a type of lipid

heart disease: any disorder of the heart or its blood supply, including heart attack, atherosclerosis, and coronary artery disease

cancer: uncontrolled cell growth

hypertension: high blood pressure

neural: related to the nervous system

efficacy: effectiveness

Bibliography

American Dietetic Association (1999). "Functional Foods—Position of the ADA." *Journal of the American Dietetic Association* 99:1278–1285. Also available from <http://www.eatright.org>

Mazza, G., ed. (1998). *Functional Foods: Biochemical and Processing Aspects.* Lancaster, PA: Technomic Publishing.

Wildman, Robert E. C., ed. (2001). *Handbook of Nutraceuticals and Functional Foods.* Boca Raton, FL: CRC Press.

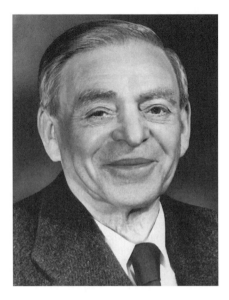

Dr. Casimir Funk, who discovered that substances in food could prevent or cure certain diseases. He called those substances "vitamines." *[AP/Wide World Photos. Reproduced by permission.]*

vitamin: necessary complex nutrient used to aid enzymes or other metabolic processes in the cell

scurvy: a syndrome characterized by weakness, anemia, and spongy gums, due to vitamin C deficiency

niacin: one of the B vitamins, required for energy production in the cell

rickets: disorder caused by vitamin D deficiency, marked by soft and misshapen bones and organ swelling

vitamin D: nutrient needed for calcium uptake and therefore proper bone formation

amine: compound containing nitrogen linked to hydrogen

hormone: molecules produced by one set of cells that influence the function of another set of cells

pituitary gland: gland at the base of the brain that regulates multiple body processes

cancer: uncontrolled cell growth

diabetes: inability to regulate level of sugar in the blood

ulcer: erosion in the lining of the stomach or intestine due to bacterial infection

drugs: substances whose administration causes a significant change in the body's function

Funk, Casimir

American biochemist
1884–1967

Casimir Funk was born in Warsaw, Poland. The son of a dermatologist, Funk earned a doctorate degree at the University of Bern, Switzerland, at the young age of twenty. He then worked at the Pasteur Institute in Paris, the Wiesbaden Municipal Hospital in Germany, the University of Berlin, and the Lister Institute in London.

Funk emigrated to the United States in 1915 and held several industrial and university positions in New York. He became a naturalized U.S. citizen in 1920. With funding provided by the Rockefeller Foundation, Funk returned to Warsaw in 1923 to serve as the director of the Biochemistry Department of the State Institute of Hygiene. Funk moved to Paris in 1927 and became a consultant to a pharmaceutical company and founded Casa Biochemica, a privately funded research institution.

At the outbreak of World War II in 1939, Funk returned to the United States to work as a consultant for the United States Vitamin Corporation. He became the president of the Funk Foundation for Medical Research in 1940.

Funk's work with what are now called **vitamins** began when he recognized that certain food factors were needed to prevent nutritional-deficiency diseases, such as beriberi (vitamin B_1 deficiency), **scurvy** (vitamin C deficiency), pellagra (**niacin** deficiency), and **rickets** (**vitamin D** deficiency). He suggested that these unidentified substances were all in a class of organic compounds called **amines**, which are vital to life, so he named them vitamines (vital amines). Although they turned out not to be amines, Funk's proposal (and the coining of the term *vitamine*) has been called a stroke of genius. He later confirmed the existence of vitamins B_1, B_2, C, and D, and he stated that they were necessary for normal health and the prevention of deficiency diseases.

In his work to find the specific factor that prevented beriberi, Funk eventually isolated nicotinic acid (niacin, or vitamin B_1) from rice. Although it did not cure beriberi, scientists later discovered that it cured pellagra. Funk also worked with the B-vitamin thiamine, determining its molecular structure and developing a method for synthesizing it.

In his later research, Funk studied animal **hormones** and contributed to the knowledge about hormones of the **pituitary** and sex glands, emphasizing the importance of balance between hormones and vitamins. Funk also investigated the biochemistry of **cancer**, **diabetes**, and **ulcers**. He improved manufacturing methods for many commercial **drugs** and developed several new commercial products in his laboratories. He died in Albany, New York, on November 20, 1967. SEE ALSO BERIBERI; PELLAGRA; VITAMINS, FAT SOLUBLE; VITAMINS, WATER-SOLUBLE.

Karen Bryla

Bibliography

Abbott, David (1984). *The Biographical Dictionary of Scientists: Chemists.* New York: P. Bedrick.

Jukes, T. H. (1989). "Historical Perspectives: The Prevention and Conquest of Scurvy, Beri-Beri, and Pellagra." *Preventive Medicine* 18:877–883.

Koppman, Lionel (1986). *Guess Who's Jewish in American History.* New York: Steimatzky.

Internet Resource

"Casimir Funk." Available from <http://www.encyclopedia.com>

Generally Recognized as Safe (GRAS)

G

In 1959, the U.S. Food and Drug Administration (FDA) established a list of seven hundred food substances that were exempt from the then new requirement that manufacturers test **food additives** before putting them on the market. The Generally Recognized as Safe, or GRAS, list acknowledged that many additives had existing scientific evidence of long and safe use in food. Among the additives on the list are sugar, salt, spices, and **vitamins**. Manufacturers can petition for GRAS status for new additives if the substances meet the criteria cited above. GRAS list additives are continually reevaluated based on current scientific evidence. SEE ALSO ARTIFICIAL SWEETENERS; BIOTECHNOLOGY; FOOD SAFETY; FUNCTIONAL FOODS.

Susan T. Borra

food additive: substance added to foods to improve nutrition, taste, appearance, or shelf-life

vitamin: necessary complex nutrient used to aid enzymes or other metabolic processes in the cell

Genetically Modified Foods

Genetic modification employs recombinant **deoxyribonucleic acid** (rDNA) technology to alter the **genes** of **microorganisms**, plants, and animals. Genetic modification is also called biotechnology, gene splicing, recombinant DNA technology, or genetic engineering. Contemporary genetic modification was developed in the 1970s and essentially transfers genetic material from one organism to another. The modification of organisms has existed for centuries in the form of plant-breeding techniques (such as cross-fertilization) used to produce desired traits. With genetic modification, however, isolated genes are inserted into plants for a desired trait with a much quicker result than occurs when cross-breeding plants, which can take years. These isolated genes do not have to come from similar species in order to be functional; theoretically, genes can be transferred among all microorganisms, plants, and animals.

genetic: inherited or related to the genes

deoxyribonucleic acid: DNA, the molecule that makes up genes

gene: DNA sequence that codes for proteins, and thus controls inheritance

microorganisms: bacteria and protists; single-celled organisms

Examples of Genetically Modified Foods

Crops may be modified to increase resistance to pests and disease, increase adaptability to environmental conditions, improve flavor or nutritional profile, delay ripening, or increase shelf life. Many common crops are genetically modified, such as corn, canola, flax, potatoes, tomatoes, squash, and soybeans. Corn and potatoes may be modified with a gene to produce an **endotoxin** that protects them against the corn-borer pest and the potato beetle, respectively. A soybean can be genetically modified with a gene from a bacterium to make it herbicide resistant. By inserting two genes from daffodil and one gene from a bacterium, rice can be enriched with beta-carotene.

endotoxin: toxic substance produced and stored within the plant tissue

In the early 1990s, genetically modified tomatoes (Flavr Savr by Calgene, Inc.) were deemed safe by the U.S., Canadian, and British governments and introduced into the market. These tomatoes were bred to stay firm after

245

harvest so they could remain on the vine longer and ripen to full flavor. However, the tomatoes were so delicate that they were difficult to transport without damage, and the product was pulled from the market in 1997.

Recombinant bovine growth hormone (rBGH), also known as recombinant bovine somatotropin (rBST), is another example of a product that has not been very successful. Recombinant BGH (Posilac by Monsanto Company) is a genetically engineered version of a growth hormone that increases milk output in dairy cows by as much as 10 to 30 percent. In 1999 the United Nations Food Safety Agency unanimously declared the use of rBGH unsafe after confirming reports of excess levels of the naturally occurring insulin-like growth factor one (IGF-1), including its highly potent variants, in rBGH milk and concluding that these posed major risks of **cancer**. Health Canada also banned the use of rBGH in milk production in 1999, but the hormone is still permitted in the U.S. milk supply.

Safety of Genetically Modified Foods

Biotechnology has moved at such a rapid pace that the safety of genetically modified foods has become a concern. At this time, there are no long-term, large-scale tests to prove their safety—or lack thereof. Unforeseen consequences may arise from widespread genetic modification of the food supply, including:

- *Allergic reaction*. If a gene producing a **protein** that causes an allergic reaction is engineered into corn, for example, an individual who is allergic to that protein may experience an allergic reaction to the corn. Despite the fact that food-regulating agencies require companies to report whether altered food contains any suspect proteins, unknown allergens could potentially slip through the system.

- *Increased toxicity*. Genetic modification may enhance natural plant **toxins** in unexpected ways. When a gene is switched on, besides having the desired effect, it may also stimulate the production of natural toxins.

- *Resistance to **antibiotics***. As part of the genetic modification of organisms, marker genes are used to determine if the desired gene has been successfully embedded. Marker genes typically provide resistance to antibiotics. Even though marker genes are genetically scrambled before use to reduce the potential for this danger, their use could contribute to the growing problem of antibiotic resistance.

- *Herbicide-resistant weeds*. Once modified crops are planted, genes may travel via airborne, waterborne, or animal-borne seeds and pollen to weedy relatives, creating "superweeds" that are able to resist herbicides.

- *Harm to other organisms*. Nontargeted species may inadvertently be harmed by a genetically modified plant producing endotoxins intended for a specific pest. For example, nearly all insect-resistant plants contain a gene from the bacterium *Baciullus thuringiensis* (Bt), which results in the production of a natural endotoxin that is toxic to all insects. The Bt endotoxin is widely used by organic and conventional farmers because it is a relatively harmless, natural pesticide. However, genetically modified plants such as Bt corn, cotton, potatoes, rice, and tomatoes constantly produce the Bt endotoxin, and thus speed up the spread of Bt resistance among pests that feed on these

cancer: uncontrolled cell growth

allergic reaction: immune system reaction against a substance that is otherwise harmless

protein: complex molecule composed of amino acids that performs vital functions in the cell; necessary part of the diet

toxins: poisons

antibiotic: substance that kills or prevents the growth of microorganisms

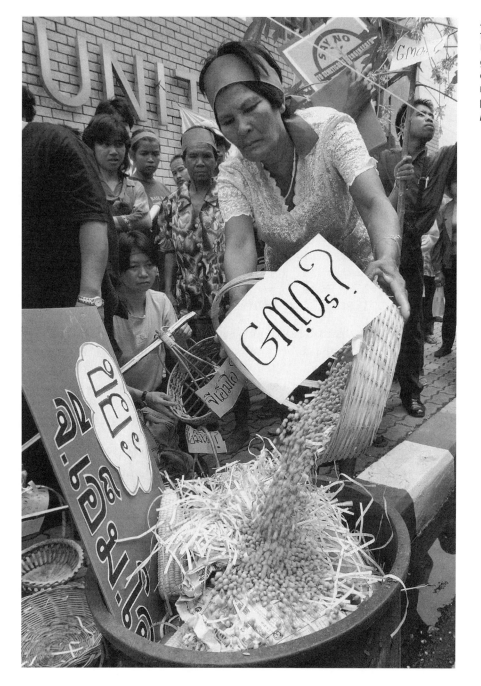

A protest of genetically modified foods in front of the regional headquarters of the United Nations in Thailand. Critics of genetically modified foods cite concern over the possibility that modified foods might have unexpected and dangerous properties. *[© AFP/Corbis. Reproduced by permission.]*

plants. They may also reduce insect diversity and population numbers among harmless and beneficial insects.

- *Pesticide-resistant insects and the demise of safe pesticides.* Most of the common genetically modified crops contain a gene that produces a protein which is toxic to a specific pest. However, exposing pests to toxins may stimulate resistance by the pests and render the pesticides useless.

Typically, when a new crop is created, whether by traditional methods or genetic modification, breeders conduct field testing for several seasons to make sure only desirable changes occur. Appearance, growth characteristics, and taste of the food are checked, and analytical tests to determine changes in **nutrients** and safety are performed. According to the U.S. Department

nutrient: dietary substance necessary for health

247

of Agriculture, there is no evidence that any genetically modified foods now on the market pose any human health concerns or are in any way less safe than crops produced through traditional breeding. In 2002, however, the European Union updated and strengthened existing regulations and labeling laws for genetically modified foods in the European markets.

The Food and Agriculture Organization (FAO) of the United Nations recognizes that genetic engineering has the potential to help increase productivity in agriculture, forestry, and fisheries. However, the FAO urges caution to reduce the risks associated with transferring toxins from one organism to another, of creating new toxins, or of transferring allergenic compounds from one organism to another. The FAO acknowledges potential risks to the environment, including outcrossing (crossing unrelated organisms), which could lead to the evolution of more aggressive weeds, pests with increased resistance to diseases, or environmental stresses that upset the ecosystem balance.

Labeling of Genetically Modified Foods

According to the Institute of Food Technologists, genetically modified foods should not be labeled because "labels are likely to mislead consumers by implying a warning.... Moreover, labeling rDNA-engineered foods would not be economically prudent." In the European Union, concern about the safety of genetically modified organisms, fanned by years of political activism, has resulted in regulations that keep many genetically modified foods out of the European market. These regulations include requirements for tracing the genetic origin of each food ingredient, and for labeling the resulting products accordingly. Fueled by consumer protest and demand, lawmakers in China and Canada have recently begun discussing stricter labeling laws as well.

Conclusion

Genetic modification of foods is an area of biotechnology that is developing very rapidly, with many potential applications for improving the quantity and quality of the food supply. As with any new food technology, however, the safety of the products derived from this technology must be carefully assessed. Consumer concerns will likely continue to fuel the debate. SEE ALSO BIOTECHNOLOGY; FOOD SAFETY; FUNCTIONAL FOODS; PESTICIDES.

M. Elizabeth Kunkel
Barbara H. D. Luccia

Bibliography

Institute of Food Technologists (2000). "Genetically Modified Organisms: A Backgrounder." *Food Technology* 54:42–45.

International Food Information Council (2000). *Food Biotechnology: A Communications Guide to Improving Understanding.* Washington, DC: Author.

Internet Resources

Food and Agriculture Organization of the United Nations (2000). "FAO Statement on Biotechnology." Available from <http://www.fao.org/biotech>

United States Department of Agriculture (2002). "Agricultural Biotechnology." Available from <http://www.usda.gov/agencies>

World Health Organization (2002). "Foods Derived from Modern Biotechnology." Available from <http://www.who.int>

The Acceptance of Genetically Modified Foods

In the United States, only limited objections have been raised to genetically modified foods, which can be more nutritious, disease-resistant, flavorful, or cheaper than natural foods. In Europe, by contrast, consumers and governments have focused on the potential dangers of genetic modification, which include unforeseen resistance to antibiotics and herbicides, the spread of dangerous allergens, and damage to livestock, public health, and the environment. Health disasters such as the mad cow outbreak have left many European consumers with a distrust of corporations and regulatory bodies and a determination to understand where their food comes from. While some genetically modified crops are allowed in Europe, the European Union has instituted strict regulatory requirements for labeling and traceability and has effectively placed a moratorium on approving new crops. These regulations have caused friction with the U.S. government by limiting the import of U.S. agricultural products, many of which are genetically modified and none of which are required to carry labeling. The American Farm Bureau Federation estimates that U.S. corn producers alone would be able to export $300 billion more corn if the ban were lifted.

—*Paula Kepos*

Glisson, Francis

English scholar, physician, and scientist
1597–1677

Francis Glisson was born in Rampisham, England, and attended Cambridge University, with which he had a long relationship. During his life he acted as a dean, senior fellow, and professor at the university. He also had a private medical practice.

The Royal College of Physicians of London admitted Glisson as a candidate in 1634, the same year he received his medical degree from Cambridge. Within the Royal College he played the roles of fellow, councilor, and president. He also belonged to the "Invisible College," a small group of professionals who met weekly in 1645 to promote investigation into natural and experimental philosophy. Later it became the Royal Society. Around that same time, a group of fellows of the Royal College began to exchange notes on **rickets**, intending to publish a book on the topic. Glisson was assigned to investigate the basic nature of rickets. His investigation skills proved to be strong, and he impressed his coworkers so much that they gave him the responsibility of drafting the entire book, with the assistance of seven contributors.

Tractatus de rachitid, sive morbo puerili (A Treatise of the Rickets), was published in 1650. It is not clear if any of the anatomical and clinical descriptions of rickets were solely Glisson's work. He claimed responsibility for sole authorship for chapters three through fourteen, where he wrote clearly about the nature of the disease. In March of 1660, Glisson became an early member of the Royal Society. In his second book, *Anatomia hepatis (Anatomy of the Liver)*, Glisson identified and described the outer capsule of connective tissue that surrounds the liver and its blood supply (now called Glisson's Capsule). In his third book, *Tractatus de ventriculo et intestini (A Treatise of the Stomach and Intestines)*, Glisson coined the term *irritability*, referring to the body's ability to sense an irritant and try to rid itself of it.

Though primarily known for his pioneering work on rickets, Francis Glisson contributed to the body of knowledge in general anatomy and **physiology** of the digestive organs. In the opening paragraph of *A Treatise of the Rickets*, he wrote that infantile rickets was "an entirely new disease, that was never described by any of the ancient or modern writers." He was able to show that infantile **scurvy** was a separate disease from rickets, although the two usually occur together. SEE ALSO NUTRITIONAL DEFICIENCY; RICKETS.

Slande Celeste

Internet Resource

Vanderbilt University Medical Center. "Rickets and Vitamin D." Available from <http://www.mc.vanderbilt.edu>

Francis Glisson was a major contributor to an early pediatric text titled *A Treatise of the Rickets*. His work accurately described both rickets and infantile scurvy, but did not recognize the dietary causes of the diseases. [Science Photo Library/Photo Researchers, Inc. Reproduced by permission.]

rickets: disorder caused by vitamin D deficiency, marked by soft and misshapen bones and organ swelling

physiology: the group of biochemical and physical processes that combine to make a functioning organism, or the study of same

scurvy: a syndrome characterized by weakness, anemia, and spongy gums, due to vitamin C deficiency

Global Database on National Nutrition Policies and Programmes

Hunger and **malnutrition** occur throughout the world, though the knowledge and resources exist to eliminate them. The challenge lies in changing

malnutrition: chronic lack of sufficient nutrients to maintain health

political will, developing realistic policies, and taking determined actions both nationally and internationally. These are the basic beliefs of the Global Database on National Nutrition Policies and Programmes (GDNNPP). GDNNPP was created by the World Health Organization (WHO) in 1995 to monitor and evaluate the progress of implementation of the 1992 World Declaration and Plan of Action for Nutrition, which states that all people should have access to safe and nutritious food and be free from hunger.

GDNNPP plays a large role in improving nutrition status globally by compiling data from six regions of the world: Africa, the Americas (in conjunction with the Pan-American Health Organization), the Eastern Mediterranean, Europe, South-East Asia, and the Western Pacific. Policies and programs vary from country to country according to population needs.

GDNNPP provides a global review and comparative analysis of national nutrition policies and plans of action. It identifies the priority nutrition issues of various countries, as well as key elements for developing and implementing effective and sustainable nutrition policies and programs. It also evaluates each country's progress in developing, strengthening, and implementing national nutrition policies and programs, and it serves as a guide to creating better national nutrition policies and programs through authoritative standards and guidelines, research, and collaboration. GDNNPP is designed to help enforce the health objectives, strategies, and activities of the WHO, which also provides technical and financial support to participating WHO countries.

Delores C. S. James

Internet Resources

Pan American Health Organization. "Nutrition and Food Protection: Current Health Topics." Available from <http://www.paho.org>

World Health Organization. "Global Database on National Nutrition Policies and Programmes." Available from <http://www.who.int/nut_pol.htm>

Glycemic Index

carbohydrate: food molecule made of carbon, hydrogen, and oxygen, including sugars and starches

diabetes: inability to regulate level of sugar in the blood

glucose: a simple sugar; the most commonly used fuel in cells

The glycemic index (GI) is a ranking of **carbohydrate** foods individuals with **diabetes** use to manage their disease. This ranking is based on the rate carbohydrates affect blood **glucose** levels relative to glucose or white bread. Generally, the glycemic index is calculated by measuring blood glucose levels following the ingestion of a carbohydrate. This blood glucose value is compared to the blood glucose value acquired following an equal carbohydrate dose of glucose or white bread. Glucose is absorbed into the bloodstream faster than any other carbohydrate, and is thus given the value of 100. Other carbohydrates are given a number relative to glucose. Foods with low GI indices are released into the bloodstream at a slower rate than high GI foods.

absorption: uptake by the digestive tract

A number of factors influence the digestion and **absorption** rate of food, including ripeness, particle size, the nature of the starch, the degree of processing and preparation, the commercial brand, and the characteristics of the diabetic patient, and these factors naturally affect each food's glycemic index position or rank. In addition, differences exist in the glycemic indeces of foods due to the choice of reference food, the timing of blood sampling, or the computational method used to calculate the glycemic index.

GLYCEMIC INDEX OF COMMON FOODS

Food item	GI (Glucose = 100)	GI (Bread = 100)	Serving size (grams or milliliters)
Beverages			
Coca Cola, soft drink (Atlanta, GA, USA)	63	90	250 ml
Apple juice, unsweetened	40	57	250 ml
Orange juice (mean of Canada, Australia, & USA)	52	74	250 ml
Breads			
Bagel, white, frozen (Lender's Bakery, Montreal Canada)	72	103	70 g
Wonder, enriched white bread	73	105	30 g
Healthy Choice Hearty 7 Grain Wheat bread (Con Agra Inc., USA)	55	79	30 g
Dairy Products and Alternatives			
Ice cream, regular flavor, not specified (mean of Canada, Italy, & USA)	61	87	50 g
Milk, full-fat (mean of Italy, Sweden, USA, Australia, and Canada)	27	38	250 g
Milk, skim (Canada)	32	46	250 g
Fruit and Fruit Products			
Apples, raw (mean of Denmark, New Zealand, Canada, USA, and Italy)	38	52	120 g
Banana, raw (mean of Canada, USA, Italy, Denmark, and South Africa)	52	74	120 g
Grapefruit, raw (Canada)	25	36	120 g
Pasta and Noodles			
Macaroni and cheese, boxed (Kraft General Foods Canada, Inc., Don Mills, Canada)	64	92	180 g
Spaghetti, white or type not specified, boiled 10-15 min (mean of Italy, Sweden, and Canada)	44	64	180 g
Ravioli, durum wheat flour, meat-filled, boiled (Australia)	39	56	180 g
Vegetables			
Green peas, frozen, boiled (mean of Canada and India)	48	68	80 g
Carrots, not specified (Canada)	92	131	80 g
Baked potato, without fat (mean of Canada and USA)	85	121	150 g

SOURCE: Adapted from Foster-Powell et al.

The objectives of **diet** management in diabetic patients are to reduce **hyperglycemia**, prevent **hypoglycemic** episodes, and reduce the risk of complications. For people with diabetes, the glycemic index is a useful tool in planning meals to achieve and maintain glycemic control. Foods with a low glycemic index release sugar gradually into the bloodstream, producing minimal fluctuations in blood glucose. High GI foods, however, are absorbed quickly into the bloodstream causing an escalation in blood glucose levels and increasing the possibility of hyperglycemia. The body compensates for the rise in blood sugar levels with an accompanying increase in **insulin**, which within a few hours can cause hypoglycemia. As a result, awareness of the glycemic indices of food assists in preventing large variances in blood glucose levels.

Experts disagree regarding the use of the glycemic index in athletes' diets and in exercise performance. Insufficient evidence exists supporting the benefit of low glycemic meals prior to prolonged exercise. Nonetheless,

diet: the total daily food intake, or the types of foods eaten

hyperglycemia: high level of sugar in the blood

hypoglycemic: related to low level of blood sugar

insulin: hormone released by the pancreas to regulate level of sugar in the blood

glycogen: storage form of sugar

a low GI pre-event meal may be beneficial for athletes who respond negatively to carbohydrate-rich foods prior to exercise or who cannot consume carbohydrates during competition. Athletes are advised to consume carbohydrates of moderate to high GI during prolonged exercise to maximize performance, approximately 1 gram per minute of exercise. Following exercise, moderate to high GI foods enhance **glycogen** storage. SEE ALSO CARBOHYDRATES; DIABETES MELLITUS; EXCHANGE SYSTEM.

Julie Lager

Bibliography

Burke, Louise M.; Collier, Gregory R.; and Hargreaves, Mark (1998). "Glycemic Index—A New Tool in Sport Nutrition?" *International Journal of Sport Nutrition* 8:401–415.

Foster-Powell, Kaye; Holt, Susanna H. A.; and Brand-Miller, Janette C. (2002). "International Table of Glycemic Index and Glycemic Load Value." *American Journal of Clinical Nutrition* 76:5–56.

Gretebeck, Randall J.; Gretebeck, Kimberlee A.; and Tittelbach, Thomas J. (2002). "Glycemic Index of Popular Sport Drinks and Energy Foods." *Journal of the American Dietetic Association* 102(3):415–416.

Ludwig, David S. (2002). "The Glycemic Index: Physiological Mechanisms Relating to Obesity, Diabetes, and Cardiovascular Disease." *Journal of the American Medical Association* 287(18):2414–2423.

Willette, Walter; Manson, JoAnn; and Liu, Simin (2002). "Glycemic Index, Glycemic Load, and Risk of Type 2 Diabetes." *American Journal of Clinical Nutrition* 76 (suppl.):274S–281S.

Wolever, Thomas; Jenkins, David J. A.; Jenkins, Alexandra L.; and Josse, Robert G. (1991). "The Glycemic Index: Methodology and Clinical Importance." *American Journal of Clinical Nutrition* 54:846–854.

Internet Resources

National Institute of Diabetes and Digestive and Kidney Diseases. "Diabetes." Available from <http://www.niddk.nih.gov>

National Library of Medicine. "Diabetes." Available from <http://medlineplus.gov>

diet: the total daily food intake, or the types of foods eaten

hormone: molecules produced by one set of cells that influence the function of another set of cells

metabolism: the sum total of reactions in a cell or an organism

stillbirth: giving birth to a dead fetus

miscarriage: loss of a pregnancy

cretinism: arrested mental and physical development

fortified: altered by addition of vitamins or minerals

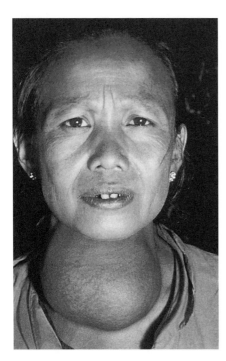

An example of grade III (large and visible) goiter. Most cases of goiter in the developing world are due to an iodine deficiency. Unable to meet the body's hormonal needs, the thyroid becomes enlarged to compensate. [© Lester V. Bergman/Corbis. Reproduced by permission.]

Goiter

A goiter is a noncancerous enlargement of the thyroid gland in the front of the neck. Many conditions can cause goiter, but the most common is a lack of sufficient iodine in the **diet**, which is usually a result of the soil in which food is grown being iodine-poor—a condition that occurs in many mountainous regions away from the sea. Iodine is required for the production of thyroid **hormones**, which regulate the body's **metabolism**.

About 740 million people have goiters, but the percentage varies greatly by region (eastern Mediterranean: 32%; Africa: 20%: Europe: 15%; Southeast Asia: 12%; western Pacific: 8%; the Americas: 5%). Surveying communities for goiters is one of the best ways of detecting iodine deficiency, which, if not treated, can cause **stillbirths**, **miscarriages**, **cretinism**, mental impairments, deafness, and dwarfism.

Iodine deficiency is the most common preventable cause of brain damage and mental retardation, affecting about 50 million people worldwide. However, these disorders have been tremendously reduced simply by using table salt **fortified** with iodine.

Adults require at least 20 micrograms of iodine daily, but 150 micrograms is recommended. Seafoods are excellent sources, while the iodine content of other foods varies depending on animal feed and soil. Iodism (iodine poisoning) is a rare condition that results in weakness, swollen salivary glands, a metallic taste in the mouth, and a runny nose. SEE ALSO MINERALS.

Donna Staton
Marcus Harding

Bibliography

Food and Nutrition Board (2002). *Dietary Reference Intakes for Vitamin A, Vitamin K, Arsenic, Boron, Chromium, Copper, Iodine, Iron, Manganese, Molybdenum, Nickel, Silicon, Vanadium and Zinc.* Washington, DC: National Academy Press.

UNICEF (1998). *The State of the World's Children 1998.* Oxford: Oxford University Press.

Internet Resource

International Council for the Control of Iodine Deficiency Disorders. "About IDD." Available from <http://www.people.virginia.edu/~jtd/iccidd>

Goldberger, Joseph

American physician
1874–1929

Often considered a significant contributor to the field of **nutrition** science, Joseph Goldberger was born to a Jewish family in Girald, Austria-Hungary. When he was six years old, Goldberger and his family emigrated to the United States, settling on Manhattan's East Side.

Goldberger enrolled in City College in New York at the age of sixteen, determined to study engineering. At the end of his second year, Goldberger decided to switch to medicine after attending a lecture at Bellevue Hospital Medical College. In 1895, he obtained his medical degree from Bellevue and began private practice in a small Pennsylvania city. Bored after two years, Goldberger decided to take a competitive exam to enter the Marine Hospital Service, and he joined its ranks in 1899. The Marine Hospital Service, responsible for caring for sick merchant seamen and for fighting epidemics, was renamed the Public Health Service in 1902.

Goldberger married Mary Farrar in 1906. Because his marriage to a non-Jewish woman was unusual in his day, there were religious-based objections from both families.

During his time at the Public Health Service, Goldberger specialized in **preventive medicine**, **infectious diseases**, and nutrition. He fought tropical fevers, **typhus**, **typhoid**, and other infectious outbreaks throughout the United States and the Caribbean. In 1914, impressed with Goldberger's success, the Surgeon General of the United States appointed him to study the disease pellagra, which was becoming prevalent in the southern United States. Pellagra is characterized by skin rashes, mouth sores, diarrhea, and, if untreated, mental deterioration.

At the time, pellagra was thought to be an infectious disease. However, as Goldberger traveled throughout the South observing those with pellagra, he never contracted the disease. He noticed that poor people were more likely to get pellagra, and that their **diet** was restricted to cornbread, molasses, and

nutrition: the maintenance of health through proper eating, or the study of same

preventive medicine: treatment designed to prevent disease, rather than waiting for it to occur before intervening

infectious diseases: diseases caused by viruses, bacteria, fungi, or protozoa, which replicate inside the body

typhus: bacterial disease transmitted by infected rodents

typhoid: fever-causing bacterial infection due to Salmonella typhi; transmitted by contaminated food or water

diet: the total daily food intake, or the types of foods eaten

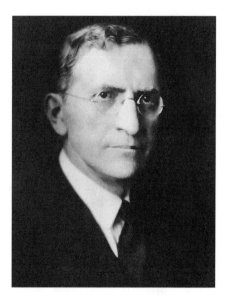

Joseph Goldberger. In 1914 the U.S. Surgeon General appointed Goldberger to fight pellagra, a disease that was sickening thousands of poor Southerners. Goldberger correctly theorized that the disease is caused by malnutrition.
[Bettman/Corbis. Reproduced by permission.]

a little pork fat. Institutions such as prisons, asylums, and orphanages also had higher levels of pellagra, and residents of these institutions also had limited diets. Based on this evidence, Goldberger concluded that pellagra had a dietary cause and was not infectious.

In 1915, Goldberger conducted a study with inmates at a Mississippi prison, who received a pardon in exchange for their participation. Inmates at this prison had a fairly balanced diet, and the volunteers were given the poor Southern diet that Goldberger associated with pellagra. Within months, the volunteers developed pellagra—and the pellagra symptoms disappeared when they were fed meat, fresh vegetables, and milk. Goldberger and his researchers also tried to catch the disease from infected inmates, but they were unsuccessful. This conclusive evidence proved Goldberger's theory that pellagra is caused by dietary factors and cannot be transmitted from one person to another.

Due to political and social circumstances, however, Goldberger had difficulty convincing others of this theory. In 1926, he reported that the lack of one of the **B vitamins** was responsible for pellagra, though he was unable to identify the specific vitamin.

Goldberger died of kidney **cancer** in 1929, at the age of fifty-four. In 1937, Conrad Elvehjem at the University of Wisconsin discovered that nicotinic acid, better known as **niacin** (vitamin B_3), prevented and healed pellagra. SEE ALSO PELLAGRA.

Karen Bryla

B vitamins: a group of vitamins important in cell energy processes

cancer: uncontrolled cell growth

niacin: one of the B vitamins, required for energy production in the cell

Bibliography

Akst, Daniel (2001). "Forgotten Plague." *American Heritage*, December/January, 72–79.

Koppman, Lionel (1986). *Guess Who's Jewish in American History.* New York: Steimatzky.

Internet Resources

National Institutes of Health, Museum of Medical Research. "Dr. Joseph Goldberger and the War on Pellagra." Available from <http://www.nih.gov/od/museum>

Science Odyssey. "People and Discoveries: Pellagra Shown to Be a Dietary Disease." Available from <http://www.pbs.9org/wgbh>

Vanderbilt University Medical Center, Eskind Biomedical Library Historical Collection. "Pellagra." Available from <http://www.mc.vanderbilt.edu>

Graham, Sylvester

American reformer
1794–1851

Sylvester Graham, a Presbyterian minister and reformer, is best known for his creation of the Graham cracker. He also put forth the idea that moderation is beneficial, and that certain foods and behaviors are detrimental to both physical and spiritual health. It is not enough to practice moderation in all things, he claimed, because some things are simply not good, either for spiritual or physical reasons, or both. These theories made Graham a central figure in the health reform movement of the 1800s.

Graham was born on July 5, 1794, in West Suffield, Connecticut. His father, the clergyman John Graham, was seventy-two years of age at the time of his birth. Within two years, his father was dead, and Graham was raised by various relatives.

Graham worked as a farm-hand, clerk, and teacher before preparing for the ministry. He married Sarah Earl in 1826. In 1830 he was made general agent for the Pennsylvania Temperance Society, and he began to study human **physiology**, **diet**, and regimen. He then launched himself on a lecture career that took him up and down the Atlantic Coast.

He advocated bread at least twelve hours old, made of the whole of the wheat, and coarsely ground. He also recommended hard mattresses, open bedroom windows, cold shower baths, loose and light clothing, daily exercise, vegetables and fruits, rough (whole-grain) cereals, pure drinking water, and cheerfulness at meals. He taught that temperance included both physical and moral reform.

In 1832, Graham edited Luigi Cornaro's *Discourse on a Sober and Temperate Life*. This discourse was translated into many languages and first published in the United States in 1788, after which it went through at least twelve editions. Cornaro wrote of three social evils: adulation and ceremony, heresy, and intemperance. Intemperance was, to Cornaro, the principal vice, and he wrote that a person should choose "to live in accordance with the simplicity of nature, to be satisfied with very little, to follow the ways of holy self-control and divine reason, and to accustom himself to eat nothing but that which is necessary to sustain life."

In 1837, Sylvester Graham wrote his *Treatise on Bread and Bread Making*, which advocated the use of Graham flour, made from coarsely ground whole-wheat kernels, and instructed wives to bake their own bread. Perhaps as a result of his impact on their business, which was reduced by the making of homemade bread, he was attacked by a mob of bakers. Meanwhile, Graham flour showed up in barrels and Graham boarding houses sprang up to minister to the new demands.

Graham influenced others to take up the cause of health reform. John Harvey Kellogg, while working as an apprentice typesetter, was exposed to a compilation of articles on health, including Graham's *Health, or How to Live*, a series of six pamphlets published by the Seventh-day Adventist Church, and he became intensely interested in Graham's dietetic and sanitary reforms. In his spare moments Kellogg read all of Graham's writings. Ralph Waldo Emerson made reference to Sylvester Graham as the "poet of bran and pumpkins." Graham died in 1851.

Louise E. Schneider

physiology: the group of biochemical and physical processes that combine to make a functioning organism, or the study of same

diet: the total daily food intake, or the types of foods eaten

Bibliography

Sabate, Joan (2001). *Vegetarian Nutrition*. Boca Raton, FL: CRC Press.

Schwartz, Richard W. (1970). *John Harvey Kellogg, MD*. Nashville, TN: Southern Publishing Association.

Shryock, Richard H. (1931). "Sylvester Graham and the Popular Health Movement, 1830–1870." *Mississippi Valley Historical Review* XVIII:172–183.

Whorton, James C. (1987). "Traditions of Folk Medicine." *Journal of the Medical Association* 257:1632–1640.

Grazing

The term grazing is used to describe the eating of small, frequent meals, or mini-meals, throughout the day, typically every three to four hours. Grazing does not mean constantly eating snack foods, but rather is a concept of

nutrient: dietary substance necessary for health

energy: technically, the ability to perform work; the content of a substance that allows it to be useful as a fuel

gastrointestinal: related to the stomach and intestines

indigestion: reduced ability to digest food

acid reflux: splashing of stomach acid into the throat

diet: the total daily food intake, or the types of foods eaten

chronic: over a long period

fat: type of food molecule rich in carbon and hydrogen, with high energy content

consuming one's daily food intake, including all necessary **nutrients**, over five or six (or more) small meals, rather than two or three large ones. Frequent eating can be a great way to maintain one's **energy** level. This is also a beneficial eating pattern for individuals with **gastrointestinal** problems such as **indigestion** and **acid reflux**. Without a focus on healthy choices, however, grazing can become an easy way to overeat, and could possibly lead to weight gain. SEE ALSO DIETARY TRENDS, AMERICAN; EATING HABITS.

Susan Mitchell

Internet Resource

American Dietetic Association. <http://www.eatright.org>

Greeks and Middle Easterners, Diet of

The "Mediterranean **diet**" gained much recognition and worldwide interest in the 1990s as a model for healthful eating habits. The diet is based on the traditional dietary patterns of Crete, a Greek island, and other parts of Greece and southern Italy. The diet has become a popular area of study due to observations made in 1960 of low incidences of **chronic** disease and high life-expectancy rates attributed to the populations who consumed a traditional Mediterranean diet. This healthful diet model goes far beyond the use of particular ingredients and recipes. It attains its full meaning in the context of climate, geography, customs, and the way of life of Mediterranean peoples.

The Mediterranean Basin

In efforts to understand the Mediterranean diet, it is necessary to first learn about the many countries that border the Mediterranean Sea. The diet is closely tied geographically to areas of olive oil cultivation in the Mediterranean Basin. It can be defined by diets of the early 1960s in Greece, southern Italy and other Mediterranean regions in which olive oil was the principal source of dietary **fat**. The olive remains the most typical Mediterranean tree because it has adapted to the regional climate of long, very hot, dry summers and mild, damp winters.

The lands surrounding the Mediterranean Sea contain some of the oldest cultures on Earth. Greece, as well as other countries of Europe, North Africa, and some Middle Eastern nations, played a central role in the expansion of empires and cross-cultural exchanges over the centuries. Over 2,000 years ago trade by means of sea routes allowed Greek, Roman, Phoenician, Carthaginian, Arab, and Oriental products and traditions to intermix, resulting in mutual enrichment and an evolution of what is now incorporated into the Mediterranean diet. However, many different diets exist throughout the Mediterranean region, and there is no such thing as just one Mediterranean diet. Variations of this diet have traditionally existed in the North African countries of Morocco and Tunisia, parts of Turkey, and other Middle Eastern countries such as Lebanon and Syria.

Traditional Eating Habits

Traditional eating habits of Mediterranean countries, and those countries along the basin, include olives, fish, lamb, wheat, rice, chick peas and other

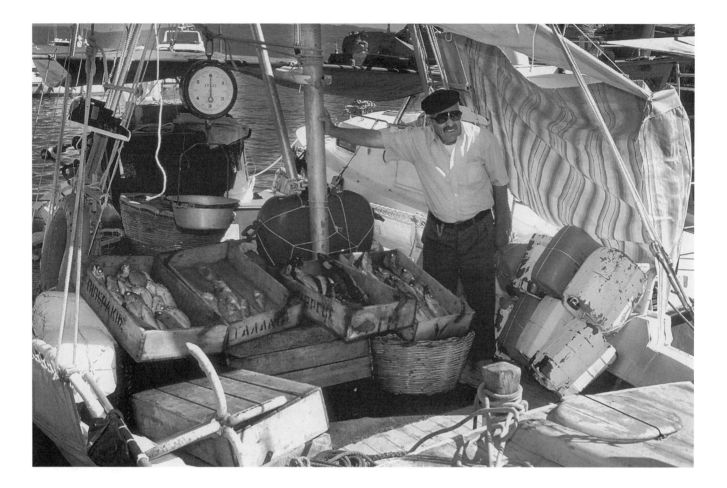

In ancient times, sea trade brought many of the world's cultural and culinary achievements to the nations around the Mediterranean Sea. More recently, the Mediterranean diet—which features low-cholesterol foods such as vegetables and fish, and includes very little meat—has been recognized as one of the world's healthiest. *[Photograph by Annebicque Bernard. Corbis. Reproduced by permission.]*

legumes, pistachios, dates, cheese, and yogurt. Bread typically accompanies each meal.

Traditional food consumption includes the following:

- *Dairy products.* Most dairy products are eaten in fermented forms, such as yogurt and cheese. Whole milk is used in desserts and puddings. Feta cheese, traditionally made of sheep or goat's milk, is the most commonly consumed cheese.

- *Meats.* Lamb is the most widely eaten meat. Pork is eaten only by Christians, not by Muslims or Jews. Many Middle Easterners will not combine dairy products or shellfish with the meal. Kosher beef, kosher poultry, lox (brine-cured cold-smoked salmon, much of which is slightly saltier than other smoked salmon), and sardines are also common foods. Legumes such as black beans, chick peas (garbanzo beans), lentils, navy beans, fava beans, and red beans are used in many dishes.

- *Breads and Cereals.* Some form of wheat or rice accompanies each meal. Pita and matzoh (unleavened bread) are common. Filo dough, which is used to make baklava, is also used in many dishes.

- *Fruits.* Fruits tend to be eaten as dessert or as snacks. Fresh fruit is preferred. Fruits made into jams and compotes (a cooked preparation of fruit in syrup) are eaten if fresh fruit is not available. Lemons and concentrated lemon juice are commonly used for flavoring.

legumes: beans, peas, and related plants

- *Vegetables.* Potatoes and eggplant are the most commonly consumed vegetables. Fruit and vegetables are preferred raw or mixed in a salad. Vegetables are often stuffed with rice or meats. Green and black olives are present in many dishes, and olive oil is most frequently used in food preparation.

Food Preparation and Storage

Grilling, frying, grinding, and stewing are the most common ways of preparing meats in countries bordering the Mediterranean Basin. A whole, roasted lamb or leg of lamb is a special dish prepared for festive gatherings. Spices and seasonings are essential in the preparation of Middle Eastern dishes. Common spices and herbs include dill, garlic, mint, cinnamon, oregano, parsley, leek, and pepper.

Many Middle Eastern nations, such as Turkey, Syria, and Lebanon, have predominantly Muslim populations. Eating *halal* is obligatory for every Muslim. *Halal* is an Arabic word meaning "lawful" or "permitted," and refers to Islamic law regarding the diet. Animals such as cows, sheep, goats, deer, moose, chickens, ducks, and game birds are *halal*, but they must be *zabihah* (slaughtered according to Islamic method) in order to be suitable for consumption. Halal foods are those that are:

- Free from any component or ingredient taken or extracted from an unlawful animal or ingredient that Muslims are prohibited from consuming.

- Processed, manufactured, prepared, or stored with apparatus, equipment and/or machinery that has been cleansed according to Islamic law.

- Free from contamination when prepared or processed with anything considered unclean.

Present-Day Eating Habits

Today, the Mediterranean region is characterized by a high increase in modernization. The traditional diet of the Mediterranean region has been affected by modernization, particularly in the area of agricultural production for trade. The countries of North Africa and the Middle East struggle the most with modernization problems. This has led to an increase in the dependence on costly food imports from outside the region. While the Greek economy remains rooted in agriculture and the government places a strong emphasis on agricultural reforms, Middle Eastern nations face constraints such as high rates of urbanization, leading to the loss of vital agricultural land.

Modernization has created significant changes in food consumption patterns in the countries of the Mediterranean region. The factors affecting the traditional dietary customs of the region are economy, environment, society and culture, disasters (e.g., war, drought), the expansion of food industries, and advertising campaigns promoting certain foods (e.g., soda, candy bars). **Fast-food** restaurant chains are also altering traditional diets. The expansion of fast food has resulted in the population consuming **processed foods** such as sweets and snack foods, which were never a part of their nutritional sustenance.

fast food: food requiring minimal preparation before eating, or food delivered very quickly after ordering in a restaurant

processed food: food that has been cooked, milled, or otherwise manipulated to change its quality

Halal food products	Food products not halal
Milk (from cows, sheep, camels, and goats)	Pork and pork by-products
Honey	Animals improperly slaughtered or dead before slaughtering
Fish	Animals killed in the name of anyone other than Allah (God)
Plants that are not an intoxicant	Alcohol and intoxicants
Fresh or naturally frozen vegetables	Carnivorous animals, birds of prey, and land animals without external ears
Fresh or dried fruits	Blood and blood by-products
Legumes and nuts such as peanuts, cashew nuts, pistachios, hazelnuts, and walnuts	Foods contaminated with any of the above products
Grains such as wheat, rice, rye, barley, and oats	

SOURCE: Adapted from <http://www.ifanca.org/halal.htm>

Culture

Mediterranean and Middle Eastern culture is centered on a strong patriarchal family. This has lessened in recent years, but family ties are still strong. Customs and family traditions influence **nutrition** greatly.

Food is an integral part of family celebrations, special days of honor, and festivals. In the Middle Eastern nation of Israel, kosher dietary laws concerning the selection, preparation, and eating of food remains influential in Jewish life. The Jewish laws of *kashrut*, or keeping kosher, determines which foods are kosher and which are non-kosher. Many ancient practices and **rituals**, handed down from generation to generation, are observed.

Many people from Mediterranean and Middle Eastern cultures observe Islam and Eastern Orthodox religions, which influence the kinds of food chosen and how the foods are combined. Fasting from sunrise to sunset is a Muslim religious obligation practiced during the sacred month of Ramadan. Muslims do not eat any form of pork, or any meat that has been slaughtered without mentioning God's name. Muslims cannot drink alcoholic beverages or foods flavored with alcohol—which differs from Greek and other Mediterranean cultures, where wine is a large part of the diet. Middle Easterners also have a high incidence of **lactose intolerance**, and therefore fresh milk is not widely consumed.

Nutrition and Disease

The wide use of olive oil in food preparation throughout the Mediterranean region contributes to a diet high in monounsaturated **fatty acids** and cultures commonly known for lower **blood pressure** among their populations. Recent research has produced scientific proof that a Mediterranean diet (which includes olive oil) is not only generally healthful, but that consuming olive oil can actually help lower harmful low density lipoprotein (LDL) **cholesterol** (often referred to as "bad" cholesterol). Olive oil contains **antioxidants** that discourage **artery** clogging and chronic diseases, including **cancer**.

The Mediterranean diet offers a practical and effective strategy that is relatively easy to adopt and more likely to be successful over the long term than most heart-healthy nutrition plans. In April 2001, the American Heart Association (AHA) published a science advisory stating that some components

nutrition: the maintenance of health through proper eating, or the study of same

ritual: ceremony or frequently repeated behavior

lactose intolerance: inability to digest lactose, or milk sugar

fatty acids: molecules rich in carbon and hydrogen; a component of fats

blood pressure: measure of the pressure exerted by the blood against the walls of the blood vessels

cholesterol: multi-ringed molecule found in animal cell membranes; a type of lipid

antioxidant: substance that prevents oxidation, a damaging reaction with oxygen

artery: blood vessel that carries blood away from the heart toward the body tissues

cancer: uncontrolled cell growth

cardiovascular: related to the heart and circulatory system

saturated fat: a fat with the maximum possible number of hydrogens; more difficult to break down than unsaturated fats

trans-fatty acids: type of fat thought to increase the risk of heart disease

heart disease: any disorder of the heart or its blood supply, including heart attack, atherosclerosis, and coronary artery disease

of the Mediterranean diet may be beneficial when used in conjunction with the association's traditional diets for the prevention and treatment of **cardiovascular** disease.

In the Mediterranean diet, not all fat is regarded as bad, however. In fact, the focus of the diet is not to limit total fat consumption, but rather to make wise choices about the type of fat in the diet. The Mediterranean diet is low in **saturated fat**, which is found mostly in meat and dairy products, vegetable oils such as coconut and palm oils (tropical oils), and butter. The diet views two types of protective fats, omega-3 fatty acids and monounsaturated fats, as healthful and places no restrictions on their consumption. Omega-3 fatty acids are found in fatty fish (e.g., sardines, salmon, tuna) and in some plant sources (e.g., pistachios, walnuts and other tree nuts, flaxseed, various vegetables). Monounsaturated fat is abundant in olive oil, nuts, and avocados.

Because the Mediterranean diet emphasizes eating whole, natural foods, it is extremely low in **trans-fatty acids**, which are increasingly recognized as important contributors to **heart disease**. These fats are found in hard margarine and deep-fried and processed snacks and food, including fast food and commercially baked products. They are similar to saturated fats and are known to raise levels of LDL cholesterol. Eating a diet incorporating the traditional foods of the Mediterranean, such as a variety of fruits and vegetables, has been shown to decrease the risk of heart disease. Five important dietary factors may contribute to the cardioprotective effect of this eating pattern. These are the inclusion of fish rich in omega-3 fatty acids, olive oil, nuts, and moderate amounts of alcohol, and the exclusion of trans-fatty acids.

Conclusion

Many common characteristics exist among the countries along the Mediterranean Basin, but each country has adapted to the geography and developed its own customs. The common core, however, can be seen in the diets of these countries. It is important to remember that the Mediterranean diet emphasizes eating whole, unprocessed foods that are extremely low in harmful LDL cholesterol. Recent studies indicate that the use of natural, monounsaturated oils such as olive oil, a balanced intake of vegetables and fish, and a low intake of red meats provides a natural defense against cardiovascular disease. Although more research is needed, the Mediterranean way of eating is potentially an ideal diet to improve the health of people by warding off illnesses.

Mohammed-Reza Forouzesh

Bibliography

Achterberg, Cheryl L.; McKenzie, J.; and Arosemena, F. (1996). *Multicultural Pyramid Packet*, Vol. 1. University Park, PA: Penn State Nutrition Center, College of Health and Human Development, Pennsylvania State University.

Giugliano, Dario; Sedge, Michael; and Sepe, Joseph (2000). *The Mediterranean Diet: Its Origins and Myths*. Reddick, FL: Idelson-Gnocchi.

Haber, B. (1997). "The Mediterranean Diet: A View from History." *American Journal of Clinical Nutrition* 66:1053S–1057S.

Keys, A. (1980). *Seven Countries: A Multivariate Analysis of Death and Coronary Heart Disease*. Cambridge, MA: Harvard University Press.

Osbourne, C. (1988). *Middle Eastern Food and Drink*. New York: Bookwright Press.

Rimm, E. B., and Ellison, R. C. (1995). "Alcohol in the Mediterranean Diet." *American Journal of Clinical Nutrition* 61:1378S–1382S.

Simopoulos, A. P., and Visoli, F. (2000). "Mediterranean Diets." In *World Review of Nutrition and Dietetics*, Vol. 87. Switzerland: Karger Publishers.

Spiller, G. A., and Bruce, B. (2002). *The Mediterranean Diet: Constituents and Health Promotion.* Boca Raton, FL: CRC Press.

Internet Resources

Curtis, B. M, and O'Keefe, J. H. Jr. (2002). "Understanding the Mediterranean Diet." *Post Graduate Medicine* 112(2). Available from <http:www.postgradmed.com>

"Health Benefits of Olive Oil and the Mediterranean Diet." Available from <http://www.mediterraneandiet.gr>

Islamic Food and Nutrition Council of America. "What Is Halal?" Available from <http://www.ifanca.org/halal.htm>

Islamic Halal Food Monitor of Canada. "A Brief Look at Dietary Laws for Muslims." Available from <http://www.eat-halal.com>

Oldways Preservation and Exchange Trust. "The Mediterranean Diet Pyramid." Available from <http://www.oldwayspt.org>

Nolan, J. E. "Cultural Diversity: Eating in America—Middle Eastern." Available from <http://ohioline.osu.edu>

The Green Revolution

The Green Revolution (GR) refers to the use of high-yield variety (HYV) seeds, which were invented by the crop geneticist Norman Borlaugh. HYVs are normally used as a part of a technological package that also includes biochemical inputs such as water, fertilizers, and pesticides, and often mechanical inputs. The GR, which started in the 1960s, is the last of the four agricultural revolutions in the world. It has been used in more than one hundred poor countries and has made possible a "revolutionary" increase in food production. The origin of the Green Revolution can be traced to the early twentieth century and the Malthusian fear that world food production would eventually fail to feed the growing population. This would result in a "red revolution" by the hungry. The implications of the GR for agrarian change, and especially for smaller farmers and laborers, have been widely debated.

Some scholars argue that since HYVs produce more food per acre, they have land-augmenting effects, and thus benefit smaller landholders. However, GR inputs are expensive, and smaller owners cannot make appropriate investments to increase output and reduce production costs as larger farmers can. So they incur losses and go into debt, which they have to clear up by selling their land. This is the classic mechanism of agrarian change from below. Larger landowners also lease land from smaller ones, who cannot afford to buy the inputs, causing "reverse tenancy" and an increased concentration of operational (as opposed to owned) land. Also, as cultivation with the use of hired labor and HYVs becomes more profitable, erstwhile landlords often evict their tenants, enhancing proletarianization and encouraging agrarian capitalism.

HYVs mature sooner than traditional seed varieties, and thus allow multiple cropping, increasing the demand for labor per acre. This increased food production leads to increased demand for harvesting, threshing, and post-harvest labor (e.g., for food processing), and creates the possibility for increased wages in GR areas. However, multiple cropping encourages capitalist farmers to resort to mechanization in order to complete farm operations on time, and this can erode employment opportunities.

The GR has also been shown to have increased regional disparity between wealthier, irrigated areas and poorer drier areas, and to have caused **ecological** problems such as water depletion and toxicity.

Raju Das

Bibliography

Das, Raju J. (2002). "The Green Revolution and Poverty: A Theoretical and Empirical Examination of the Relation Between Technology and Society." *Geoforum* 33(1):55–72.

Lipton, Michael. (1989). *New Seeds and Poor People.* Baltimore: Johns Hopkins University Press.

Shiva, Vandana (1991). *The Violence of the Green Revolution: Third World Agriculture, Ecology, and Politics.* London: Zed Books.

ecological: related to the environment and human interactions with it

Growth Charts

Growth charts are used by pediatricians, dietitians, nurses, and parents to assess the growth of infants, children, and adolescents. In the United States, growth charts are created by the Centers for Disease Control and Prevention (CDC) and assess weight, height, and **body mass index** (BMI). Each chart consists of a series of percentile curves that are used to compare the body measurements of children to others their age and gender. For example, a five-year-old girl whose weight falls in the 25th percentile weighs the same as or more than 25 percent of other five-year-old girls—and less than 75 percent of other five-year-old girls.

Amy N. Marlow

body mass index: weight in kilograms divided by square of the height in meters times 100; a measure of body fat

Growth Hormone

Human growth hormone (HGH) stimulates the growth of bones and affects the **metabolism** of **carbohydrate**, **protein**, and **fat**. It is secreted by the **pituitary gland**, which is located in the brain. Whereas HGH is produced in the body, genetic engineering has resulted in the development of recombinant human growth hormone (rHGH), which is used to treat stunted growth in children. Bovine somatotropin (BST) is a naturally occurring protein hormone in cows that increases milk production when administered as a supplement. BST is not biologically active in humans and is broken down into inactive **amino acids** and peptides when consumed. Therefore, milk from cows treated with BST is believed to be as safe and nutritious as milk from untreated cows.

Supplemental HGH is used by athletes, particularly body builders and power lifters, to increase muscle mass and decrease body fat. Individuals who are HGH-deficient and take supplemental HGH will see an increase in muscle mass and decreased body fat, whereas those with normal HGH levels will see an increase in lean body mass from an increase in the size of heart,

metabolism: the sum total of reactions in a cell or an organism

carbohydrate: food molecule made of carbon, hydrogen, and oxygen, including sugars and starches

protein: complex molecule composed of amino acids that performs vital functions in the cell; necessary part of the diet

fat: type of food molecule rich in carbon and hydrogen, with high energy content

pituitary gland: gland at the base of the brain that regulates multiple body processes

amino acid: building block of proteins, necessary dietary nutrient

liver, and kidneys, and from fluid retention, but there will be no increase in muscle mass. Excessive use can cause acromegaly (an increase in the size of the bones of the hand, feet, and jaw), as well as muscle weakness, **arthritis**, impotence, and **diabetes**. Since HGH increases the size of the liver, kidneys, and heart, its use can predispose the individual to **chronic** diseases. HGH is classified as an **anabolic** hormone, and its ability to increase muscle and decrease fat confers an unfair athletic advantage on the user. The use of HGH is thus banned by the International Olympic Committee (IOC), the National Collegiate Athletic Association (NCAA), and many professional sporting organizations. SEE ALSO ERGOGENIC ACIDS; SPORTS NUTRITION.

Leslie Bonci

arthritis: inflammation of the joints

diabetes: inability to regulate level of sugar in the blood

chronic: over a long period

anabolic: promoting building up

Bibliography

Rosenbloom, Christine, ed. (2000). *Sports Nutrition: A Guide for the Professional Working with Active People*, 3rd edition. Chicago: American Dietetic Association.

Williams, M. (1998). *The Ergogenics Edge*. Champaign, IL: Human Kinetics.

Health

Health is a measure of quality of life that is difficult to define and measure. In the 1940s, the World Health Organization (WHO) defined health as a "state of complete physical, mental, and social well-being and not merely the absence of disease or infirmity." At the first International Conference on Health Promotion in Ottawa, Canada (1986), the Ottawa Charter for Health Promotion built on the WHO's concept and further defined health as "a resource for everyday life ... a positive concept emphasizing social and personal resources, as well as physical capabilities." Good health enables one to function independently within a changing environment. SEE ALSO HEALTH COMMUNICATION; HEALTH EDUCATION; HEALTH PROMOTION; HEALTHY PEOPLE 2000 REPORT.

Delores C. S. James

Bibliography

World Health Organization (1948). *Official Records of the World Health Organization, No 2: Proceedings and Final Acts of the International Health Conference Held in New York from 19 June to 22 July 1946*. New York: United Nations, WHO Interim Commission.

Internet Resource

World Health Organization (1986). *Ottawa Charter for Health Promotion*. Available from <http://www.who.int/hpr>

Health Claims

As part of the Nutrition Labeling and Education Act of 1990 (NLEA), the Food and Drug Administration (FDA) and the United States Department of Agriculture (USDA) implemented regulations defining what terms may be used to describe the level of a **nutrient** in a food, as well as what claims could be made about the relationship between a nutrient or a food and the risk of a disease or health-related condition. Prior to the implementation of

nutrient: dietary substance necessary for health

263

these regulations, there were no guidelines for food manufacturers to use when making statements about the nutritional value of a food product. Consequently, consumers had difficulty comparing foods based solely on the nutritional content of the products. The NLEA served to level the playing field for manufacturers of nutritionally focused food products by providing a consistent definition of claims to assist consumers when shopping for food products.

Nutrient Content Claims

calcium: mineral essential for bones and teeth

cholesterol: multi-ringed molecule found in animal cell membranes; a type of lipid

fiber: indigestible plant material that aids digestion by providing bulk

calorie: unit of food energy

Nutrient content claims, such as "high in **calcium**" or "lite," are a form of advertising used to highlight the levels of key nutrients, **cholesterol, fiber,** or **calories** in the products being labeled. The claim is usually placed on the front side of the package so it is visible to the shopper wanting to make quick comparisons among food products. As a result of NLEA, the FDA strictly regulates nutrient content claims. The regulations spell out which nutrient content claims are allowed and under what circumstances they can be used. There are eleven core terms: "free," "low," "lean," "extra lean," "high," "good source," "reduced," "less," "light," "fewer," and "more." In addition, there is a multitude of synonyms that may be used for each of these terms.

"Healthy"

fat: type of food molecule rich in carbon and hydrogen, with high energy content

saturated fat: a fat with the maximum possible number of hydrogens; more difficult to break down that unsaturated fats

iron: nutrient needed for red blood cell formation

protein: complex molecule composed of amino acids that performs vital functions in the cell; necessary part of the diet

vitamin: necessary complex nutrient used to aid enzymes or other metabolic processes in the cell

mineral: an inorganic (non-carbon-containing) element, ion, or compound

Food labeling regulations allow manufacturers to make a "healthy" claim on the label. Due to the types of foods that are regulated by each agency, however, the FDA's definition of "healthy" is different from the USDA's definition. Under the FDA, "healthy" may be used if the food is low in **fat** and **saturated fat** and has a limited amount of sodium and cholesterol. In addition, single-item foods must provide at least 10 percent of one or more of vitamin A, vitamin C, **iron**, calcium, **protein**, and fiber. Raw, canned, or frozen fruits and vegetables and certain cereal-grain products do not necessarily need to meet this criteria. These foods can be labeled "healthy" if they do not contain ingredients that change the nutritional profile and, in the case of enriched grain products, if they conform to the standards of identity, which call for certain required ingredients (**vitamins, minerals**, protein, or fiber). Meal-type products (those large enough to be considered a meal [6 ounces]) must provide 10 percent of the Daily Value of two or three of these ingredients, in addition to meeting the other criteria. The sodium content cannot exceed 360 mg (milligrams) for individual foods and 480 mg for meal-type foods.

Health Claims

Health claims describe a relationship between a food substance and a disease or health-related condition. Due to the nature of such claims and the complexity of the science upon which such claims are made, the FDA carefully regulates health claims. Under the provisions of NLEA, the FDA has approved twelve specific health claims, and also provided a framework for additional specific claims to be approved as nutritional science evolves. Since NLEA, other processes have been established that allow food manufacturers a more efficient process to obtain approval for making a health claim. The Food and Drug Administration Modernization Act (FDAMA) was passed in 1997. Under FDAMA, upon successful submission of a "notification," a health claim may be made for a food based on an authoritative state-

---

NUTRIENT CONTENT CLAIMS

Claim	Definition	Nutrient
"Free"	No amount of or only trivial amounts.	Fat Saturated Fat Cholesterol Sodium Sugars Calories
"Very Low"	Not an overall definition.	Sodium
"Low"	May be used on foods that can be eaten frequently without exceeding dietary guidelines. Amount varies depending on the nutrient.	Fat Saturated Fat Sodium Cholesterol Calorie
"Lean" and "Extra Lean"	Used to describe fat in meat, poultry, seafood, and game meats.	Fat
"High"	May be used if the food contains 20% or more of the Daily Value per serving.	Vitamins and Minerals Dietary Fiber Protein
"Good Source"	May be used if the food contains 10% to 19% of the Daily Value per serving.	Vitamins and Minerals Dietary Fiber Protein
"Reduced"	Nutritionally altered to contain at least 25% less of a nutrient, or of calories, than the reference food. Reduced claim cannot be made if it is already labeled low.	Fat Saturated Fat Sodium Cholesterol Calorie
"Less"	Contains 25% less of a nutrient, or of calories, than the reference food.	Fat Saturated Fat Sodium Cholesterol Calorie
"Light"	One-third fewer calories, or half the fat, of the reference food. If the food derives 50% or more of calories from fat, the reduction must be 50%.	Calories Fat
"Light in Sodium"	Sodium has been reduced by at least 50%.	Sodium
"More"	Contains at least 10% of the Daily Value of the nutrient present in reference food. "Fortified," "enriched," "added," "extra," and "plus" are all synonyms of "more."	Vitamins and Minerals Dietary Fiber Protein

ment of a scientific body of the U.S. government or the National Academy of Sciences. The passage of this law has provided an opportunity for additional health claims, and for food manufacturers to efficiently communicate to consumers information about the relationship between foods and health.

General requirements for making a health claim. All products carrying a health claim must meet general requirements for levels of nutrients that may be associated with the risk of **chronic** disease. Food products with high levels of total fat, saturated fat, cholesterol, or sodium are not allowed to make a health claim. For individual foods, these levels are 13 grams of fat, 4 grams of saturated fat, 60 mg of cholesterol, and 480 mg of sodium per standardized serving. For meal products, the levels are 26 grams of fat, 8 grams of saturated fat, 120 mg of cholesterol, and 960 mg of sodium per label serving size. The levels for a main dish product are 19.5 grams of fat, 6 grams of saturated fat, 90 mg of cholesterol, and 720 mg of sodium per label serving size.

chronic: over a long period

Types of health claims. Health claims can be made through third-party references (such as the National Cancer Institute), statements, symbols (such as a heart), and vignettes or descriptions. In all cases, the claim must meet

diet: the total daily food intake, or the types of foods eaten

heart disease: any disorder of the heart or its blood supply, including heart attack, atherosclerosis, and coronary artery disease

the requirements for authorized health claims. The claim cannot state the degree of risk reduction and can only use "may" or "might" in discussing the food–disease relationship and it must indicate other factors that play a role in the specified disease. The claim must also be presented in relationship to the overall **diet**. For example, it might say: "While many factors affect **heart disease**, diets low in saturated fat and cholesterol may reduce the risk of this disease."

Nutrition is a dynamic science. FDA and USDA food-labeling regulations are designed to be flexible enough to evolve with the science, yet they also provide the consistency consumers need to make sound food choices in the supermarket. Through NLEA, food manufacturers have an equal opportunity by which to market food products. Additionally, consumers have credible food labels so they make informed food choices based on the nutritional attributes of a food product. SEE ALSO FOOD LABELS; REGULATORY LABELS.

Karen Hare

Health Communication

Health communication is the discipline that studies and develops appropriate communication strategies to inform individuals and communities about ways to enhance health. It is used at all levels of disease prevention and health promotion and can contribute to improving health and delaying disease, disability, and death. Health communication can be used to: (1) improve patient-provider relationships, (2) assist individuals to search for and use reputable health information and services, (3) enable individuals to adhere to provider recommendations, (4) develop and evaluate public health messages and campaigns, (5) assess health images in the media, (6) and distribute information to those at risk. SEE ALSO HEALTH; HEALTH EDUCATION; HEALTH PROMOTION.

Delores C. S. James

Bibliography

U.S. Department of Health and Human Services (2000). *Healthy People 2010, Conference Edition, in Two Volumes.* Washington, DC: U.S. Public Health Service.

Health Education

lifestyle: set of choices about diet, exercise, job type, leisure activities, and other aspects of life

Health education is the discipline dedicated to designing, implementing, and evaluating health programs and materials that improve the health of individuals, families, and communities. Health education is one of the tools of health promotion. A goal of health education is to provide individuals with the knowledge, skills, and motivation to make healthier **lifestyle** choices. Health education takes place in a variety of settings, such as schools; health care facilities; businesses; nonprofit organizations; and local, state, and federal health agencies. A certified health education specialist (CHES) is a person who has met the standards of competence established by the National Commission for Health Education Credentialing and has successfully passed the CHES examination. SEE ALSO HEALTH; HEALTH COMMUNICATION; HEALTH PROMOTION.

Delores C. S. James

Internet Resource

National Commission for Health Education Credentialing. "What Is a Certified Health Education Specialist?" Available from <http://www.nchec.org>

Health Promotion

Achieving optimal health is not the sole responsibility of the individual. Health promotion enables individuals to improve their health and delay disease, disability, and death. Health-promoting activities include healthful eating, adequate physical activity, **stress** management, not smoking, and adequate sleep. On a societal level, health promotion focuses on achieving equity in health among all ethnic and socioeconomic groups. Health disparities can be reduced or eliminated by providing culturally relevant health information, programs, and services; improving access to health care; creating public policy that promotes health; creating healthy environments; and providing other opportunities for making healthy choices. SEE ALSO HEALTH; HEALTH COMMUNICATION; HEALTH EDUCATION.

Delores C. S. James

stress: heightened state of nervousness or unease

Internet Resource

World Health Organization (1986). *Ottawa Charter for Health Promotion.* Available from <http://www.who.int/hpr>

Healthy Eating Index

Nutrition plays a vital role in the prevention of **chronic** diseases such as **coronary heart disease**, **hypertension**, and **diabetes**. The Healthy Eating Index (HEI) is a measure of the overall quality of an individual's **diet**. It was developed by the U.S. Department of Agriculture (USDA) to assess how well American diets comply with the *2000 Dietary Guidelines for Americans* and the *Food Guide Pyramid*.

The HEI measures the intake of ten dietary components to provide a single score out of a possible 100 points. A diet with a score greater than 80 is considered "good," one with a score of 51-80 is considered "fair," and one with a score of less than 51 is considered "poor." Each component contributes equally to the overall score.

Components 1–5 assess how well an individual's diet complies with the *Food Guide Pyramid* serving recommendations for the Grain, Vegetable, Fruit, Milk, and Meat Groups. Recommended servings for each food group are calculated based on diets containing 1,600, 2,200, and 2,800 **calories** per day. Components 1–5 have a maximum of 50 points, with 10 coming from each food group. A score of zero is assigned to a group if no items from that category are consumed. Intermediate scores are calculated proportionately to the number of servings consumed.

Component 6 assesses total **fat** consumption as a percentage of total caloric intake. Ten points are given if fat intakes are less than or equal to 30 percent of total calories. Zero points are given if the proportion of fat

nutrition: the maintenance of health through proper eating, or the study of same

chronic: over a long period

coronary heart disease: disease of the coronary arteries, the blood vessels surrounding the heart

hypertension: high blood pressure

diabetes: inability to regulate level of sugar in the blood

diet: the total daily food intake, or the types of foods eaten

calorie: unit of food energy

fat: type of food molecule rich in carbon and hydrogen, with high energy content

By applying the Healthy Eating Index (HEI) to data gathered by various consumer surveys, the USDA is able to assess the quality of Americans' diets. Recent HEI results suggest that Americans need to eat more fruit. *[Royalty-Free/Corbis. Reproduced by permission.]*

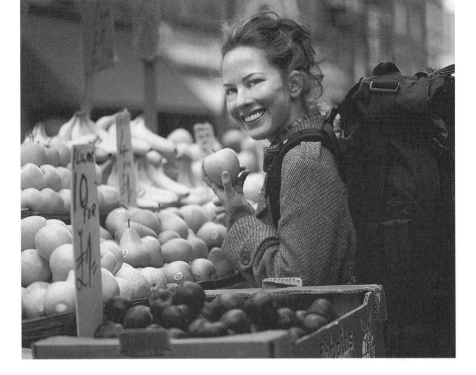

saturated fat: a fat with the maximum possible number of hydrogens; more difficult to break down that unsaturated fats

cholesterol: multi-ringed molecule found in animal cell membranes; a type of lipid

to total calories is 45 percent or higher. Intakes between 30 percent and 45 percent are scored proportionately.

Component 7 assesses **saturated fat** consumption as a percentage of total caloric intake. Ten points are given to saturated fat intakes of 10 percent or less of total calories. Zero points are given if the saturated fat intake is 15 percent or more of total calories. Scores between the two cutoff values are calculated proportionately.

Component 8 assesses total **cholesterol** intake. It is recommended that individuals consume no more than 300 milligrams of cholesterol daily. Ten points are given if cholesterol intake is less than or equal to 300 milligrams. Zero points are given when intake reaches 450 milligrams or more. Values between the two cutoff points are scored proportionately.

Component 9 assesses total sodium intake. Individuals should ideally consume no more than 2,400 milligrams of sodium daily. Ten points are given at an intake level of 2,400 milligrams or less. Zero points are given at a level of 4,800 milligrams or more. Scores between the two levels of intake are scored proportionately.

Component 10 assesses variety in the diet. While there is agreement that individuals should eat a variety of foods daily, there is no consensus of how to measure variety. The HEI measures variety by adding together the number of "different" foods eaten in amounts sufficient to contribute at least one-half of a serving in a food group. Ten points are given if at least half a serving of eight or more different types of food items are eaten daily. Zero points are given if at least half a serving of three or fewer different foods were eaten in a day. Intermediate intakes are calculated proportionately.

The USDA periodically applies the HEI to data from the national food consumption surveys. The most recent HEI uses data from the National

Health and Nutrition Examination Survey (NHANES). Previous data were based on the Continuing Survey of Food Intakes by Individuals (CSFII). Current data are based on 24-hour dietary recalls of representative samples. The HEI is computed for Americans two years of age and older. The findings indicated that:

- HEI scores have improved slightly since 1989, but did not change significantly from 1996 to 2000.

- The mean HEI score for 1999-2000 was 63.8.

- Most Americans need to improve their diet, especially in the Fruit Group and Milk Group.

- HEI scores improved with education.

- HEI is only modestly affected by income.

- Non-Hispanic blacks, low-income groups, and those with a high school diploma (or less education) had lower-quality diets.

- Women tend to have higher scores than men.

The HEI is a practical tool for assessing dietary quality, and results from the index can provide insights on how to improve eating patterns. Different strategies need to be developed to reach different segments of the population. The USDA Center for Nutrition and Public Policy has developed an interactive, self-assessment version of the Healthy Eating Index, which can be found on its Web site. SEE ALSO DIETARY GUIDELINES FOR AMERICANS; FOOD GUIDE PYRAMID.

Delores C. S. James

Bibliography

Basiotis, P.; Carlson, A.; Gerrior, S.; Juan, W.; and Lino, M. (2002). *The Healthy Eating Index 1999–2000.* Washington, DC: U.S. Department of Agriculture.

U.S. Department of Health and Human Services (2000). *Healthy People 2010, Conference Edition, in Two Volumes.* Washington, DC: U.S. Public Health Service.

Internet Resources

Center for Nutrition and Public Policy. "The Interactive Healthy Eating Index." Available from <http://147.208.9.133/default.asp>

U.S. Department of Agriculture. "The Healthy Eating Index." Available from <http://www.nalusda.gov/fnic>

Healthy People 2010 Report

In the mid-1970s, the United States government began to focus on national health issues, particularly disease prevention and health promotion. The first document to focus on the nation's health was the *Report of the President's Committee on Health Education* (1973). This was followed by the enactment of the *National Consumer Health Information and Health Promotion Act of 1976*, which created the *Office of Disease Prevention and Health Promotion.* In 1979, this office produced the first Healthy People report, *Healthy People: The Surgeon General's Report on Health Promotion and Disease Prevention,* which focused on reducing mortality rates and increasing independence among older adults.

Healthy People 2010 describes ten leading health indicators (LHIs) that reflect important health concerns for U.S. citizens. The LHIs, which include physical activity, mental health, and substance abuse, among others, are accompanied by a set of objectives designed to improve Americans' health.
[I.Q. Solutions. Reproduced by permission.]

HEALTHY PEOPLE 2010

Understanding and Improving Health

obesity: the condition of being overweight, according to established norms based on sex, age, and height

diabetes: inability to regulate level of sugar in the blood

In 1990, *Healthy People 2000* was published. This report contained twenty-two priority areas and 319 health objectives to be achieved by the year 2000. The overall goals were to increase years of healthy life, reduce health disparities, and improve access to preventive health services. These goals were set partly on the basis of the original 1979 goals, as well as to address the health of high-risk populations, racial and ethnic disparities, and to involve more community organizations in formulating the objectives.

While the nation has achieved many of the *Healthy People 2000* objectives, such as reducing mortality rates, reducing unintentional injuries, and increasing immunization rates, other health issues became more critical between 1990 and 2000. For example, smoking increased among the young-adult population, specifically in girls; HIV infection due to risky sexual behavior continued to be a concern, specifically among African-American women; **obesity** rose 50 percent between 1980 and 2000, and there was an increase in the percentage of people with **diabetes** and mental health disorders. All of these emerging issues prompted the next set of objectives to focus more closely on individual **lifestyle** behavior change and community health.

Healthy People 2010, released in January 2000, has twenty-eight focus areas and 467 objectives, with the overall goals of eliminating health disparities and increasing the quality and years of healthy life.

Healthy People 2010 expands on the *Healthy People 2000* objectives, while also addressing emerging issues such as obesity and mental health. For example, obesity has been linked to many other health concerns such as **high blood pressure**, diabetes, **cancer**, and **heart disease**. Therefore, one objective of *Healthy People 2010* is to promote health and reduce **chronic** disease associated with **diet** and weight. This objective will focus on weight status and growth; food and **nutrient** consumption; **iron** deficiency and **anemia**; schools, worksites, and **nutrition** counseling; and food security.

The Healthy People 2010 objectives will be used by state agencies, such as health departments, in planning health promotion and disease prevention programs. Local health agencies will also use the guidelines when planning health programs. For example, schools will use the nutrition objectives in school nutrition programs; private companies will use the physical activity objectives to plan worksite **wellness** programs; and various organizations will join together in planning health fairs.

Through the collaborative effort of all people in the nation using the *Healthy People 2010* guidelines, there can be a significant improvement in the length and quality of life for all. SEE ALSO HEALTH EDUCATION; HEALTH PROMOTION, NATIONAL INSTITUTES OF HEALTH.

Pauline A. Vickery

lifestyle: set of choices about diet, exercise, job type, leisure activities, and other aspects of life

high blood pressure: elevation of the pressure in the bloodstream maintained by the heart

cancer: uncontrolled cell growth

heart disease: any disorder of the heart or its blood supply, including heart attack, atherosclerosis, and coronary artery disease

chronic: over a long period

diet: the total daily food intake, or the types of foods eaten

nutrient: dietary substance necessary for health

iron: nutrient needed for red blood cell formation

anemia: low level of red blood cells in the blood

nutrition: the maintenance of health through proper eating, or the study of same

wellness: related to health promotion

Bibliography

Green, L., and Ottoson, J. (1999). *Community and Population Health*, 8th edition. Boston: WCB/McGraw-Hill.

U.S. Department of Health and Human Services (1991). *Healthy People 2000: National Health Promotion and Disease Prevention Objectives.* Washington, DC: U.S. Government Printing Office.

U.S. Department of Health and Human Services, 2001. *Healthy People 2010.* Washington, DC: U.S. Government Printing Office.

Internet Resources

U.S. Department of Health and Human Services. *Healthy People 2010.* Available from <http://www.health.gov/healthypeople>

U.S. Department of Health and Human Services. "Healthy People 2010: Fact Sheet." Available from <http://www.health.gov/hpcomments>

Heart Disease

The heart, which is about the size of a human fist, is the body's largest, strongest, and most important muscle. The heart continuously pumps blood through the body, helps regulate and prolong health, and controls the flow (circulation) of blood to the lungs, organs, muscles, and tissues in the body.

Heart disease is a leading cause of debilitation and death worldwide in men and women over age sixty-five. In many countries heart disease is viewed as a "second epidemic," replacing **infectious diseases** as the leading cause

heart disease: any disorder of the heart or its blood supply, including heart attack, atherosclerosis, and coronary artery disease

infectious diseases: diseases caused by viruses, bacteria, fungi, or protozoa, which replicate inside the body

of death. It is especially devastating in countries that do not have adequate health care. There are many types of diseases and disorders that affect the heart.

Congenital Heart Disease

Congenital cardiac anomaly (CAA), also known as congenital heart disease (CHD), refers to any structural defect of the heart or major vessels that exists from birth. It is the most common cause of infant death, other than problems of prematurity, and death is likely to occur in the first year of life. CAA may result either from **genetic** causes or from external causes such as maternal infection or exposure to other factors that affect embryonic **development**. The general problems associated with CAA include increased cardiac workload, **hypertension**, poor oxygenation of blood, and respiratory infections. There are many types of CAA, including aortic stenosis, atrial septal defect, valvular stenosis, and pulmonary stenosis.

Rheumatic Heart Disease

Rheumatic heart disease (RHD) involves damage to the heart and heart vessels caused by rheumatic fever. A susceptible person acquires a streptococcal infection, which may trigger an autoimmune reaction in the heart tissue. Rheumatic fever can cause swelling (inflammation) in the heart, joints, brain, and spinal cord. Rheumatic fever produces **fatigue** (tiredness) and the infection can damage or weaken heart valves. Problems with the heart may be evident early, or it may occur long after the infection. RHD is characterized by heart murmurs, abnormal pulse rate and rhythm, and congestive heart failure. **Acute** RHD requires aggressive treatment to prevent heart failure. **Chronic** RHD requires continuous observation. If poor cardiac function develops, it may be treated with a low-sodium **diet** and **diuretics**. Patients with deformed heart valves should be given prophylactic **antibiotics** before dental and surgical procedures.

Myocardial Infarction (MI)

Myocardial infarction (MI) is the clinical term for a **heart attack**. It is caused by occlusion (blockage) of the coronary **artery** (**atherosclerosis**) or a blood clot (coronary thrombosis), resulting in the partial or total blockage of one of the coronary arteries. When this occurs, the heart muscle (myocardium) does not receive enough **oxygen**. If the MI is mild, the heart muscle may partially repair itself. Permanent damage may occur when a portion of the heart muscle dies (called an infarction).

MI is characterized by crushing chest pains that may radiate to the left arm, neck, or upper abdomen (which may feel like acute **indigestion** or a gallbladder attack). The affected person usually has shortness of breath, ashen color, clammy hands, and faints. Treatment within one hour of the heart attack is important and usually includes chewing aspirin and administering CPR. Many individuals die each year of their first MI.

Coronary Artery Disease (CAD)

Coronary artery disease (CAD) refers to any one of the conditions that affect the coronary arteries and reduces blood flow and **nutrients** to the heart.

genetic: inherited or related to the genes

development: the process of change by which an organism becomes more complex

hypertension: high blood pressure

fatigue: tiredness

acute: rapid-onset and short-lived

chronic: over a long period

diet: the total daily food intake, or the types of foods eaten

diuretic: substance that depletes the body of water

antibiotic: substance that kills or prevents the growth of microorganisms

heart attack: loss of blood supply to part of the heart, resulting in death of heart muscle

artery: blood vessel that carries blood away from the heart toward the body tissues

atherosclerosis: build-up of deposits within the blood vessels

oxygen: O_2, atmospheric gas required by all animals

indigestion: reduced ability to digest food

nutrient: dietary substance necessary for health

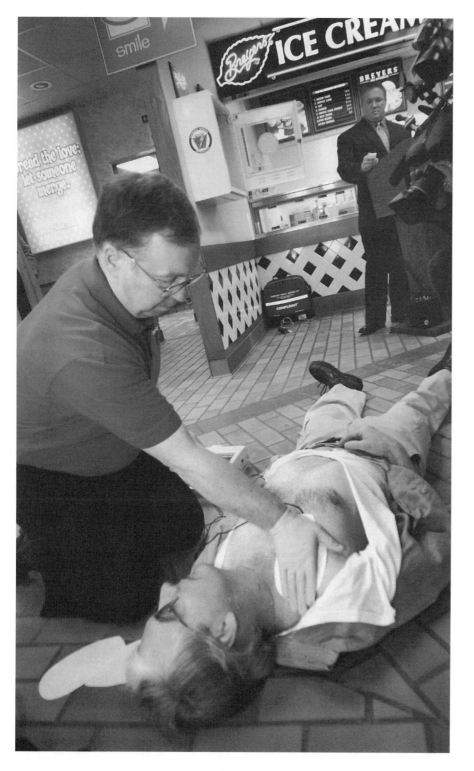

According to the American Heart Association, heart disease is the most common cause of cardiac arrest, and 95 percent of cardiac arrest patients die before they reach the hospital. That high mortality rate has prompted the placement of portable defibrillators in places such as schools, airplanes, police cars, and in this service plaza along the Pennsylvania Turnpike. *[Photograph by Keith Srakocic. AP/Wide World Photos. Reproduced by permission.]*

It is the leading cause of death worldwide for both men and women. The most common kind of CAD is atherosclerosis, which results in narrowing and hardening of the arteries. Coronary atherosclerosis is at epidemic proportions worldwide.

Traditionally, CAD was seen as a disease of aging and was observed primarily in the elderly. However, atherosclerosis is now occurring more often in younger populations. One out of every three individuals worldwide,

estrogen: hormone that helps control female development and menstruation

menopause: phase in a woman's life during which ovulation and menstruation ends

lipid: fats, waxes, and steroids; important components of cell membranes

cholesterol: multi-ringed molecule found in animal cell membranes; a type of lipid

triglyceride: a type of fat

trans-fatty acids: type of fat thought to increase the risk of heart disease

obesity: the condition of being overweight, according to established norms based on sex, age, and height

diabetes: inability to regulate level of sugar in the blood

stress: heightened state of nervousness or unease

calorie: unit of food energy

fiber: indigestible plant material which aids digestion by providing bulk

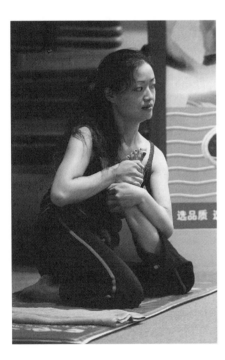

Chronic stress is a risk factor for heart disease, and acute stress can trigger heart attacks. Regular yoga or other exercise may help prevent both conditions by releasing stress and strengthening the heart muscle. *[AP/Wide World Photos. Reproduced by permission.]*

and one in five in the United States, dies from heart disease each year. In the United States, CAD has declined more rapidly in whites than in blacks. CAD affects women ten years later than men, mostly due to the protective production of **estrogen**. After **menopause**, a woman is two times more susceptible to heart disease than women who have not reached menopause.

Risk factors. Controlled risk factors associated with CAD include hypertension; cigarette smoking; elevated blood **lipids** (e.g. **cholesterol**, **triglyceride**); a high-fat diet (especially saturated fats and **trans-fatty acids**); physical inactivity; **obesity**; **diabetes**; and **stress**. Lifestyle changes can assist in prevention of CAD. Uncontrolled risk factors include a family history of CAD, gender (higher in males), and increasing age.

Tobacco use is one of the leading contributors to heart disease. Smoking increases the risk of heart attacks (and increases the risk of lung diseases) by decreasing oxygen flow to the heart and lungs. Hypertension, which makes the heart work harder than normal, can be caused by poor diet, excessive dietary salt, lack of exercise, smoking, and chronic stress. Adult-onset diabetes mellitus may result from poor dietary habits and lack of exercise over a lifetime. Uncontrolled diabetes can lead to heart failure. Exercise can reduce the risk for CAD by increasing coronary blood flow, and it has shown positive effects on blood flow to the heart (myocardial perfusion). Long-term benefits of exercise include lower incidences of coronary heart failure and increased cardiac function in normal subjects.

Prevention. Health professionals recommend that dietary fat be reduced to 30 percent or less of total **calories**. The diet also should have no more than 10 percent of its calories from saturated fats, no more than 300 milligrams (mg) of cholesterol daily, no more than 2,400 mg of sodium, and at least 3,500 mg of potassium. A plant-based diet consisting primarily of whole grains, fruits, and vegetables is recommended. Eating at least 25 grams of **fiber** and five servings of fruits and vegetables daily may reduce the risk for heart disease.

Individuals who consume alcohol should do so in moderation. Moderation is defined as two drinks for women and one drink for men daily. Alcohol is a very addictive substance, however, and should not be used as a primary means of prevention. Caffeine in moderation has no adverse effect; however, excessive intake may make the heart pump faster. Increased heart rate stresses the heart and may cause long-term damage to blood vessels.

Establishing good exercise and dietary habits early in childhood is important to prevent heart disease. Regular activity and proper **nutrition** decreases **reactivity** to stress and makes the heart stronger and more efficient. At least thirty minutes of moderate exercise daily is recommended to prevent heart disease. Stress management helps to prevent **high blood pressure**, which is a major contributor to heart disease. Techniques such as yoga, deep breathing, and **meditation** may prevent coronary disease by improving resistance to stress. SEE ALSO ARTERIOSCLEROSIS; ATHEROSCLEROSIS; CARDIOVASCULAR DISEASES; EXERCISE.

Teresa Lyles

Bibliography

Goldberg, I. J.; Mosca, L.; Piano, M. R.; and Fisher, E. A. (2001). "Wine and Your Heart: A Science Advisory for Healthcare Professionals from the Nutrition Committee, Council on Epidemiology and Prevention, and Council on Cardiovascular Nursing of the American Heart Association." *Circulation* 103:472–475.

Insel, P. M., and Roth, W. T. (2004). "Cardiovascular Disease and Cancer." In *Core Concepts in Health*, 9th (brief) edition. New York: McGraw-Hill.

Mosby's Medical, Nursing, and Allied Health Dictionary, 6th edition (2003). St. Louis, MO: American Dietetic Association.

Internet Resources

American Heart Association. "Congenital Heart Defects in Children Fact Sheet." Available from <http://www.americanheart.org>

American Heart Association/American Stroke Association. "Heart Disease and Stroke Statistics—2003 Update." Available from <http://www.americanheart.org>

"Description of Congenital Heart Defects." Available from <http://www.congenital heartdefects.com/typesofcad.html>

"Heart Attack." Available from <http://www.heartcenteronline.com/myheartdr>

Hispanics and Latinos, Diet of

The United States Census Bureau defines *Hispanics* as those who indicate their origin to be Mexican, Puerto Rican, Cuban, Central or South American (e.g., Dominican, Nicaraguan, Colombian) or other Hispanic origin. This designation is made independently of racial classification. According to the 2002 U.S. Census, 13.3 percent of the U.S. population (or over 37 million Americans) identified themselves as being of Hispanic origin. This number exceeds the number of non-Hispanic blacks, or African Americans, in the United States, making Hispanics the largest minority subpopulation within the nation. The three major subgroups that make up the Hispanic population are Mexican Americans, Puerto Ricans, and Cubans. By far the largest of these is the Mexican-American population, which represents at least two-thirds of all Hispanics.

Ethnic and racial **diversity** within the U.S. increased dramatically during the latter part of the twentieth century, with much of the large-scale immigration coming from Asia and Latin America. From 1980 to 2000 the Hispanic population within the United States doubled. More than 40 percent of Hispanics were living in the western part of the country at the end of the century. In 2000, New Mexico had a higher proportion of Hispanics in its population than any other state, with 42 percent of its population being of Hispanic origin. The high growth rate among Hispanics is attributable to higher fertility rates than those observed in other ethnic groups, and to increases in immigration, especially in border states such as California and Texas. Compared to the non-Hispanic white population, the Hispanic population in the United States is younger, less educated, economically disadvantaged, and more likely to live in larger households. However, there are significant differences among the Hispanic subpopulations, with those of Mexican origin being relatively less advantaged and those of Cuban origin being relatively more advantaged in terms of education and income.

Characteristics of the Hispanic Diet

The contemporary diet of Hispanics in the United States is heavily influenced by the traditional dietary patterns of their countries of origin, as well

nutrition: the maintenance of health through proper eating, or the study of same

reactivity: characteristic set of reactions undergone due to chemical structure

high blood pressure: elevation of the pressure in the bloodstream maintained by the heart

meditation: stillness of thought, practiced to reduce tension and increase inner peace

diversity: the variety of cultural traditions within a larger culture

as by the dietary practices of the adopted communities in which they live. As such, there are many regional differences between Hispanic subgroups, both in terms of the composition of the diet and the means of food preparation. Despite the heterogeneous ancestral backgrounds of Hispanic Americans, many Hispanics still retain core elements of the traditional Hispanic diet, including a reliance on grains and beans and the incorporation of fresh fruits and vegetables in the diet. Family life has traditionally occupied a central place in Hispanic culture, and this has influenced dietary behaviors through home preparation of meals and the practice of families eating together.

Information about what Hispanics in the United States eat has been compiled through national surveys conducted by the U.S. Department of Agriculture (USDA). Among the highlights of these data are that Hispanics tend to eat more rice, but less pasta and ready-to-eat cereals, than their non-Hispanic white counterparts. With the exception of tomatoes, Hispanics are also less likely to consume vegetables, although they have a slightly higher consumption of fruits. Compared to non-Hispanic whites, Hispanics are more than twice as likely to drink whole milk, but much less likely to drink low-fat or skim milk. Hispanics are also more likely to eat beef, but less likely to eat processed meats such as hot dogs, sausage, and luncheon meats. Hispanics are more likely to eat eggs and **legumes** than non-Hispanic whites, and less likely to consume fats and oils or sugars and candy.

Analysis of the **macronutrient** content of the diet reveals that Hispanics, especially Mexican Americans, have a lower intake of total fat and a higher intake of dietary **fiber** compared to non-Hispanic white populations, with much of the dietary fiber coming from legumes. In general, Mexican Americans and other Hispanic subgroups are low in many of the same micronutrients as the general population, with intakes of vitamin E, **calcium**, and **zinc** falling below Recommended Daily Allowances.

Acculturation and the Hispanic Diet

Just as Hispanics have altered American cuisine, American culture has also altered the diet of Hispanic Americans. As with many other immigrant groups in the United States, the lifestyle of Hispanic Americans is undergoing a transition away from one based on the traditional values and customs of their ancestry, as they begin to adopt the values and behaviors of their adopted country. With regard to health behaviors, this process of acculturation is typically characterized by a more **sedentary** lifestyle and a change in dietary patterns. The effects of acculturation on the Hispanic diet are illustrated in national dietary survey data that show that Hispanic Americans who continue to use Spanish as a primary language eat somewhat more healthful diets than those who use English as a primary language. These healthier eating behaviors include lower consumption of fat, **saturated fat**, and **cholesterol**. Additional analysis of these survey data reveals that these dietary differences do not appear to be the result of greater nutritional knowledge or greater awareness of food-disease relationships.

The degradation of diet quality that occurs as Hispanic Americans become acculturated into the mainstream U.S. population occurs in the context of improvements in, rather than degradation of, economic status. For example, first-generation Mexican-American women, despite being of lower

legumes: beans, peas, and related plants

macronutrient: nutrient needed in large quantities

fiber: indigestible plant material that aids digestion by providing bulk

calcium: mineral essential for bones and teeth

zinc: mineral necessary for many enzyme processes

sedentary: not active

saturated fat: a fat with the maximum possible number of hydrogens; more difficult to break down that unsaturated fats

cholesterol: multi-ringed molecule found in animal cell membranes; a type of lipid

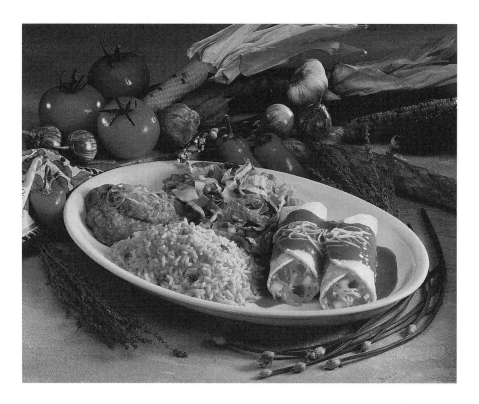

The traditional Hispanic diet includes plenty of grains and legumes. It is somewhat lower in fat and cholesterol than the diets of non-Hispanic whites in the U.S. *[Royalty-Free/Corbis. Reproduced by permission.]*

socioeconomic status than second-generation Mexican American or non-Hispanic white women, tend to have higher intakes of **protein**, **vitamins** A and C, folic acid, and calcium than these other groups. The diets of second-generation Mexican American women more closely resemble those of non-Hispanic white women of similar socioeconomic status.

The process of acculturation and the changing nature of the Hispanic diet has serious implications for the state of Hispanic health. The **prevalence** of type 2 **diabetes** mellitus is two to three times higher in Hispanic Americans than in non-Hispanic whites, with an estimated 10 percent of adults over the age of twenty and 25 to 30 percent of those over the age of fifty affected. The prevalence of the disease is especially high among Mexican Americans. Diabetes, a disease characterized by high levels of **glucose** in the blood, is a major cause of death and disability in the United States. Compared to nondiabetic individuals, those with the disease are also at two to four times higher risk of developing **cardiovascular** disease, the leading cause of death in the country. Accompanying this increased risk of diabetes among Hispanics is a marked increase in the risk of **obesity**.

Much of the increased risk of diabetes experienced by Hispanic Americans is believed to be attributable to the changing lifestyle that accompanies the acculturation process, including the changing quality of the Hispanic diet and the adoption of a more sedentary lifestyle. These trends are occurring across all segments of the Hispanic population, although the extent of the changes are more pronounced in some subgroups (e.g., Mexican Americans in large urban areas) than in others. Although Hispanic Americans generally smoke less than their non-Hispanic white counterparts, the direction of Hispanic health is also threatened by an increasing frequency of cigarette smoking, particularly among younger segments of the population.

socioeconomic status: level of income and social class

protein: complex molecule composed of amino acids that performs vital functions in the cell; necessary part of the diet

vitamin: necessary complex nutrient used to aid enzymes or other metabolic processes in the cell

prevalence: describing the number of cases in a population at any one time

diabetes: inability to regulate level of sugar in the blood

glucose: a simple sugar; the most commonly used fuel in cells

cardiovascular: related to the heart and circulatory system

obesity: the condition of being overweight, according to established norms based on sex, age, and height

PERCENTAGES OF INDIVIDUALS CONSUMING SPECIFIED FOODS, FROM A ONE-DAY DIETARY RECALL

Food item	Mexican Americans	Other Hispanics	Non-Hispanic whites
Cereals and pasta			
Ready-to-eat cereals	26.2	23.9	30.3
Rice	14.7	29.0	6.1
Pasta	3.7	6.6	8.3
Vegetables			
Dark green vegetables	3.2	5.2	9.6
Deep yellow vegetables	9.3	8.6	14.2
Tomatoes	46.2	40.1	39.1
Green beans	3.4	6.3	8.1
Citrus	29.1	29.6	26.1
Other (noncitrus) fruits	43.8	37.7	40.4
Whole milk	37.5	31.3	15.2
Low fat milk	17.6	19.4	30.3
Beef	25.9	25.3	20.5
Processed meats (hot dogs, sausages, luncheon meats)	23.5	24.2	32.7
Eggs	29.8	24.4	16.9
Legumes	30.6	23.5	11.8
Fats and oils (table fats and salad dressings)	36.9	44.0	59.0
Sugars and candy	46.0	49.3	54.7

SOURCE: U.S. Dept. of Agriculture, Agricultural Research Service.

nutrition: the maintenance of health through proper eating, or the study of same

Approaches for improving the health of Hispanics need to be broad-based and to consider the complexities of a variety of lifestyle factors. **Nutrition** education programs aimed at improving the quality of the Hispanic diet are currently based on a combination of preserving some elements of the traditional Hispanic diet—including a reliance on beans, rice, and tortillas—and a change in others—such as reduced consumption of high-fat dairy products and less use of fat in cooking. SEE ALSO CENTRAL AMERICANS AND MEXICANS, DIETS OF; SOUTH AMERICANS, DIET OF.

Braxton D. Mitchell

Bibliography

Aldrich L, and Variyam, J. N. (2000). "Acculturation Erodes the Diet Quality of U.S. Hispanics." *Food Review* 23:51–55.

Flegal, K. M.; Ezzati, T. M.; Harris, M., et al. (1991). "Prevalence of Diabetes in Mexican Americans, Cubans, and Puerto Ricans from the Hispanic Health and Nutrition Examination Survey, 1982–1984." *Diabetes Care* 14(Suppl 3):628–638.

Guendelman, S., Abrams, B. (1995). "Dietary Intake among Mexican-American Women: Generational Differences and a Comparison with White Non-Hispanic Women." *American Journal of Public Health* 85:20–25.

Harris, M. I.; Flegal, K. M.; Cowie, C. C., et al. (1998). "Prevalence of Diabetes, Impaired Fasting Glucose, and Impaired Glucose Tolerance in U.S. Adults: The Third National Health and Nutrition Examination Survey (NHANES), 1988–94." *Diabetes Care* 21:518–524.

Hobbs, F., and Stoops, N. (2000). *Demographic Trends in the 20th Century.* U.S. Census Bureau, Census 2000 Special Reports, Series CENSR-4. Washington, DC: U.S. Government Printing Office.

Romero-Gwynn, E.; Gwynn, D. L.; Grivetti, R., et al. (1993). "Dietary Acculturation among Latinos of Mexican Descent." *Nutrition Today* (July/Aug.):6–11.

U.S. Census Bureau (1999). *The Hispanic Population in the United States: Population Characteristics.* Washington, DC: U.S. Government Printing Office.

Internet Resource

U.S. Department of Agriculture, Agricultural Research Service (1999). "Data Tables: Food and Nutrient Intake by Hispanic Origins and Race, 1994-1996." Available from <http://www.barc.usda.gov/bhnrc>

HIV/AIDS

HIV (human immunodeficiency virus) was identified in 1983 by the French scientist Luc Montagier and his staff at the Pasteur Institute in Paris. Ever since that discovery, scientists have been searching for ways to treat those infected with HIV, and to produce a vaccine to prevent its spread. While new antiviral treatments have been developed, a vaccine has yet to be found. HIV causes AIDS (acquired immunodeficiency syndrome), an unpredictable condition that may progress over many years and is characterized by a slow deterioration of the **immune system**. Once an individual becomes infected (HIV has infected the target cells) it takes a week or more before the virus is spread throughout the body's blood and **lymph system**. The immune system responds by turning out HIV **antibodies** in about six to eighteen weeks. The progression of HIV infection to AIDS may take several years. In the initial period, prolonged (2–4 weeks) flu-like symptoms may appear. This is followed by an **asymptomatic** period (clinical latency) that may last ten or more years. When the immune system becomes further compromised, the patient may experience **opportunistic infections**, caused by the reduced function of the immune system resulting in a plethora of nonspecific and variable signs and symptoms. The condition known as AIDS is marked by severe compromise of the immune system and the presence of one or more opportunistic infections. Some clinical signs and symptoms may include sweating, diarrhea, malaise (feeling tired), anorexia (loss of appetite), weight loss, wasting (loss of muscle tissue), chest pain, swelling of the **lymph nodes**, **fungal** infections, **neurological** disorders, body-fat accumulations, and increased blood fats. In addition to disease-induced signs and symptoms, medications used to treat HIV/AIDS may produce additional signs and symptoms.

Nutrition for HIV/AIDS

In the absence of a cure, it is important to control symptoms, support the immune system, and lower the levels of HIV circulating in the blood. To lower the level of HIV in the blood, patients take a prescribed combination of antiviral **drugs**. The role nutrition plays will vary along the disease continuum (disease progression over many years), with consideration given to the patient's age, gender, behaviors, current medication, drug history, **socioeconomic status**, and associated health concerns.

In all cases, adequate **hydration** (fluid intake) and increased **calorie** and **protein** intake are necessary to fight the infection. Proper nutrition must begin immediately to support **nutritional deficiencies** (including vitamin A and E, the **B vitamins**, magnesium, and **zinc**) that occur early in the disease process. These nutritional deficiencies contribute to decreased immunity and disease progression. Ellen Mazo and Keith Berndtson, in *The Immune Advantage*, suggest that once the patient has been diagnosed with HIV infection, more protein and complex **carbohydrates**, along with moderate amounts of fats, should be consumed. The **diet** should include lean

immune system: the set of organs and cells, including white blood cells, that protect the body from infection

lymph system: system of vessels and glands in the body that circulates and cleans extracellular fluid

antibody: immune system protein that protects against infection

asymptomatic: without symptoms

opportunistic infections: infections not normally threatening, which gain a foothold in people with weakened immune systems

lymph node: pocket within the lymph system in which white blood cells reside

fungal: of or from fungi

neurological: related to the nervous system

drugs: substances whose administration causes a significant change in the body's function

socioeconomic status: level of income and social class

hydration: degree of water in the body

calorie: unit of food energy

protein: complex molecule composed of amino acids that performs vital functions in the cell; necessary part of the diet

nutritional deficiency: lack of adequate nutrients in the diet

B vitamins: a group of vitamins important in cell energy processes

zinc: mineral necessary for many enzyme processes

carbohydrate: food molecule made of carbon, hydrogen, and oxygen, including sugars and starches

diet: the total daily food intake, or the types of foods eaten

energy: technically, the ability to perform work; the content of a substance that allows it to be useful as a fuel

metabolism: the sum total of reactions in a cell or an organism

electrolyte: salt dissolved in fluid

acute: rapid-onset and short-lived

chronic: over a long period

gastrointestinal: related to the stomach and intestines

steroids: group of hormones that affect tissue build-up, sexual development, and a variety of metabolic processes

intestines: the two long tubes that carry out the bulk of the processes of digestion

mucosa: moist exchange surface within the body

oral-pharyngeal: related to mouth and throat

nutritional requirements: the set of substances needed in the diet to maintain health

intravenous: into the veins

meat, fish, beans, seeds and nuts, whole-grain breads and cereals, and fruits and vegetables. Moderate amounts of fat for **energy** and calories can be acquired through foods such as nuts, avocado dip, peanut butter, and seeds.

The diet should include each of the five major food groups (dairy, vegetable, meat, fruit, and bread). The sixth group (fats and sugars) should be used sparingly. Patients with a poor appetite should eat six or more small meals throughout the day, rather than three large ones. In prolonged cases of appetite depression, a physician may prescribe an appetite stimulant (e.g., megesterol acetate). It is important to keep all foods refrigerated, to avoid eating rare meats, to practice proper hand washing, and to use soap and hot water to clean sinks and utensils. Food-borne illnesses pose serious threats for HIV/AIDS patients.

HIV/AIDS Complications

Some symptoms will require additional attention beyond general nutritional recommendations. For example, diarrhea will rapidly reduce the water content of the body, causing severe alterations in the body's **metabolism** and **electrolyte** balance. Electrolytes may be replaced with products such as Pedialyte or Gatorade. Proteins and calories should be increased to prevent weight loss, and dairy products, alcohol, caffeine, and spicy and fatty foods should be avoided.

A second complication is that of weight loss and wasting. According to Derek Macallan, in *Wasting HIV Infection and AIDS*, wasting may be either **acute** (associated with a secondary disease) or **chronic** (associated with **gastrointestinal** disease), and is the result of a variety of processes, including drug use, medications, concurrent disease, and HIV itself. HIV infection causes abnormal protein and fat metabolism. During episodes of acute wasting the patient may require a prescription for **steroids**, to help support tissue maintenance and tissue development, in combination with optimal protein and calories in the diet.

Contributing to weight loss and wasting is malabsorption (the failure of nutritional substances to be absorbed in the **intestines**). Malabsorption occurs in advanced cases of HIV infection when gastrointestinal disease is present. Diseases that can cause malabsorption in HIV/AIDS patients include Kaposi's sarcoma, non-Hodgkin's lymphoma, cytomegalovirus, *Myco-bacterium avium* complex, and cryptosporidiosis. Malabsorption may require an alternative to oral nutrition.

Alternatives to Oral Nutrition

Alternative routes for nutrition must be considered in patients with fungal growth in the oral cavity, inflammation of the gums and oral **mucosa**, open sores, difficulty in swallowing, and other debilitating diseases of the **oral-pharyngeal** region and/or gastrointestinal tract. These alternatives include parenteral (PN) and enteral nutrition. PN replaces essential **nutritional requirements** via **intravenous** (IV) access. The IV may be placed in a peripheral vein or in a large central vein, depending on the medical condition of the patient and the choice of nutrition replacement therapy. The cost for PN is high, and there is a risk of severe infection; therefore it is not recommended except for brief treatment measures during known episodic cases of acute weight loss and in the absence of gastrointestinal (GI) function.

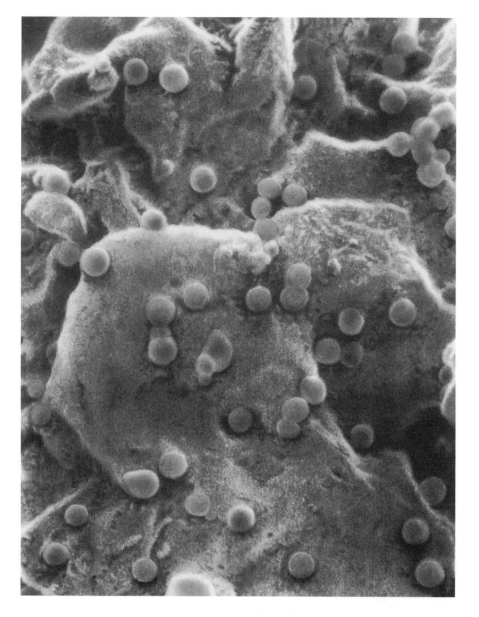

This scanning electron micrograph (SEM) shows a T-lymphocyte white blood cell, lumpy from infection. The smaller circles are AIDS viruses budding from the cell's membrane. *[Nibsc/Photo Researchers, Inc. Reproduced by permission.]*

Enteral nutrition (placing a tube into the stomach or intestine) is preferred in those patients who have difficulty in swallowing, disease of the oral-pharyngeal region, and adequate GI function. The medical risks with enteral nutrition are less than for PN, but may include injury to the GI tract and infection in the absence safe food practices.

Ethical Considerations for Care

It is strongly advised that those suspected with or diagnosed with HIV infection seek professional attention from a qualified physician and a registered dietician. For these caregivers, the development of new antiviral drugs, changes in methods of administration of existing drugs, and new information regarding nutrition require diligent and regular review. It is important for health care workers to keep an open dialogue with the patient, so that they stay aware of the patient's health status and treatment measures. Many issues regarding the amount (drugs and nutrition) and length of care for AIDS patients remain controversial and should be negotiated with the patient.

Finally, when traditional medical wisdom fails, some patients may turn to alternative medicine. There are many questionable products on the market that make extraordinary health claims, and caution is required. These products are often overpriced and marketed with misleading claims, and should therefore be considered carefully before use. SEE ALSO FOOD SAFETY; IMMUNE SYSTEM; MALNUTRITION.

Stephen Hohman

Bibliography

Lehman, Robert H. (1997). *Cooking for Life: A Guide to Nutrition and Food Safety for the HIV-Positive Community.* New York: Dell.

Macallan, Derek C. (1999). "Wasting HIV Infection and AIDS." *Journal of Nutrition* 129(1S):238–242.

Mazo, Ellen, and Berndtson, Keith (2002). *The Immune Advantage.* Emmaus, PA: Rodale.

Morrison, Gail, and Hark, Lisa (1999). *Medical Nutrition & Disease*, 2nd edition. Cambridge: MA: Blackwell Science.

"Questionable Mail Order Products" (1999). *Nutrition Forum.* 16(6):46.

Romeyn, Mary (1998). *Nutrition and HIV: A New Model for Treatment*, 2nd edition. San Francisco: Jossey-Bass.

Watson, Ronald R. (2001). *Nutrition and AIDS*, 2nd edition. Boca Raton, FL: CRC Press.

Homelessness

Homelessness is a global problem. According to a 1996 United Nations report, 500 million people worldwide were homeless or residing in low-quality housing and unsanitary conditions in 1995. The number of homeless continues to rise, however, and quantifying this population is difficult. Most homelessness rates are reported by service providers, and countries with the best-developed service systems will therefore report the highest number of homeless, a condition referred to as the service-systems paradox. Various other problems, such as double-counts, overcounts, the problem of mobility, and hidden homelessness also affect estimates.

In the United States, homelessness gained national attention in the early 1980s. While some people thought the growth in the homeless population was a result of the recession that occurred during this period, the problem has not gone away.

It is estimated that two million people per year are homeless in the United States. A report issued by the Urban Institute in 2000 stated that 2.3 million adults and children in the United States are likely to experience homelessness at least once in a year.

A way to get at the root of the problem is to understand the causes of homelessness. Worldwide, homelessness is caused by a breakdown in traditional family support systems, continued urbanization, the effects of structural adjustment programs, civil wars, and natural disasters. A shortage in affordable rental housing and an increase in poverty are thought to be two major factors contributing to the rise of homelessness in the United States. Other potential causes are the lack of affordable health care, domestic violence, mental illness, and addiction disorders. Often, individuals will have several risk factors causing them to "choose between food, shelter, and other

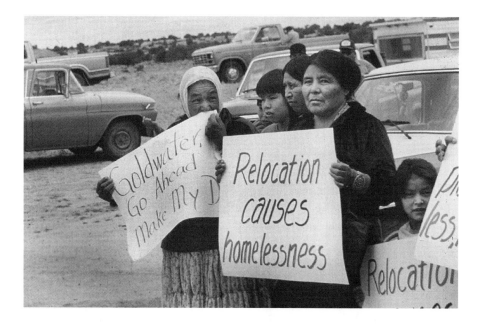

basic needs" (National Coalition for the Homeless, p. 6). Shelter is often the lowest priority, and is often unaffordable, and thus homelessness becomes a problem. Similar risk factors affect both the homeless and those who are experiencing poverty. Because homelessness and poverty are linked, efforts to improve poverty will inevitably decrease homelessness.

Economics of Poverty and Undernutrition

Looking at a nation's poverty data is one way to judge its economic well-being. In the United States in 2001, 32.9 million people were living below the poverty line, which was $9,034 for an individual (for a family of three, the poverty threshold in 2001 was a salary of $14,128, while for a family of four it was $18,104). However, the poverty rate dropped a half percentage point to 11.3 percent between 1999 and 2000.

Around the world, poverty is pervasive: one billion people lived in poverty in 2001. Poverty and hunger are undeniably linked, so that solving the hunger problem by feeding people, without attacking the poverty problem, does not address the root cause of poverty.

In 1999, 31 million households (10.1%) in the United States were on the verge of hunger, while 3 percent of households were hungry. Even more startling, between 750 and 800 million people around the world were hungry in 1996. Of these, 550 million were in Asia, while 170 million were in sub-Saharan Africa. Along with hunger comes undernutrition, which can pose serious health threats.

Consequences of Long-Term Undernutrition among Homeless Children

The Institute of Medicine has estimated the number of homeless children in the United States to be approximately 100,000 each night. Almost half of these children are younger than six years of age. Although this is a growing population, few studies have examined the effect of undernutrition on homeless children. However, recent studies have found that a poor **diet**

diet: the total daily food intake, or the types of foods eaten

283

chronic: over a long period

obesity: the condition of being overweight, according to established norms based on sex, age, and height

incidence: number of new cases reported each year

fatigue: tiredness

anemia: low level of red blood cells in the blood

gastric: related to the stomach

ulcer: erosion in the lining of the stomach or intestine due to bacterial infection

gastrointestinal: related to the stomach and intestines

cardiovascular: related to the heart and circulatory system

hypertension: high blood pressure

hypercholesterolemia: high levels of cholesterol in the blood

acute: rapid-onset and short-lived

infectious diseases: diseases caused by viruses, bacteria, fungi, or protozoa, which replicate inside the body

diabetes: inability to regulate level of sugar in the blood

malnutrition: chronic lack of sufficient nutrients to maintain health

nutrient: dietary substance necessary for health

in early childhood has implications for long-term health and cognitive development.

Homeless children suffer several medical problems due to undernutrition, including **chronic** and recurring physical ailments, and higher rates of fever, cough, colds, diarrhea, and **obesity**. In addition, a greater **incidence** of infections, **fatigue**, headaches, and **anemia**, as well as impaired cognitive development and visual motor integration, has been documented in homeless children.

Homeless adults also suffer several medical problems due to undernutrition. Common problems include anemia, dental problems, **gastric ulcers**, other **gastrointestinal** complaints, **cardiovascular** disease, **hypertension**, **hypercholesterolemia**, **acute** and chronic **infectious diseases**, **diabetes**, and **malnutrition**.

Government Programs to Reduce Hunger and Undernutrition

According to the United States Census Bureau, 5 million adults and 2.7 million children lived in hungry households in 1999. To combat hunger and the undernutrition problem, the United States government funds and administers several food programs, including the Food Stamp Program; the National School Lunch Program; the School Breakfast Program; the Special Supplemental Nutrition Program for Women, Infants and Children; the Child and Adult Care Food Program; the Emergency Food Assistance Program; and the Community Food and Nutrition Program.

The Food Stamp Program provides coupons for low-income families that enable them to buy food. The coupons are dispersed on a monthly basis, with the purpose of reducing hunger and malnutrition.

Through the National School Lunch Program (NSLP), schools can be reimbursed for providing nutritious meals to children. A nutritious school lunch provides children with one-third or more of their Recommended Dietary Allowance (RDA) for **nutrients**.

Similar to the NSLP, the School Breakfast Program offers reimbursements to schools for providing breakfast to students. This breakfast provides one-fourth or more of their RDA for nutrients. In addition, meals and snacks are provided for children at risk for hunger through the Summer Food Service Program for Children. The food is usually provided during educational and recreational activities, and one-third of the children's RDA is provided through this program.

The Special Supplemental Nutrition Program for Women, Infants and Children (WIC) has a mission to improve the diets of women, infants, and children by providing monthly food packages that include certain foods.

Federal funds are provided to public and nonprofit child-care centers, family and group child-care homes, and after-school programs for meals and snacks to the populations they serve through the Child and Adult Care Food Program (CACFP). The programs are required to follow the nutrition standards set by USDA when providing meals.

Through the Emergency Food Assistance Program (TEFAP), food is distributed through emergency food shelters. The food is provided through surplus commodities purchased by the United States Department of Agriculture (USDA). Low-income families are served as well.

Finally, the Community Food and Nutrition Program (CFNP) is the source of federal funding for programs providing hunger relief and improving nutrition for low-income individuals. The funding is provided on the local, state, and national levels.

Organizations Providing Community-Based Solutions to Homelessness

Several community-based solutions to homelessness have been developed, such as emergency shelters, transitional housing, permanent housing for formerly homeless individuals, voucher distribution for housing, food pantries, soup kitchens and meal distribution programs, mobile food programs, physical and mental health, alcohol and/or drug, HIV/AIDS, and outreach programs, drop-in centers, and migrant housing.

Examples of organizations seeking to provide solutions to hunger and homelessness include the Food Research and Action Center, America's Second Harvest, the Center on Hunger and Poverty, Bread for the World, World Hunger Year, and the Food Industry Crusade Against Hunger. These organizations provide coordination and support to antihunger networks of food banks and food assistance programs, education of the public, and encouragement to policy makers for the expansion and protection of programs aiding the homeless.

Deficits in the Diet

Many homeless people rely on shelters and soup kitchens for their food intake. However, these sites may not provide an adequate diet. "Most shelters rely on private donations, a local food bank, and surplus commodity distributions. Because the nutritional quality and quantity of these resources vary greatly over time, meals may be nutritionally limited, even though the quantity of the food served may be acceptable to the recipient" (Wolgemuth et al., 1992, p. 834). Furthermore, easily stored and prepared foods do not provide the best nutritional value. These items are typically "high in salt, **fat**, preservatives, and empty **calories** (i.e., calories with little or no nutritional value), and low in variety, **fiber**, and **protein**" (Strasser et al., 1991, p. 70).

Due to the food sources of the homeless, deficits in the diet have been documented in numerous studies. The **B vitamins**, vitamin C, **zinc**, **calcium**, thiamine, folic acid, magnesium, and **iron** are all commonly found to be deficient in the homeless. Iron deficiencies are particularly common among the homeless, leading to high rates of anemia. In addition, the food that is likely to be offered at most local shelters and soup kitchens is high in salt, fat, and **cholesterol**, contributing to a high incidence of hypertension among the homeless.

Clearly, the homeless are a widely varied population, and responses to homelessness must also be varied in nature. Several such responses are needed. These include: prevention of homelessness through improving the housing stock; improving outreach through increased soup kitchens, emergency responses, and night shelters; and creating supportive housing to

fat: type of food molecule rich in carbon and hydrogen, with high energy content

calorie: unit of food energy

fiber: indigestible plant material that aids digestion by providing bulk

protein: complex molecule composed of amino acids that performs vital functions in the cell; necessary part of the diet

B vitamins: a group of vitamins important in cell energy processes

zinc: mineral necessary for many enzyme processes

calcium: mineral essential for bones and teeth

iron: nutrient needed for red blood cell formation

cholesterol: multi-ringed molecule found in animal cell membranes; a type of lipid

help homeless persons reintegrate into society. Interagency coordination to improve services and the provision of enterprise development and skills training to improve the economic survival of the homeless are also needed. Finally, federal and local governments must be involved in efforts to help the homeless through policy development. This multifaceted approach will ensure a more effective response to homelessness. SEE ALSO FOOD INSECURITY; NUTRITIONAL DEFICIENCY; WIC PROGRAM.

Pauline A. Vickery
Heidi Williams
Nadia Lugo

Bibliography

Carrillo, T. E.; Gilbride, J. A.; and Chan, M. M. (1990). "Soup Kitchen Meals: An Observation and Nutrient Analysis." *Journal of the American Dietetic Association* 90(7):989–991.

Dalaker, J. (2001). *Poverty in the United States: 2000.* Washington, DC: U.S. Census Bureau.

Hwang, S. W. (2001). "Homelessness and Health." *Canadian Medical Association Journal* 164(2):229–233.

Kelly, E. (1998). "Nutrition Among Homeless Children." *Public Health Reports* 113:287.

Luder, E.; Ceysens–Okada, E.; Koren-Roth, A.; and Martinez-Weber, C. (1990). "Health and Nutrition Survey in a Group of Urban Homeless Adults." *Journal of the American Dietetic Association* 90(10):1387–1392.

Oliviera, N. L., and Goldberg, J. P. "The Nutrition Status of Women and Children Who Are Homeless." *Nutrition Today* 37(2):70–77.

Strasser, J. A.; Damrosch, S.; and Gaines, J. (1991). "Nutrition and the Homeless Person." *Journal of Community Health Nursing* 8(2):65–73.

Wiecha, J. L.; Dwyer, J. T.; and Dunn-Strohecker, M. (1991). "Nutrition and Health Services Needs Among the Homeless." *Public Health Reports* 106(4):364–374.

Wolgemuth, J. C.; Myers-Williams, C.; Johnson, P.; and Henseler, C. (1992). "Wasting Malnutrition and Inadequate Nutrient Intakes Identified in a Multiethnic Homeless Population." *Journal of the American Dietetic Association* 92(7):834–839.

Internet Resources

Action Against Hunger (2002). "Hunger FAQ: Who Is Hungry?" Available from <http://www.aah-usa.org>

Burt, M. R.; Aron, L. Y.; Douglas, T.; Valente, J.; Lee, E.; and Iwen, B. (1999). "An Overview of Homeless Clients." Available from <http://www.huduser.org/publications>

Food Research and Action Center. "Federal Food Programs." Available from <http://www.frac.org>

Global Issues. "Causes of Poverty: Hunger and Poverty." Available from <http://www.globalissues.org>

National Coalition for the Homeless (2002). "Facts about Homelessness." Available from <http://www.nationalhomeless.org>

United Nations (1995). "Global Report on Human Settlements." Available from <http://www.un.org>

United Nations (2000). "Strategies to Combat Homelessness." Available from <http://www.unhabitat.org>

Urban Institute (2000). "Millions Still Face Homelessness in a Booming Economy: New Estimates Reveal a Large and Changing Homeless Population Served by Growing Diverse Network." Available from <http://www.urban.org>

U.S. Census Bureau. "Poverty 2001." Available from <http://www.census.gov/hhes>

U.S. Department of Housing and Urban Development. *Homelessness: Programs and the People They Serve.* Available from <http://www.huduser.org/publications>

World Hunger Year. "Hunger, Poverty and Homelessness in the U.S." Available from <http://www.worldhungeryear.org>

Hunger

Hunger is the **physiological** drive to find and eat food. According to the World Health Organization (WHO), hunger is the world's major health risk. Globally, one in three people suffer from **chronic** hunger, which is a result of a lack of food security. Food insecurity means people do not have access at all times to nutritionally adequate food. There are three dimensions to food insecurity: a lack of (1) purchasing power (lack of money or resources), (2) accessibility (ability to get food), and (3) availability (amount of food). In the United States, hunger is caused by poverty, whereas in developing countries it is caused by poverty, war, civil unrest, or an undeveloped economy. SEE ALSO DISASTER RELIEF ORGANIZATIONS; FOOD INSECURITY; MEALS ON WHEELS; NUTRITIONAL DEFICIENCY.

Delores C. S. James

physiological: related to the biochemical processes of the body

chronic: over a long period

Internet Resources

Brundtland, Gro Harlem. "World Food Summit Plenary Address." Available from <http://www.who.int/dg>

World Health Organization. "Fifty Facts from the World Health Report 1998: Global Health Situation and Trends 1955–2025." Updated 2001. Available from <http://www.who.int/whr2001>

Hyperglycemia

Hyperglycemia, or high blood sugar, is the result of either too little **insulin** or of the body's inefficient use of insulin. Indicators of hyperglycemia include frequent urination, thirst, high levels of sugar in the urine, and high blood sugar. Failure to address hyperglycemia results in **dehydration** and **ketoacidosis**. Over the long term, hyperglycemia causes **heart disease**, foot problems, blindness, kidney disease, and nerve damage.

For diabetics, frequent blood **glucose** testing and **diet** management are critical to preventing hyperglycemia. Regular self-monitoring of blood glucose levels determines the degree of adjustment in insulin and diet. A registered dietician can conduct a nutritional assessment that will reveal nutritional needs critical to preventing and treating **chronic** complications of **diabetes**. This assessment, based on personal, cultural, and **lifestyle** preferences, is the foundation for a diabetic's dietary plan. For meal planning, the diabetic exchange system provides a quick method for estimating and maintaining the proper balance of **carbohydrates**, fats, **proteins**, and **calories**. In the exchange system, foods are categorized into groups, with each group comprised of foods with similar amounts of carbohydrate, protein, **fat**, and calories. Based on the individual's diabetes treatment plan and goals, any food on the list can be exchanged with another food within the same group.

Exercise improves physical fitness, assists in weight control, and provides **psychological** benefits. For those with diabetes, physical activity

insulin: hormone released by the pancreas to regulate level of sugar in the blood

dehydration: loss of water

ketoacidosis: accumulation of ketone bodies along with high acid levels in the body fluids

heart disease: any disorder of the heart or its blood supply, including heart attack, atherosclerosis, and coronary artery disease

glucose: a simple sugar; the most commonly used fuel in cells

diet: the total daily food intake, or the types of foods eaten

chronic: over a long period

diabetes: inability to regulate level of sugar in the blood

lifestyle: set of choices about diet, exercise, job type, leisure activities, and other aspects of life

carbohydrate: food molecule made of carbon, hydrogen, and oxygen, including sugars and starches

protein: complex molecule composed of amino acids that performs vital functions in the cell; necessary part of the diet

calorie: unit of food energy

fat: type of food molecule rich in carbon and hydrogen, with high energy content

psychological: related to thoughts, feelings, and personal experiences

cholesterol: multi-ringed molecule found in animal cell membranes; a type of lipid

blood pressure: measure of the pressure exerted by the blood against the walls of the blood vessels

reduces **cholesterol** levels, lowers **blood pressure**, decreases body fat, and increases sensitivity to insulin. Exercise further contributes to blood glucose control and reduces the risk factors for diabetes-related complications. With meal planning, exercise has the ability to control type 2 diabetes without medications. SEE ALSO DIABETES MELLITUS; EXCHANGE SYSTEM; HYPOGLYCEMIA; INSULIN.

Julie Lager

Bibliography

American Diabetes Association (2003). "Hyperglycemia Crises in Patients with Diabetes Mellitus." *Diabetes Care* 26(4):S109–S117.

Kitabach, Abbas E.; Umpierrez, Guillermo E.; Murphy, Mary Beth; Barrett, Eugene, J.; Kreisberg, R. A.; Malone, J. I.; and Wall, B. M. (2001). "Management of Hyperglycemic Crises in Patients with Diabetes." *Diabetes Care* 24(1):131–153.

Internet Resources

American Diabetes Association. "Hyperglycemia." Available from <http://www.diabetes.org>

National Institute of Diabetes and Digestive and Kidney Diseases. "Diabetes." Available from <http://www.niddk.nih.gov>

WebMD. "Complications of Diabetes: Hyperglycemia." Available from <http://webmd.com>

Hypertension

blood pressure: measure of the pressure exerted by the blood against the walls of the blood vessels

artery: blood vessel that carries blood away from the heart toward the body tissues

Blood pressure is the force with which blood pushes against the **artery** walls as it travels through the body. Like air in a balloon, blood fills arteries to a certain capacity—and just as too much air pressure can cause damage to a balloon, too much blood pressure can harm healthy arteries. Blood pressure is measured by two numbers—systolic pressure and diastolic pressure. Systolic pressure measures cardiac output and refers to the pressure in the arterial system at its highest. Diastolic pressure measures peripheral resistance and refers to arterial pressure at its lowest. Blood pressure is normally measured at the brachial artery with a sphygmomanometer (pressure cuff) in millimeters of mercury (mm Hg) and given as systolic over diastolic pressure.

A blood pressure reading thus appears as two numbers. The upper number is the systolic pressure, which is the peak force of blood as the heart pumps it. The lower number is the diastolic pressure, which is the pressure when the heart is filling or relaxing before the next beat. Normal blood pressure for an adult is 120/70 (on average), but normal for an individual varies with the height, weight, fitness level, age, and health of a person.

What Is Hypertension?

stroke: loss of blood supply to part of the brain, due to a blocked or burst artery in the brain

Hypertension, or high blood pressure, is defined as a reading of 140/90 on three consecutive measurements at least six hours apart. The definition varies for pregnant women, where hypertension is defined as 140/90 on two consecutive measurements six hours apart. Consistently high blood pressure causes the heart to work harder than it should and can damage the coronary arteries, the brain, the kidneys, and the eyes. Hypertension is a major cause of **stroke**.

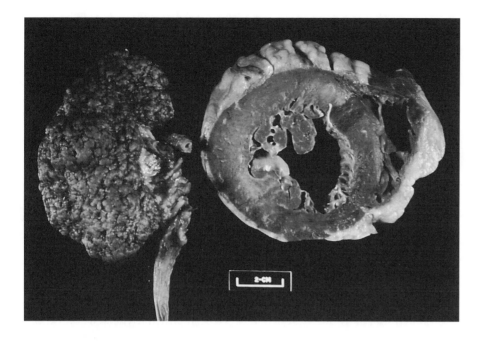

A kidney (left) and a cross-section of a heart (right) that were affected by hypertension. The heart shows signs of advanced atherosclerosis, one possible complication arising from hypertension. *[Photograph by Dr. E. Walker. Photo Researchers, Inc. Reproduced by permission.]*

Types of Hypertension

Hypertension is classified as either *primary* (or *essential*) *hypertension* or *secondary hypertension*. Primary hypertension has no specific origin but is strongly associated with lifestyle. It is responsible for 90 to 95 percent of diagnosed hypertension and is treated with **stress** management, changes in **diet**, increased physical activity, and medication (if needed). Secondary hypertension is responsible for 5 to 10 percent of diagnosed hypertension. It is caused by a preexisting medical condition such as congestive heart failure, kidney failure, liver failure, or damage to the endocrine (**hormone**) system.

Pregnancy-induced hypertension (PIH) may appear in otherwise healthy women after the twentieth week of pregnancy. It is more likely to occur in women who are **overweight** or **obese**. PIH may be mild or severe, and it is accompanied by water retention and **protein** in the urine. About 5 percent of PIH cases progress to preeclampsia. Preeclampsia is characterized by dizziness, headache, visual disturbance, abdominal pain, facial **edema**, poor appetite, **nausea**, and vomiting. Severe preeclampsia affects the mother's blood system, kidneys, brain, and other organs. In rare cases, the woman can die. Preeclampsia is more likely to occur during first pregnancies, multiple fetuses, in women with existing hypertension, and in women younger than twenty-five years old or over thirty-five years old. If convulsions occur with PIH, it is called eclampsia. PIH disappears within a few weeks after birth.

Causes of Hypertension

Many prescription and **over-the-counter drugs** can cause or exacerbate hypertension. For example, corticosteroids and immunosuppressive drugs increase blood pressure in most solid-organ transplant recipients. Medication taken for pain and inflammation such as nonsteroidal anti-inflammatory drugs (NSAIDs) and cyclooxygenase-2 (COX-2) inhibitors may raise blood pressure since their antiprostaglandin properties affect the kidneys.

stress: heightened state of nervousness or unease

diet: the total daily food intake, or the types of foods eaten

hormone: molecules produced by one set of cells that influence the function of another set of cells

overweight: weight above the accepted norm based on height, sex, and age

obese: above accepted standards of weight for sex, height, and age

protein: complex molecule composed of amino acids that performs vital functions in the cell; necessary part of the diet

edema: accumulation of fluid in the tissues

nausea: unpleasant sensation in the gut that precedes vomiting

over-the-counter: available without a prescription

drugs: substances whose administration causes a significant change in the body's function

Tobacco products (cigarettes, cigars, smokeless tobacco) contain nicotine, which temporarily increases blood pressure (for about thirty minutes or less). The blood pressure of smokers should be rechecked after thirty minutes if initial readings are high. Nicotine patches that are used for smoking cessation do not appear to increase blood pressure.

There does not appear to be a direct relationship between caffeine and **chronic** hypertension, even though caffeine intake can cause an **acute** (rapid but brief) increase in blood pressure. This may be due to the fact that **tolerance** to caffeine develops rapidly.

Chronic overuse of alcohol is a potentially reversible cause of hypertension. Five percent of hypertension is due to alcohol consumption and 30 to 60 percent of alcoholics have hypertension. Alcohol-induced hypertension is more likely to occur in women than men.

Diet and Hypertension

Sodium intake has been a primary target for hypertension control, though it is ranked fourth as the lifestyle factor associated with hypertension. About 50 percent of individuals appear to be "sodium sensitive." This means that excessive sodium intake tends to increase blood pressure in these groups of people, and they do not appear to excrete excessive amount of salt via the kidneys. Sodium-sensitive individuals include the elderly, obese individuals, and African Americans. The Dietary Guidelines for Americans recommend that adults consume no more than 2,400 milligrams of sodium daily. There are a number of ways to limit sodium in the diet, including:

- Do not use salt at the table
- Check food labels for sodium content
- Choose unprocessed foods
- Limit processed meats and cheeses
- Limit pickled meats and vegetables
- Limit salty snacks
- Limit intake of soy sauce, BBQ sauce, and other condiments and foods that may be high in sodium

Potassium supplements (2–4 grams daily) have been shown to moderately decrease blood pressure. Fruits and vegetables are excellent sources of potassium. The Dietary Guidelines for Americans recommend that adults consume at least 3,500 milligrams of potassium daily. A diet high in fruits and vegetables has been linked to a decreased risk of both hypertension and stroke. Foods high in omega-3 **fatty acids** have positive effects on hypertension and **cardiovascular** disease by relaxing arteries and thinning the blood. In addition, several studies have demonstrated that individuals with hypertension may benefit from daily doses of **calcium** (800 mg) or magnesium (300 mg).

The DASH Eating Plan

Research has shown that a diet that is low in sodium but rich in calcium, potassium, and magnesium can decrease blood pressure, especially among African Americans. This eating plan is called the DASH (Dietary Approach

chronic: over a long period

acute: rapid-onset and short-lived

tolerance: development of a need for increased amount of drug to obtain a given level of intoxication

fatty acids: molecules rich in carbon and hydrogen; a component of fats

cardiovascular: related to the heart and circulatory system

calcium: mineral essential for bones and teeth

to Stop Hypertension) eating plan and it is as effective in decreasing blood pressure as some medications commonly used to treat hypertension. The DASH eating plan is based on 2,000 **calories** a day with 18 percent of the calories coming from protein, 55 percent from **carbohydrates**, and 27 percent from fats. The eating plan contains less **fat** than the Food Guide Pyramid, more fruits and vegetables, and includes a serving of nuts.

Pharmacological Treatment of Hypertension

Hypertension is commonly treated with medication, and a combination of two or more drugs is common. Patients are usually given a diuretic to help them excrete excess fluids. However, most **diuretics** also cause excretion of potassium in the urine, and individuals on diuretics should monitor their potassium intakes. Drugs used to control hyertension include beta-blockers (e.g., atenolol [Tenorim]) which act to slow heart rate and cause some vaso-dilation (widening of the lumen, or interior, of blood vessels). Drugs that contain calcium channel blockers (e.g., amlopidine [Norvasc]) or angiotensin-converting **enzyme** (ACE) inhibitors also cause vasodilation.

Lifestyle Treatment of Hypertension

Most of the risk factors for primary hypertension are preventable, and lifestyle modification may prevent as well as treat the condition. Secondary hypertension can be managed by treating the underlying cause. Individuals in the high normal and stage 1 hypertension categories should attempt to lower blood pressure through diet and lifestyle changes before going on a regimen of medications. Recommendations include:

- Eliminate tobacco

- Control stress

- Maintain weight at 15 percent or less of desirable weight

- Restrict alcohol intake to no more than two drinks a day for men and one for women (one drink equals 12 ounces of beer, 5 ounces of wine, or 1.5 ounces 80-proof whiskey)

- Restrict sodium intake to 1.5 to 2.5 grams per day (4 to 6 tsp salt)

- Exercise five to seven days a week for sixty minutes per session

- Increase intake of fruits and vegetables

- Increase intake of low-fat dairy products

SEE ALSO CARDIOVASCULAR DISEASES; HEART DISEASE.

Delores C. S. James

calorie: unit of food energy

carbohydrate: food molecule made of carbon, hydrogen, and oxygen, including sugars and starches

fat: type of food molecule rich in carbon and hydrogen, with high energy content

diuretic: substance that depletes the body of water

enzyme: protein responsible for carrying out reactions in a cell

Bibliography

Anderson, Douglas M., et al. (2003). *Mosby's Medical, Nursing, and Allied Health Dictionary*, 6th edition. St. Louis, MO: Mosby.

Worthington-Roberts, B., and Williams, S. (1997). *Nutrition in Pregnancy and Lactation*, 6th edition. Madison, WI: Brown and Benchmark.

Internet Resources

Onusko, E. (2003). "Diagnosing Secondary Hypertension." *American Family Physician* 67:67–74. Also available from <http://www.aafp.org/afp>

National Heart, Lung, and Blood Institute. "Facts about the DASH Eating Plan." Available from <http://www.nhlbi.gov/health>

Hypoglycemia

glucose: a simple sugar; the most commonly used fuel in cells

blood pressure: measure of the pressure exerted by the blood against the walls of the blood vessels

insulin: hormone released by the pancreas to regulate level of sugar in the blood

hormone: molecules produced by one set of cells that influence the function of another set of cells

diabetes: inability to regulate level of sugar in the blood

Hypoglycemia, or abnormally low blood sugar, is caused by the impaired response (or failure) of the liver to release **glucose** as blood sugar levels decrease. The imbalance in the rate of glucose released from the liver and its use by other body tissues can result in the following hypoglycemic symptoms: hunger, nervousness, dizziness, confusion, sleepiness, difficulty speaking, feeling anxious or weak, irritability, sweating, loss of consciousness, and increased **blood pressure**. In diabetic individuals, too much **insulin**, limited or delayed food intake, a sudden increase in exercise, and excessive alcohol ingestion cause *fasting hypoglycemia*. *Reactive hypoglycemia*, however, occurs about four hours after a meal. The cause is unknown, but experts speculate that deficiencies in the release of glucagon (**hormone** released by the pancreas to increase blood glucose levels) and sensitivity to epinephrine (hormone released by the adrenal glands) contribute to hypoglycemia.

Normal blood sugar levels range from 70 to 110 mg/dl (milligrams per deciliter) upon waking and 70 to 140 mg/dl following meals. For those with **diabetes**, blood glucose levels before meals should be between 90 mg/dl and 130 mg/dl. One to two hours after a meal, blood glucose values should be less than 180 mg/dl. A blood sugar level of 70 mg/dl or less is defined as hypoglycemia. Severe hypoglycemia occurs when values are less than 40 mg/dl. Diagnosis of hypoglycemia requires fasting blood glucose values of less than 50mg/dl or of blood glucose values less than 70 mg/dl after ingesting food or drink. Treatment for hypoglycemia involves administering sugar in the form of glucose tablets, fruit juice, regular soft drinks, milk, hard candy, honey, or sugar. Hypoglycemia is prevented with regular meals and limiting alcohol and caffeine intake. SEE ALSO DIABETES MELLITUS; INSULIN.

Julie Lager

Bibliography

Cryer, Philip E.; Fisher, Joseph N.; and Shamoon, Harry (1994). "Hypoglycemia." *Diabetes Care* 17(7):734–755.

Internet Resources

American Diabetes Association. "Tight Diabetes Control." Available from <http://www.diabetes.org>

National Institute of Diabetes and Digestive and Kidney Diseases. "Hypoglycemia." Available from <http://www.niddk.nih.gov>

National Library of Medicine. "Diabetes." Available from <http://www.medlineplus.gov/>

Glossary

absorption: uptake by the digestive tract

acid reflux: splashing of stomach acid into the throat

acidity: measure of the tendency of a molecule to lose hydrogen ions, thus behaving as an acid

acidosis: elevated acid level in the blood

acupuncture: insertion of needles into the skin at special points to treat disease

acute: rapid-onset and short-lived

adequate intake: nutrient intake that appears to maintain the state of health

adipose tissue: tissue containing fat deposits

aerobic: designed to maintain adequate oxygen in the bloodstream

allergen: a substance that provokes an allergic reaction

allergic reaction: immune system reaction against a substance that is otherwise harmless

allergy: immune system reaction against substances that are otherwise harmless

amenorrhea: lack of menstruation

Americanized: having adopted more American habits or characteristics

amine: compound containing nitrogen linked to hydrogen

amino acid: building block of proteins, necessary dietary nutrient

anabolic: promoting building up

anaerobic: without air, or oxygen

anaphylaxis: life-threatening allergic reaction, involving drop in blood pressure and swelling of soft tissues especially surrounding the airways

anemia: low level of red blood cells in the blood

angioplasty: reopening of clogged blood vessels

anorexia nervosa: refusal to maintain body weight at or above what is considered normal for height and age

anthropometric: related to measurement of characteristics of the human body

antibiotic: substance that kills or prevents the growth of microorganisms

antibody: immune system protein that protects against infection

antioxidant: substance that prevents oxidation, a damaging reaction with oxygen

anxiety: nervousness

appendicitis: inflammation of the appendix

aqueous: water-based

artery: blood vessel that carries blood away from the heart toward the body tissues

arthritis: inflammation of the joints

assisted-living: facility that provides aid in meal preparation, cleaning, and other activities to help maintain independent living

asthma: respiratory disorder marked by wheezing, shortness of breath, and mucus production

asymptomatic: without symptoms

atherosclerosis: build-up of deposits within the blood vessels

atole: a porridge made of corn meal and milk

atoms: fundamental particles of matter

ayurvedic: an Indian healing system

B vitamins: a group of vitamins important in cell energy processes

bacteria: single-celled organisms without nuclei, some of which are infectious

bactericidal: a substance that kills bacteria

bacteriostatic: a state that prevents growth of bacteria

basal metabolic rate: rate of energy consumption by the body during a period of no activity

basal metabolism: level of body energy consumption and chemical processes in the absence of exertion

behavioral: related to behavior, in contrast to medical or other types of interventions

bile: substance produced in the liver which suspends fats for absorption

binge: uncontrolled indulgence

bioavailability: availability to living organisms, based on chemical form

biochemical: related to chemical processes within cells

biodiversity: richness of species within an area

biological: related to living organisms

biotin: a portion of certain enzymes used in fat metabolism; essential for cell function

biotoxin: poison made by living organisms

blood clotting: the process by which blood forms a solid mass to prevent uncontrolled bleeding

blood pressure: measure of the pressure exerted by the blood against the walls of the blood vessels

body mass index: weight in kilograms divided by square of the height in meters times 100; a measure of body fat

bone marrow: dividing cells within the long bones that make the blood

botanical: related to plants

botulism: poisoning from the bacterium Clostridium botulinum

bowel: intestines and rectum

brain allergy: allergy whose symptoms affect brain function

bulimia: uncontrolled episodes of eating (bingeing) usually followed by self-induced vomiting (purging)

calcium: mineral essential for bones and teeth

calorie: unit of food energy

cancer: uncontrolled cell growth

candidal: related to the yeast Candida

candidiasis: a yeast infection

carbohydrate: food molecule made of carbon, hydrogen, and oxygen, including sugars and starches

carbohydrate metabolism: breakdown and use of sugars and starches in the body

carcinogen: cancer-causing substance

cardiovascular: related to the heart and circulatory system

cardiovascular disease: disease affecting the heart and/or circulatory system

caries: cavities in the teeth

carotenoid: plant-derived molecules used as pigments

carrageenan: a thickener derived from red seaweed

catabolism: breakdown of complex molecules

catalyze: cause to happen more rapidly

cataract: clouding of the lens of the eye

cellulose: carbohydrate made by plants; indigestible by humans

chiropractic: manipulation of the spine and other bones for healing

cholera: bacterial infection of the small intestine causing severe diarrhea, vomiting, and dehydration

cholesterol: multi-ringed molecule found in animal cell membranes; a type of lipid

chronic: over a long period

chronic disease: diseases that occur over a long period, in contrast to acute diseases

clinical: related to hospitals, clinics, and patient care

cloning: creation of an exact genetic copy of an organism

congenital: present from birth

Congregate Dining: a support service that provides a meal at a central location on a specified day

constipation: difficulty passing feces

consumerism: reliance on buying, rather than making, items necessary for living

contraindicated: not recommended

convenience food: food that requires very little preparation for eating

coronary heart disease: disease of the coronary arteries, the blood vessels surrounding the heart

cretinism: arrested mental and physical development

crossbreeding: breeding between two different varieties of an organism

cuisine: types of food and traditions of preparation

cytoplasm: contents of a cell minus the nucleus

deamination: removal of an NH2 group from a molecule

dehydration: loss of water

dementia: loss of cognitive abilities, including memory and decision making

dentition: formation of the teeth

deoxyribonucleic acid: DNA, the molecule that makes up genes

dependence: a condition in which attempts to stop use leads to withdrawal symptoms, including irritability and insomnia

depression: mood disorder characterized by apathy, restlessness, and negative thoughts

DETERMINE: checklist used to identify nutritionally at-risk individuals

development: the process of change by which an organism becomes more complex

diabetes: inability to regulate level of sugar in the blood

diet: the total daily food intake, or the types of foods eaten

dietary assessment: analysis of nutrients in the diet

Dietary Reference Intakes: set of guidelines for nutrient intake

diphtheria: infectious disease caused by Cornybacterium diphtheriae, causing damage to the heart and other organs

disaccharide carbohydrate: molecule composed of two linked sugars

diuretic: substance that depletes the body of water

diversity: the variety of cultural traditions within a larger culture

diverticulosis: presence of abnormal small sacs in the lining of the intestine

DNA: deoxyribonucleic acid; the molecule that makes up genes, and is therefore responsible for heredity

drugs: substances whose administration causes a significant change in the body's function

dyslipidemia: disorder of fat metabolism

dysmorphia: the belief that one's body is different (fatter, thinner, etc.) than it really is

eating disorder: behavioral disorder involving excess consumption, avoidance of consumption, self-induced vomiting, or other food-related aberrant behavior

ecological: related to the environment and human interactions with it

eczema: skin disease causing itching and flaking

edema: accumulation of fluid in the tissues

efficacy: effectiveness

electrolyte: salt dissolved in fluid

elemental: made from predigested nutrients

elimination diet: diet in which particular foods are eliminated to observe the effect

endotoxin: toxic substance produced and stored within the plant tissue

enema: substance delivered via the rectum

energy: technically, the ability to perform work; the content of a substance that allows it to be useful as a fuel

enrichment: addition of vitamins and minerals to improve the nutritional content of a food

enteric: pertaining to the intestine; delivered via a tube into the intestine

entrepreneur: founder of a new businesses

environment: surroundings

environmental illness: illness due to substances in the environment

enzymatic: related to use of enzymes, proteins that cause chemical reactions to occur

enzyme: protein responsible for carrying out reactions in a cell

epinephrine: hormone that promotes "fight or flight;" also called adrenaline

epithelial cell: sheet of cells lining organs throughout the body

Escherichia coli: common bacterium found in human large intestine

essential fatty acids: particular molecules made of carbon, hydrogen, and oxygen that the human body must have but cannot make itself

estradiol: female hormone; a type of estrogen

estrogen: hormone that helps control female development and menstruation

etiology: origin and development of a disease

eukaryots: organisms whose cells contain nuclei

failure to thrive: lack of normal developmental progress or maintenance of health

famine: extended period of food shortage

fast food: food requiring minimal preparation before eating, or food delivered very quickly after ordering in a restaurant

fat: type of food molecule rich in carbon and hydrogen, with high energy content

fat-soluble: able to be dissolved in fats, including the membranes of cells

fatigue: tiredness

fatty acids: molecules rich in carbon and hydrogen; a component of fats

fermentation: reaction performed by yeast or bacteria to make alcohol

fiber: indigestible plant material that aids digestion by providing bulk

folate: one of the B vitamins, also called folic acid

food additive: substance added to foods to improve nutrition, taste, appearance, or shelf-life

food poisoning: illness caused by consumption of spoiled food, usually containing bacteria

fortification: addition of vitamins and minerals to improve the nutritional content of a food

fortified: altered by addition of vitamins or minerals

free radical: highly reactive molecular fragment, which can damage cells

functional food: food whose health benefits are claimed to be higher than those traditionally assumed for similar types of foods

fungal: of or from fungi

galactosemia: inherited disorder preventing digestion of milk sugar, galactose

gamma rays: very high energy radiation, more powerful than x rays

gastric: related to the stomach

gastric mucosa: lining of the stomach

gastrointestinal: related to the stomach and intestines

gastrointestinal system: the digestive tract (mouth to anus) plus associated organs

gastrointestinal tract: the continuous tube through which food passes including throat, stomach, and intestines

gene: DNA sequence that codes for proteins, and thus controls inheritance

gene expression: use of a gene to make the protein it encodes

genetic: inherited or related to the genes

genetic engineering: manipulation of genes to change the characteristics of a living organism

globalization: development of world-wide economic system

glucagon: hormone that promotes release of sugar from the liver to raise the level of blood sugar

glucose: a simple sugar; the most commonly used fuel in cells

gluten: a protein found in wheat

glycerol: simple molecule that forms a portion of fats

glycogen: storage form of sugar

glycolysis: cellular reaction that begins the breakdown of sugars

growth factor: protein that stimulates growth of surrounding cells

growth hormone: hormone produced by the pituitary gland that increases the rate of growth

growth spurts: periods of rapid growth

guar gum: a thickener made from a tropical bean

Harris-Benedict equation: a formula for calculating a person's minimum energy expenditure

HDL: high density lipoprotein, a blood protein that carries cholesterol

health-promotion: related to advocacy for better health, preventive medicine, and other aspects of well-being

heart attack: loss of blood supply to part of the heart, resulting in death of heart muscle

heart disease: any disorder of the heart or its blood supply, including heart attack, atherosclerosis, and coronary artery disease

heavy metal: lead, chromium, and other metals found in the middle section of the periodic table of the elements

hemoglobin: the iron-containing molecule in red blood cells that carries oxygen

hemorrhoids: swollen blood vessels in the rectum

hepatitis: liver inflammation

hepatitis B: viral disease affecting the liver

herbal: related to or made from herbs

high blood pressure: elevation of the pressure in the bloodstream maintained by the heart

high potency: a claim about vitamin or mineral content, defined as 100% or more of the Recommended Daily Intake

homeostasis: regulation of the proper internal state

hookworm: parasitic nematode that attaches to the intestinal wall

hormone: molecules produced by one set of cells that influence the function of another set of cells

hydration: degree of water in the body

hydrolyze: to break apart through reaction with water

hygiene: cleanliness

hype: advertising and brash claims

hypercholesterolemia: high levels of cholesterol in the blood

hyperglycemia: high level of sugar in the blood

hyperlipidemia: high levels of lipids (fats or cholesterol) in the blood

hypertension: high blood pressure

hypertrophy: excess increase in size

hypoglycemia: low blood sugar level

hypoglycemic: related to low level of blood sugar

immune system: the set of organs and cells, including white blood cells, that protect the body from infection

immunocompromised: having a weakened immune system

immunologic: related to the immune system, which protects the body from infection

incidence: number of new cases reported each year

incisor: chisel-shaped tooth used for cutting; one of the types of primary teeth

indigestion: reduced ability to digest food

infectious diseases: diseases caused by viruses, bacteria, fungi, or protozoa, which replicate inside the body

informed consent: agreement to a procedure after understanding the risks

injera: spongy flat bread

insoluble: not able to be dissolved in water

insulin: hormone released by the pancreas to regulate level of sugar in the blood

internship: training program

interstitial: between the tissues

intestines: the two long tubes that carry out the bulk of the processes of digestion

intravenous: into the veins

iron: nutrient needed for red blood cell formation

isoflavones: estrogen-like compounds in plants

job sharing: splitting a single job among two or more people

junk food: food with high fat and sugar content, without correspondingly high amounts of protein, vitamins, or minerals

keto-acid: an acid compound containing the reactive CO group

ketoacidosis: accumulation of ketone bodies along with high acid levels in the body fluids

ketones: chemicals produced by fat breakdown; molecule containing a double-bonded oxygen linked to two carbons

ketosis: build-up of ketone bodies in the blood, due to fat breakdown

kidney stones: deposits of solid material in kidney

killer-cell: type of white blood cell that helps protect the body from infection

kinetic: related to speed of reaction

Krebs cycle: cellular reaction that breaks down numerous nutrients and provides building blocks for other molecules

kwashiorkor: severe malnutrition characterized by swollen belly, hair loss, and loss of skin pigment

lactic acid: breakdown product of sugar in the muscles in the absence of oxygen

lactose intolerance: inability to digest lactose, or milk sugar

learned behaviors: actions that are acquired by training and observation, in contrast to innate behaviors

leavening: yeast or other agents used for rising bread

legumes: beans, peas, and related plants

lifestyle: set of choices about diet, exercise, job type, leisure activities, and other aspects of life

lipid: fats, waxes, and steroids; important components of cell membranes

lipoprotein: blood protein that carries fats

listeriosis: infectious disease caused by Listeria bacteria

long-term care facilities: hospitals or nursing homes in which patients remain for a long time for chronic care, rather than being treated and quickly discharged

lymph node: pocket within the lymph system in which white blood cells reside

lymph system: system of vessels and glands in the body that circulates and cleans extracellular fluid

lymphatic system: group of ducts and nodes through which fluid and white blood cells circulate to fight infection

macrobiotic: related to a specific dietary regimen based on balancing of vital principles

macronutrient: nutrient needed in large quantities

macular degeneration: death of cells of the macula, part of the eye's retina

malabsorption: decreased ability to take up nutrients

malaise: illness or lack of energy

malaria: disease caused by infection with Plasmodium, a single-celled protozoon, transmitted by mosquitoes

malignant: spreading to surrounding tissues; cancerous

malnourished: lack of adequate nutrients in the diet

malnutrition: chronic lack of sufficient nutrients to maintain health

marasmus: extreme malnutrition, characterized by loss of muscle and other tissue

meditation: stillness of thought, practiced to reduce tension and increase inner peace

menopausal: related to menopause, the period during which women cease to ovulate and menstruate

menopause: phase in a woman's life during which ovulation and menstruation end

menstrual cycles: the build-up and sloughing off of the lining of the uterus in women commencing at puberty and proceeding until menopause

metabolic: related to processing of nutrients and building of necessary molecules within the cell

metabolic activities: sum total of the body's biochemical processes

metabolism: the sum total of reactions in a cell or an organism

metabolism-free radical: highly reactive molecular fragment, which are created through metabolism, or processing of nutrients

metabolite: the product of metabolism, or nutrient processing within the cell

metabolize: processing of a nutrient

microflora: microscopic organisms present in small numbers

micronutrient: nutrient needed in very small quantities

microorganisms: bacteria and protists; single-celled organisms

mineral: an inorganic (non-carbon-containing) element, ion, or compound

miscarriage: loss of a pregnancy

mitochondria: small bodies within a cell that harvest energy for use by the cell

molar: grinding tooth toward the rear of the mouth

molecule: combination of atoms that form stable particles

monocultural: from a single culture

monoglyceride: breakdown product of fats

morbidity: illness or accident

mucosa: moist exchange surface within the body

muscle wasting: loss of muscle bulk

mycotoxin: poison produced by a fungus

myoglobin: oxygen storage protein in muscle

nandrolone: hormone related to testosterone

nausea: unpleasant sensation in the gut that precedes vomiting

needs assessment: formal procedure for determining needs

nervous system: the brain, spinal cord, and nerves that extend throughout the body

neural: related to the nervous system

neural tube defects: failures of proper development of the spinal cord

neurological: related to the nervous system

neuropathy: malfunction of nerve cells

neurotransmitter: molecule released by one nerve cell to stimulate or inhibit another

NHANES: National Heath and Nutrition Examination Survey

niacin: one of the B vitamins, required for energy production in the cell

nitrite: NO_2, used for preservatives

nitrogen: essential element for plant growth

nonpathogenic: not promoting disease

nonpolar: without a separation if charge within the molecule; likely to be hydrophobic

nutrient: dietary substance necessary for health

nutrient deficiencies: lack of adequate nutrients in the diet

nutrition: the maintenance of health through proper eating, or the study of same

nutritional deficiency: lack of adequate nutrients in the diet

nutritional requirements: the set of substances needed in the diet to maintain health

obese: above accepted standards of weight for sex, height, and age

obesity: the condition of being overweight, according to established norms based on sex, age, and height

opacity: impermeability to light

opportunistic infections: infections not normally threatening, which gain a foothold in people with weakened immune systems

oral-pharyngeal: related to mouth and throat

osteoarthritis: inflammation of the joints

osteoblast: cell that forms bone

osteomalacia: softening of the bones

osteopathic: related to the practice of osteopathy, which combines standard medical therapy with manipulation of the skeleton to correct problems

osteoporosis: weakening of the bone structure

over-the-counter: available without a prescription

overweight: weight above the accepted norm based on height, sex, and age

oxidative: related to chemical reaction with oxygen or oxygen-containing compounds

oxygen: O_2, atmospheric gas required by all animals

paralysis: inability to move

parasite: organism that feeds off of other organisms

parasitic: feeding off another organism

parasitic diseases: diseases caused by parasites, including amebic diseases, Giardia, roundworms, and others

pasteurization: heating to destroy bacteria and other microorganisms, after Louis Pasteur

pathogen: organism that causes disease

pH: level of acidity, with low numbers indicating high acidity

phenylketonuria: inherited disease marked by the inability to process the amino acid phenylalanine, causing mental retardation

phospholipid: a type of fat used to build cell membranes

phosphorus: element essential in forming the mineral portion of bone

physiological: related to the biochemical processes of the body

physiology: the group of biochemical and physical processes that combine to make a functioning organism, or the study of same

phytate: plant compound that binds minerals, reducing their ability to be absorbed

phytochemical: chemical produced by plants

phytoestrogen: plant-derived estrogen compound

pituitary gland: gland at the base of the brain that regulates multiple body processes

plaque: material forming deposits on the surface of the teeth, which may promote bacterial growth and decay

plasma: the fluid portion of the blood, distinct from the cellular portion

plateaus: periods during which growth is greatly reduced

pluralistic: of many different sources

pneumonia: lung infection

polar: containing regions of positive and negative charge; likely to be soluble in water

polyunsaturated: having multiple double bonds within the chemical structure, thus increasing the body's ability to metabolize it

potable: safe to drink

pre-renal: kidney disease caused by change in the blood supply to the kidney

prevalence: describing the number of cases in a population at any one time

preventive medicine: treatment designed to prevent disease, rather than waiting for it to occur before intervening

processed food: food that has been cooked, milled, or otherwise manipulated to change its quality

proscription: prohibitions, rules against

prostaglandin: hormone that helps regulate inflammation and other tissue processes

prostate: male gland surrounding the urethra that contributes fluid to the semen

protein: complex molecule composed of amino acids that performs vital functions in the cell; necessary part of the diet

protein digestion: breakdown of proteins into amino acids in the digestive tract

psoriasis: skin disorder characterized by red, dry, scaly skin

psychological: related to thoughts, feelings, and personal experiences

psyllium: bulk-forming laxative derived from the Plantago psyllium seeds

puberty: time of onset of sexual maturity

reactivity: characteristic set of reactions undergone due to chemical structure

Recommended Dietary Allowances: nutrient intake recommended to promote health

renal failure: inability of the kidneys to cleanse the blood

respiratory system: the lungs, throat, and muscles of respiration, or breathing

rice genome: the set of genes possessed by rice

rickets: disorder caused by vitamin D deficiency, marked by soft and misshapen bones and organ swelling

ritual: ceremony or frequently repeated behavior

RNA: ribonucleic acid, used in cells to create proteins from genetic information

salmonellosis: food poisoning due to Salmonella bacteria

saturated fat: a fat with the maximum possible number of hydrogens; more difficult to break down than unsaturated fats

scurvy: a syndrome characterized by weakness, anemia, and spongy gums, due to vitamin C deficiency

sedentary: not active

serotonin: chemical used by nerve cells to communicate with one another

serum: noncellular portion of the blood

serum estrone: blood level of estrone, a steroid hormone that is one of the estrogens, a type of female hormone

shock: state of dangerously low blood pressure and loss of blood delivered to the tissues

sideroblastosis: condition in which the blood contains an abnormally high number of sideroblasts, or red blood cells containing iron granules

sleep apnea: difficulty breathing while sleeping

smallpox: deadly viral disease

smog: air pollution

social group: tribe, clique, family, or other group of individuals

socioeconomic status: level of income and social class

staples: essential foods in the diet

steroid: class of hormones composed of carbon rings, necessary for sexual development and mineral balance

steroid hormones: class of hormones composed of carbon rings, necessary for sexual development and mineral balance

steroids: group of hormones that affect tissue build-up, sexual development, and a variety of metabolic

sterol: building blocks of steroid hormones; a type of lipid

stillbirth: giving birth to a dead fetus

stress: heightened state of nervousness or unease

stroke: loss of blood supply to part of the brain, due to a blocked or burst artery in the brain

subcutaneous: beneath the skin

sucrose: table sugar

temperate zone: region of the world between the tropics and the arctic or Antarctic

testosterone: male sex hormone

thalassemia: inherited blood disease due to defect in the hemoglobin protein

thermoregulate: regulate temperature

tofu: soybean curd, similar in consistency to cottage cheese

tolerance: development of a need for increased amount of drug to obtain a given level of intoxication

toxicant: harmful substance

toxins: poisons

trace: very small amount

trans-fatty acids: type of fat thought to increase the risk of heart disease

triglyceride: a type of fat

tuber: swollen plant stem below the ground

tuberculosis: bacterial infection, usually of the lungs, caused by Mycobacterium tuberculosis

tularemia: bacterial infection by Francisella tularensis, causing fever, skin lesions, and other symptoms

type II diabetes: inability to regulate the level of sugar in the blood due to a reduction in the number of insulin receptors on the body's cells

typhoid: fever-causing bacterial infection due to Salmonella typhi; transmitted contaminated food or water

typhus: bacterial disease transmitted by infected rodents

ulcer: erosion in the lining of the stomach or intestine due to bacterial infection

uncharged: neither positively nor negatively charged

undernutrition: food intake too low to maintain adequate energy expenditure without weight loss

uric: from urine

vaccine: medicine that promotes immune system resistance by stimulating pre-existing cells to become active

vegan: person who consumes no animal products, including milk and honey

viral disease: disease caused by viruses, including flu, colds, AIDS, hepatitis, and others

virus: noncellular infectious agent that requires a host cell to reproduce

vitamin: necessary complex nutrient used to aid enzymes or other metabolic processes in the cell

vitamin D: nutrient needed for calcium uptake and therefore proper bone formation

wasting: loss of body tissue often as a result of cancer or other disease

water-soluble: able to be dissolved in water

wean: cease breast-feeding

wellness: related to health promotion

white blood cell: immune system cell that fights infection

yeast allergy: allergy to yeasts used in baking or brewing

zinc: mineral necessary for many enzyme processes

Index

335